NEUROSCIENCE RESEARCH PROGRESS SERIES

LEARNING AND MEMORY DEVELOPMENTS AND INTELLECTUAL DISABILITIES

NEUROSCIENCE RESEARCH PROGRESS SERIES

Current Advances in Sleep Biology
Marcos G. Frank (Editor)
2009. ISBN: 978-1-60741-508-4

Neuroscience Research Advances
Benito Figueredo and Fidel Meléndez (Editors)
2009. ISBN: 978-1-60692-967-4

Dendritic Spines: Biochemistry, Modeling and Properties
Louis R. Baylog (Editor)
2009. ISBN: 978-1-60741-460-5

Relationship between Automatic and Controlled Processes of Attention and Leading to Complex Thinking
Rosa Angela Fabio
2009. ISBN: 978-1-60741-810-8

Neurochemistry: Molecular Aspects, Cellular Aspects and Clinical Applications
Anacleto Paços and Silvio Nogueira (Editors)
2009. ISBN: 978-1-60741-831-3

Sleep Deprivation: Causes, Effects and Treatment
Pedr Fulke and Sior Vaughan (Editors)
2009. ISBN: 978-1-60741-974-7

Color Perception: Physiology, Processes and Analysis
Darius Skusevich and Petras Matikas (Editors)
2009. ISBN: 978-1-60876-077-0

Translational Neuroscience in Animal Research: Advancement, Challenges, and Research Ethics
Jason E. Warnick and Allan V. Kalueff (Editors)
2010. ISBN: 978-1-60876-185-2

Developmental Neurotoxicity of PBDEs, Mechanisms and Implications
Henrik Alm and Birger Scholz
2010. ISBN: 978-1-61668-602-4

Developmental Neurotoxicity of PBDEs, Mechanisms and Implications
Henrik Alm and Birger Scholz
2010. ISBN: 978-1-61668-295-8 (Online Book)

Spatial Memory: Visuospatial Processes, Cognitive Performance and Developmental Effects
Jacob B. Thomas (Editor)
2010. ISBN: 978-1-61668-139-5

Spatial Memory: Visuospatial Processes, Cognitive Performance and Developmental Effects
Jacob B. Thomas (Editor)
2010. ISBN: 978-1-61668-467-9 (Online Book)

Handbook of Neuropsychiatry Research
Rebecca S. Davies (Editor)
2010. ISBN: 978-1-61668-138-8

Handbook of Neuropsychiatry Research
Rebecca S. Davies (Editor)
2010. ISBN: 978-1-61668-798-4 (Online Book)

Neural Computation and Particle Accelerators: Research, Technology and Applications
Emmerich Chabot and Horace D'Arras (Editors)
2010. ISBN: 978-1-60741-280-9

Horizons in Neuroscience Research, Volume 2
Andres Costa and Eugenio Villalba Davies (Editors)
2010. ISBN: 978-1-60876-876-9

Cultural and Linguistic Influence on Developmental Neural Basis of Theory of Mind: Whorfian Hypothesis Revisited
Chiyoko Kobayashi Frank
2010. ISBN: 978-1-60876-362-7

The Importance of Colour Perception to Animals and Man
Birgitta Dresp-Langley and Keith Langley
2010. ISBN: 978-1-60876-394-8

Learning and Memory Developments and Intellectual Disabilities
Lucas C. Eklund and Aron S. Nyman (Editors)
2010. ISBN: 978-1-60876-397-9 2010.

Dual Processing in the Visual System
Hitoshi Sasaki
2010. ISBN: 978-1-60876-399-3

(COB) Dual Processing Model of Visual Information. Cortical and Subcortical Processing
Hitoshi Sasaki
2010. ISBN: 978-1-60876-399-3

Homeostatic Role of the Parasympathetic Nervous System in Human Behavior
Aurélien Pichon and Didier Chapelot
2010. ISBN: 978-1-60876-804-2

Rehabilitation of the Shaken Soldier Syndrome
Larry E. Schutz, David Patterson, Mathu Hanson and Elizabeth A. McNamara
2010. ISBN: 978-1-61668-192-0

Rehabilitation of the Shaken Soldier Syndrome
Larry E. Schutz, David Patterson, Mathu Hanson and Elizabeth A. McNamara
2010. ISBN: 978-1-61668-492-1 (Online Book)

NEUROSCIENCE RESEARCH PROGRESS SERIES

LEARNING AND MEMORY DEVELOPMENTS AND INTELLECTUAL DISABILITIES

LUCAS C. EKLUND

AND

ARON S. NYMAN

EDITORS

Nova Science Publishers, Inc.

New York

For permission to use material from this book please contact us:
Telephone 631-231-7269; Fax 631-231-8175
Web Site: http://www.novapublishers.com

LIBRARY OF CONGRESS CATALOGING-IN-PUBLICATION DATA

Learning and memory developments and intellectual disabilities / editors, Lucas C. Eklund and Aron S. Nyman.
p. ; cm.
Includes bibliographical references and index.
ISBN 978-1-60876-397-9 (hardcover)
1. Mental retardation. 2. Mental illness. 3. Learning. 4. Memory. I. Eklund, Lucas C. II. Nyman, Aron S.
[DNLM: 1. Memory--physiology. 2. Developmental Disabilities. 3. Learning--physiology. 4. Learning Disorders. WL 102 L4353 2009]
RC570.2.L427 2009
616.85'88--dc22

2009051576

Published by Nova Science Publishers, Inc. † New York

CONTENTS

PREFACE

This book reviews behavioral and neuroimaging evidence that has revealed effects of emotion on memory and attention in individuals with and without post-traumatic stress disorder (PTSD). The authors also review the historical development of memory reconsolidation, discuss some of the important behavioral characteristics and potential mechanisms of memory reconsolidation, and consider the possible implications of this research for treatment of psychiatric conditions such as PTSD, phobias and drug addiction. Moreover, assessment of cognitive, motor, sensory and communicative functions in children with profound intellectual and multiple disabilities (PIMD) is still in its infancy. The characteristics of children PIMD are described in this book. The importance of alertness in assessment, both as a mean and as an objective, is then explained. The implications of such a complex pattern of disabilities for assessment of alertness is considered as well. In this book, the authors also examine the effects of age and knowledge of memory aging on subjective appraisals of memory in forgetful others using a person perception paradigm. The social/communication features that differentiate intellectual disabilities of three different etiologies: Low Functioning Autism, Down Syndrome and Idiopathic Intellectual Disability are explored as well. Other chapters review evidence about laboratory-based and environment-based research on spatial memory, the influence of music on various forms of memory, and evidence from literature that working memory is a major component of successful performance on an IQ test. Impairment is discussed in working memory in ID, which could also affect problem solving abilities on a non-verbally based measure, such as the Raven's Coloured Progressive Matrices (RCPM).

Chapter 1 - Out of all of the information that we experience, only a subset will become part of our memories. Attentional processes, engaged during an event's unfolding, are essential for allowing us to transform an experience into a memory, and emotion can critically modulate those attentional processes, increasing the likelihood that an emotional experience becomes part of our memory stores. This chapter reviews behavioral and neuroimaging evidence that has revealed effects of emotion on memory and attention in individuals with and without post-traumatic stress disorder (PTSD). First, we review how emotion influences the attentional processes that allow individuals with and without PTSD to transform experiences into a memory. Second, we focus on differences in the way emotional items are remembered in people with and without PTSD and how this may be linked to differences in attention at encoding. Third, we discuss current controversies regarding the uniqueness of traumatic memories in PTSD.

Chapter 2 - The current legislation, *No Child Left Behind,* mandates that students with intellectual disabilities have access to core curriculum courses. This action research investigates a comprehensive life skills program, Life Centered Career Education (LCCE), being integrated into the curriculum of high school students with intellectual disabilities. The LCCE program was utilized to educate students on Personal-Social Skills, Daily Life skills, and Occupational lessons with an academic emphasis.

Chapter 3 - In animals and in humans, cytokines are typically immune system molecules that help orchestrate the host responses to infection. Pro-inflammatory cytokines coordinate immune, physiological, metabolic and behavioral responses that are collectively termed the acute phase reaction. In addition to their role in immunoregulation of inflammatory processes, pro-inflammatory cytokines represent the major communication link between peripheral immunity and the central nervous system. Cytokines are known to play a role in the physiological and behavioral adjustments that occur during sickness, leading to "sickness behavior". One of the most salient symptoms of the sickness behavior syndrome is alteration in learning and memory processes. Studies in animals have demonstrated that acute activation of pro-inflammatory cytokine signaling in the brain in response to peripheral immune activation is associated with deficits in hippocampal-dependent memory.

Recent studies suggest that brain cytokines may also have some physiological roles in neural, neuroendocrine, and behavioral regulation in non-pathological situations. Cytokine-induced modulation of memory processes is a complex phenomenon, including both detrimental and beneficial effects, depending on the specific pro-inflammatory cytokine, its levels (particularly within the brain), and the particular condition that elicits the cytokine secretion. Some cytokines, e.g., Interleukin (IL)-1, have been shown to significantly influence memory consolidation. IL-1, IL-6 and tumor necrosis factor (TNF)-α are the main cytokines involved in learning and memory modulation. These behavioral data are consistent with the impairing effect of enhanced cytokine signaling on hippocampal long-term potentiation.

We will review the literature, including our own contribution, on human and animal model studies of the role of cytokines in learning and memory.

Chapter 4 - We examined the effects of age and knowledge of memory aging on subjective appraisals of memory in forgetful others using a person perception paradigm. Younger and older adults were tested in one of three information conditions: no information control group, grandparent seminar group, and memory aging seminar group. All completed the Knowledge Memory of Aging Questionnaire (KMAQ; Cherry, Brigman, Hawley, & Reese, 2003) at pretest and posttest to evaluate changes in memory aging knowledge. All read vignettes that described forgetful younger (in their 20's to 30's) or older characters (in their 60's to 70's). Attribution ratings on the potential causes of the forgetful behavior and memory opinion ratings were solicited. All completed the Memory Functioning Questionnaire (MFQ; Gilewski, Zelinski, & Schaie, 1990) at posttest to measure self-perceived memory ability. Both age groups showed an age-based double standard in memory appraisal. Attribution and memory opinion ratings did not vary across the information groups. Only the memory aging seminar participants showed significant pre- to posttest gains on the KMAQ. Self-perceived memory functioning was significantly correlated with perceptions of forgetful characters. These data indicate that although memory knowledge improved following instruction, perceptions of forgetfulness in older adults were not influenced by increased knowledge of normative age-associated memory changes.

Chapter 5 - Since the 1960s, research has indicated that the acquisition of new information is followed by a time-limited period of memory consolidation. During this consolidation period, the new memory exists in a labile state, where enhancing or impairing treatments are capable of modulating the subsequent strength of the memory. Considerable evidence supports the existence of a period of memory consolidation; however, following the completion of the consolidation period many scientists believed that the new long-term memory became immune to memory enhancing or impairing treatments. Over the decades, isolated studies challenged this view and suggested that old memories may sometimes become malleable again under the right circumstances. During the last 10 years a substantial body of research has developed indicating that old, previously consolidated memories may enter a state of reconsolidation when retrieved from long-term memory. In other words, the retrieval of old memories may return them to a state where they are once again susceptible to memory modulation. This chapter will review the historical development of memory reconsolidation, summarize some of the tasks, species, and treatments used in research on reconsolidation, discuss some of the important behavioral characteristics and potential mechanisms of memory reconsolidation, and consider the possible implications of this research for treatment of psychiatric conditions such as post-traumatic stress disorder, phobias, and drug addiction.

Chapter 6 - Currently Intellectual Disability (ID) is classified as a Wechsler Intelligence Scale for Children - Fourth Edition (WISC-IV) Intelligence Quotient (IQ) below 70 and an impairment in adaptive skills during the developmental period. We suggest that the the non-verbal visual matching Raven's Coloured Porgressive Matrices (RCPM) should replace the commonly used WISC-IV measure of intelligence, as a means of matching groups of ID to a Typically Developing (TD) group according to their mental age, as it is a better measure of reasoning ability in children with ID who invariably have verbally based deficits. In addition, we present evidence that RCPM mental aged matched children with Low Functioning (LF) Autism, Down Syndrome (DS) and Idiopathic ID use different problem solving strategies than TD children, to achieve the same overall performance on the RCPM. This is presumably due to group differences in brain impairments as evidenced by brain imaging studies. We also present evidence from the literature that working memory is a major component of successful performance on an IQ test and that impairment in working memory in ID could affect problem solving abilities on the RCPM. The theoretical and educational implications of the discrepancy between similar overall performance level on an intelligence test, but different use of problem solving strategies are also explored.

Chapter 7 - Research reveals background music played during learning can variously enhance or impair memory, although the conditions which determine its effect are not yet understood. Possible explanations for the differing effects of music on memory include characteristics of the music itself, such as tempo and lyrics, induced mood of the listener and personality differences. In this chapter, consideration of the type of music used to manipulate learning and memory will be reviewed, indicating that arousal may play an important moderating role, either as a means of reducing anxiety or increasing arousal to an optimum performance levels. As music is often reported to increase arousal via emotion induction or enjoyment, a well established theory of arousal-modulated memory will be argued to underly the facilitatory effects of music on memory. The methodology used within this research paradigm will be described, and adaptations will be proposed that make it amenable to investigating the effect of music induced arousal on memory. This approach provides a novel method for combining the knowledge gained from music and memory research with arousal and memory literature to further investigate the potential memory enhancing role of music.

Chapter 8 - Spatial memory is a necessary prerequisite of most everyday activities. We usually define "spatial" that information useful to locate objects and to interact with them. Therefore, it is "spatial" information about relational and metric properties, such as relative positions (e.g., left/right), distance, size, orientation, as well as dynamic properties, such as velocity and strength. Clearly, the ability to navigate in the environment requires an understanding of all these properties and a representation in memory of structured information. To organize spatial memory, egocentric (i.e. based on body's position) or allocentric (i.e. based on external positions) frames of reference are used. Although research on spatial memory has a long history, in the majority of the cases experimental settings and procedures are restricted to laboratory situations, and the results are typically generalized to real world contexts. Consequently, little is known on the characteristics of spatial memory based on bodily interactions with large-scale everyday environments. In this paper we review evidence about laboratory-based and environment-based research on spatial memory. Further, a research is presented that investigated whether familiarity with a large-scale regular environment affects the spatial frames of reference necessary to represent it in memory. It was tested the hypothesis that familiarity facilitates an allocentric representation of the environment. Familiar and unfamiliar participants had to study 5 triads of buildings by walking along a path surrounding each triad. Afterwards, they had to provide relative distance judgments in relation either to their body (egocentric) or external buildings (allocentric). Results showed that familiar participants were more accurate than unfamiliar participants in the allocentric judgments and faster on the whole. Unfamiliar participants performed similarly in both judgments and were better than familiar participants in the egocentric judgments. These findings suggest that when the environment is familiar and regular it is represented on the basis of allocentric frames of reference. The results are discussed in relation to models of spatial memory that emphasize the importance of experience and of the geometric structure.

Chapter 9 - In the research literature, Intellectual Disability (ID) is conceptualised as a set of unique cognitive deficits associated with particular genetic causes rather than simply low IQ. We add to this literature by exploring social/communication features that differentiate ID of three different etiologies: Low Functioning (LF) Autism, Down Syndrome (DS) and Idiopathic ID. A body of research suggests that slow shifting and/or disengaging visual attention in Autism is likely to be a major contributing factor to their impaired social and cognitive development. We propose that slow visual orienting ability in Autism is due to impairment in magnocellular processing of the visual system. Thus, we suggest that individuals with Autism are delayed in shifting and/or disengaging attention as evidenced by a disregard for transient stimuli in their environment, where as individuals with DS and Idiopathic ID show the opposite pattern, in that they appear to be unable to maintain attention to a task, being easily distracted by transient stimuli in their environment. The implications of this visual orienting deficit are discussed in terms of conceptualisation of Autism, visual orienting research in Autism and evidence based educational practice for children with Autism, DS and Idiopathic ID.

Chapter 10 - Lesions of hippocampal formation structures produce a severe global amnesia, encompassing verbal as well as non-verbal material. Since the first studies with medial temporal lobe amnesic patients, it was noted that they do not exhibit deficits of short-term memory despite the severe long-term memory impairment and this was taken as a strong evidence in favor of a subdivision of memory, that between long-term and short-term memory. The continuing studies with H.M. and other amnesic patients have led to an important discovery that gave rise to the notion of multiple memory systems. The crucial finding was that, in spite of their profound amnesia, amnesic patients usually are able to learn and retain a number of tasks. This has led to the important subdivision of memory between explicit (or declarative) episodic memory and implicit (or non-declarative memory. Implicit memory refers to retrieval independent of consciously processes. Explicit memory can be defined as the ability to store and consciously retrieve facts and events. Other fundamental finding was that the prefrontal cortex is involved with short-term memory, a concept that developed to a larger scope framework, that of working memory. The prefrontal cortex plays a crucial role in working memory, and, in particular, contributes to the functioning of the working memory episodic buffer in which multimodal information is maintained for a short time allowing for the binding of information to create integrated episodes. It has been traditionally accepted that the hippocampal system is not necessary for working memory, but, recently, this widely accepted neuroanatomic dissociation has been challenged by a number of studies that have disclosed a relationship between long-term memory and working memory. Working memory has been shown to contribute to episodic memory formation, and the reverse also seems to occur, that is, long-term memory contributing to working memory as well. The relativelly small deficit of episodic memory in the healthy elderly can be explained by a decline in the working memory capacity and executive functions that is observed in this age. Episodic memory impairment caused by haloperidol, an antagonist of D2 dopamine receptors widely used as an antipsychotic drug, can be fully explained by the drug's action in the working memory capacity but not in the central executive. Other line of evidence can be found in the increasing number of work employing neuroimaging and electrophysiological recording that reveals a relationship between the prefrontal cortex activity and the temporal lobe memory system. These studies lend support to the notion of large scale connection pathways between frontal and posterior brain regions underlying and linking the functioning of the multiple memory subsystems instead of independent modules for each type of memory.

Chapter 11 - When inserted into mouse brain by transgenic or knockin methods, *PS1* mutations responsible for hereditary Alzheimer's disease, despite the absence of Aβ plaques, cause anomalies in calcium homeostasis, potentiate excitotoxicity, and alter the electrophysiologic properties of neurons. Transgenic and knockin mice with presenilin mutations are slower than age-matched controls in acquisition of spatial learning in the Morris water maze, as well as non-spatial learning in object recognition and Pavlovian trace conditioning. These detrimental effects are likely mediated either by increased $A\beta_{42}$ concentrations or by the direct action of mutated *PS1*.

Chapter 12 - Assessment of cognitive, motor, sensory, and communicative functions in children with profound intellectual and multiple disabilities (PIMD) is still in its infancy. There is a lack of standardized instruments, with the instruments mainly used being checklists and observation scales. Although these lists often fail to meet the requirements of validity and reliability, they nevertheless often prove a helpful tool to determine how the person involved can best be supported.

One very specific factor entailed in assessment that is related to the complexity and severity of their disabilities is the level of alertness in a child with PIMD. The assessors are often not sure when the "best moment" to start an assessment is. In addition, they are often unaware of which conditions can help provoke and maintain optimal alertness levels for assessment. Alertness, however, is not just a way to optimize the assessment process; it can also be the objective of the assessment process itself.

An observation list has been developed to assess the level of alertness in children with PIMD in order to 1. establish the optimal period or periods during the day to offer a stimulus or an activity; and 2. to establish the pattern of alertness in a child and the contextual influences on this pattern. In the chapter, the meaning of the concept 'alertness' will be discussed. Furthermore, a description of the content of the list and its use will be presented. For this list, inter-observer and intra-observer reliability were determined by comparing the scores of three (groups of) observers: teachers, an external observer who had received additional information about the clients, and an external observer who did not know the clients at all. The results of the reliability scores for 78 situations will be presented.

The observation list seems to be a functional and sensitive instrument that provides direct support staff with the opportunity to discern individual differences in alert moments and the impact that different stimuli have on alertness. This information can be useful in clinical practice.

Chapter 13 - In the time-dependent society of today, those with limited ability to manage time will show a heightened dependence on others and more need for support, exacerbating their vulnerability. Children with developmental disorders e.g. intellectual disabilities or Autism Spectrum Disorders are reported to have problems in time perception, time orientation or time management, in this chapter all related to the suggested overarching concept: *time processing ability* (TPA). The aim of this short communication is to present a currently developed innovative assessment of TPA and its relation to daily time management (TM) in children with and without developmental disabilities, including intellectual disabilities. The new assessment of TPA; **Ki**t for **a**ssessing **Ti**me processing ability (KaTid) for children was based on current knowledge of information processing in children with cognitive disabilities e.g. using iconic symbols and concrete concepts. Using modern test statistics (Rasch analysis), the evaluation of the KaTid and a related Parent scale for estimating the daily TM presented acceptable psychometric properties. The results indicate that the items in KaTid, initially defined as time perception, time orientation and time management, all empirically support a potential uni-dimensional construct, TPA. In this TPA construct, time perception, time orientation and time management can be seen as different levels of complexity rather than as separate constructs. The Parent scale of daily TM also demonstrated acceptable psychometric properties. There is a relation between the parents' ratings of a child's daily TM and TPA in children with developmental disabilities. Thus TPA seems to be a factor related to children's daily TM that needs to be taken into consideration when planning and evaluating interventions designed to facilitate everyday functioning for children with ID. This is a step towards providing evidence-based instruments that, together with other information, can help the professional in structuring the intervention *planning* process for children with difficulties in daily TM.

Chapter 14 - People with intellectual disabilities have had a long history of exclusion and enforced dependency. As this commentary examines, the uncertainty regarding their definition and an acknowledgement that a person with an intellectual disability can be particularly vulnerable to dependency, has led to a very hidden geography for this group. From the middle of the last century, geographers examined the locational separation of people committed to the 'idiot' asylums of Victorian Britain and Canada. It was clear that the asylum had a symbolic influence in the community well beyond its rather narrow role as the place of residence. More recently geographers have traced the movement of people with intellectual disabilities to group homes, co-operative housing, residence with parents and independent housing. It was hoped that the relocation from isolated stand-alone institutions would help to get rid of, or diminish stigmatisation. However, Hall urges us to move away from assuming that marginalisation equates solely with exclusion from mainstream social activities and spaces, and constructing inclusion as a process of incorporation into these activities and spaces. This commentary therefore forces us to take a critical approach on today's geography of care, where we move beyond narrow binaries of institutionalisation/ deinstitutionalisation, isolation/integration and success/failure. We must be critical of the spaces of incorporation and not assume a place of incorporation is the best choice for a person with an intellectual disability. This is particularly the case if people with intellectual disabilities face a mix of patronisation, fear, an unwillingness to understand 'non-standard' forms of communication, and a strong sense of difference in public life.

In: Learning and Memory Developments...
Editors: L. C. Eklund, A. S. Nyman, pp. 1-32
ISBN: 978-1-60876-397-9

Chapter 1

EMOTION'S EFFECTS ON ATTENTION AND MEMORY: RELEVANCE TO POSTTRAUMATIC STRESS DISORDER

Katherine Mickley Steinmetz [*] ***and Elizabeth Kensinger***
Boston College Psychology Department.

ABSTRACT

Out of all of the information that we experience, only a subset will become part of our memories. Attentional processes, engaged during an event's unfolding, are essential for allowing us to transform an experience into a memory, and emotion can critically modulate those attentional processes, increasing the likelihood that an emotional experience becomes part of our memory stores. This chapter reviews behavioral and neuroimaging evidence that has revealed effects of emotion on memory and attention in individuals with and without post-traumatic stress disorder (PTSD). First, we review how emotion influences the attentional processes that allow individuals with and without PTSD to transform experiences into a memory. Second, we focus on differences in the way emotional items are remembered in people with and without PTSD and how this may be linked to differences in attention at encoding. Third, we discuss current controversies regarding the uniqueness of traumatic memories in PTSD.

INTRODUCTION

We are constantly bombarded by a plethora of information and experiences, only a small subset of which will actually be encoded into lasting memories. Emotion may be one subset that is likely to be selected from the barrage of information, leading to lasting memories. *Encoding* refers to this set of processes that transform aspects of an experience into a memory. As a consequence of the fact that our attentional facilities may be allocated differently towards emotional information than to nonemotional information, we may also

[*] Corresponding author: Department of Psychology, Boston College, 140 Commonwealth Ave., Chestnut Hill, MA 02467, Fax: 617-552-0523

encode that emotional information differently, and subsequently remember it differently, than nonemotional information.

The study of emotion's effects on attention and memory are especially salient in the study of post-traumatic stress disorder (PTSD), a disorder in which people are haunted by their memory of an extreme, emotional, traumatic event. However, it is unclear if people with PTSD have memories that are just extreme forms of typical emotional memory or if these trauma memories are truly unique. Thus, it is important to compare differences in traumatic memories in PTSD to emotional memories in people without PTSD in order to discover what is unique about the disorder as opposed to a typical memory for an emotional item. In this literature review, we review the current literature regarding the differences in attention and memory for emotional information in people with and without PTSD and discuss the debate concerning the uniqueness of the traumatic memory in PTSD.

ENCODING AND ATTENTIONAL PROCESSES

It is well known that emotional information is more likely to be encoded than nonemotional information. There are many different types of processes that are tied to the successful encoding of emotional information (e.g., perceptual, working memory, semantic, attentional, etc.); however, in this paper we will focus on *attention* as a key component that may lead to differences in encoding of emotional memories and that may be greatly affected in PTSD. *Attention* refers to the ability to focus processing resources on a task, an ability that requires conscious concentration and executive control (see James, 1890 for an early definition). Though attention refers to a deliberate and conscious process (see Cohen, 2005; Rensink, 2005; Yantis, 1998), the allocation of attention can often be guided by *preattentive processes*, which operate below the threshold of consciousness to efficiently and automatically bias where one's attention is allocated (Cohen, 2005; Rensink, 2005). These processes can allow some stimuli to "capture" attention or to have a prioritization in processing (Egeth & Yantis, 1997). Once attention is directed to information, there also are processes that influence the likelihood that attention is maintained on that information. *Sustained attention* refers to this set of processes. Sustained attention can occur because of *vigilance*[1] which refers to one's readiness to attend to unpredicted events in the environment (Sarter, Givens & Bruno, 2001), or because of a failure in *disengagement*, which refers to one's ability to shift his or her attention away from an item and towards something else (Koster, Crombez, Verschuere, & De Houwer, 2003). One way to look at the processes underlying sustained attention is that it may be due to a difficulty *inhibiting* the processing of an item in order to attend to other things in the environment. So, as in the often-used example of not being able to look away from a car accident, one's attention may be caught by the scene of the wreck and one may not be able to direct one's attention away from or inhibit the processing of that scene.

Because focusing attention on a piece of information boosts the likelihood of successful encoding, effects of emotion on any of these attentional components may lead to differences

[1] Vigilance is used quite liberally in the clinical literature and may simply mean an increased likelihood to detect a piece of information, which could either be caused by a constant readiness or a quick shift of attention. However, the traditional definition of vigilance focuses on the constant readiness to detect a piece of information.

in memory for emotional items as compared to nonemotional items. Therefore, it is likely that if PTSD influences how attention is allocated toward emotional information, then it would also influence how successfully emotional information is encoded. In the following section, we will explore how these varying attentional processes may be differentially affected in the processing of emotional as compared to nonemotional items in people with and without PTSD. We will also discuss neural differences in processing emotional information in people with and without PTSD in an effort to more fully understand the types of attentional processes that may be affected by the disorder.

Attentional Processing of Emotion in People without PTSD

As outlined above, for people without affective disorders, emotional arousing information[2] may affect attentional processing in a number of different ways. Emotional information may "grab" one's attention and be prioritized in processing, it may cause changes in directed attention, and it may also lead to more sustained attention due to an inability to disengage one's attention.

Preattentive Processes. There is abundant evidence that the processing of emotional information may initially be exerted at a more automatic, subconscious level. Indeed, Joseph LeDoux has hypothesized, based on extensive animal work (see LeDoux, 1996) that the amygdala - a brain area important in the detection of high arousal stimuli – is central to both automatic and controlled processing of emotional information. He proposes that when one encounters an emotional and arousing item, the automatic response is the neural "low road." This direct path from the visual thalamus to the amygdala, bypasses the visual processing areas and allows for a rapid but crude detection of the stimuli. This process is automatic and happens without conscious awareness, but allows one to rapidly evoke fight or flight mechanisms. However, with time, one is able to more deliberately process the emotional information. Via this neural "high road" information from the visual thalamus is sent for further processing in the visual cortex and then to the amygdala. Thus, even the unconscious "low road" is sufficient to activate the amygdala.

Support for the idea of preattentive processing of emotional information is found in studies that look at the processing of emotional information in individuals for whom the information does not reach conscious awareness. Blindsight patients provide a useful population in which to investigate whether there is automatic prioritized processing of emotional information because these patients have damage to their primary visual cortex and therefore do not have a conscious awareness of seeing. However, these patients do receive subcortical visual information (e.g., visual information is processed in their thalamus), and so it is possible to examine whether these subcortical (and subconscious) routes are sufficient to provide affective modulation of processing. Morris et al. (2001) found that patients with blindsight had just as much amygdala activity when emotional faces were presented in their

---

[2] Many emotion researchers have found it useful to divide emotional information by two different spectrums. One of these is *valence*, or how positive or negative something is. This may be seen as a continuum from very positive or pleasant to very negative or unpleasant. The other spectrum is *arousal*, varying from items high in arousal (e.g., exciting or agitating) to items low in arousal (e.g., calming or soothing). Any piece of emotional information can vary by these two components independently, thus something can be negative and nonarousing, positive and nonarousing or neutral and nonarousing (see Russell, 1980 for more information).

blind hemifield than when they were presented in their sighted hemifield. In other words, the amygdala was as activated even when they were unaware of being presented with emotional faces as when they could perceive the emotional faces. This indicates that effects of emotional stimuli may influence these preattentive attentional processes.

Although emotion appears to influence preattentive processes, the question remains as to whether it does so via independent mechanisms from those used to influence preattentive processes when emotion is not involved. If the mechanism is distinct, this would provide important evidence for a unique effect of emotion on preattentive processing. Patients with damage to attentional systems provide some clues. Patients with damage to the parietal cortex (most often in the right hemisphere) suffer from "neglect," lacking awareness of the opposite (left) side of space. A milder form of neglect is referred to as "extinction." During extinction, patients can perceive an object in their neglected field when it is presented in isolation, but when it is presented concurrently with an object in their attended field, they are unable to perceive any item in their neglected field. Vuilleumier & Schwartz (2001) investigated whether these patients would be more likely to notice an emotional object in their neglected field than a nonemotional object. They showed patients who exhibited extinction threatening objects (spiders) or nonthreatening objects (flowers) in their neglected field, along with a competing object in their contralateral field. The patients were more likely to detect the threatening stimuli than the non-threatening stimuli. Thus, though spatial attention was impaired due to the parietal cortex damage, there must be areas of the brain independent from the standard parietal system, which allow preattentive biasing towards emotional information (see Driver & Vuilleumier, 2001).

If preattentive processing of emotional information recruits a distinct neural network from that of nonemotional information, what areas of the brain are involved in this distinct network? In the backwards-masking paradigm, a stimulus is presented briefly (often for fewer than 30ms) and then another stimulus is presented for a longer duration (often for longer than 250ms) in order to curtail processing of that first stimulus and to prevent it from reaching conscious awareness (See Figure 1). Though participants do not consciously detect the first stimulus, their behavioral responses or neural activity can be modified by its presentation. For example, one study quickly presented images of fearful eyes[3] (with more whites of the eyes showing) or happy eyes (with little eye whites showing) to participants, quickly masking these images with another picture to prevent the eyes from consciously being detected (Whalen et al, 2004). Though these participants did not report ever detecting the eyes, they had an increase in activation of the amygdala when fearful eye whites had been presented as compared to when neutral eye whites had been presented. This result suggests that the amygdala can be activated even when participants are not consciously aware of a stimulus (and see LeDoux, 2000 for further discussion). Thus, it appears that the amygdala may be part of the network implicated in emotion-specific preattentive processing.

---

[3] It is important to distinguish the difference between fear and threat. Fearful stimuli are usually used to describe faces making a fearful expression, while threatening stimuli are more generalized negative and arousing stimuli which may cause fear in the individual. However, fear faces may be an indication of a threatening situation and thus may evoke the same attentional processes. This is especially true in anxious individuals and when the fear face is looking away – indicating that there is a threatening object in the environment - as opposed to looking at you, indicating that the person in the picture is afraid of you (Adams & Kleck, 2003).

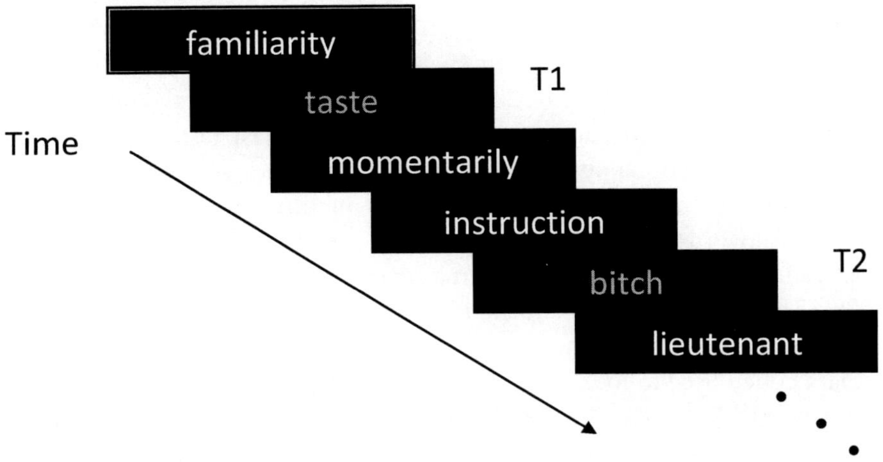

Figure 1. Rapid Serial Visual Processing (RSVP) Task. Part of one trial depicting the presentation of targets (taste = T1 and bitch = T2). Within an experiment, the number of distractors presented between the target words varies, thereby changing the interstimulus interval between the T1 and the T2. Each word is presented at around 100 ms, yeilding a lag bettween the T1 and T2 that is between 100 and 800 ms. At the end of the trial, participants are asked to recall the two target (blue) words.

This neurological evidence is also supported by behavioral evidence for prioritized processing of emotional information. Eye gaze studies can provide evidence for prioritization of emotional information. These studies are based on the idea that most of the time, eye gaze is a good proxy for attention: usually people's attention is directed to the same location where their eyes are focused (Parkhurst, Law, & Niebur, 2002). Using eye tracking, some studies have found that when an emotional (positive or negative) picture is presented next to a neutral picture, people initially look at the emotional picture (Calvo & Lang, 2004; Nummenmaa, Hyona, & Calvo, 2006). These findings may indicate automatic preattentive processes since participants looked at the emotional information very quickly (in the first 500 ms), and since even when they were instructed to ignore it, participants still looked at the emotional picture first and more often.

In summary, it seems as though emotional information may be prioritized in processing and that these preattentive processes may rely on neural networks that include the amygdala and are separate from nonemotional attentional processing networks.

Effects of Emotion on Directed Attention. How many of the effects of preattentive processing are carried over to directed attention? There has been some evidence to suggest that some conscious attention is necessary for a maximal amygdala response (Pessoa, McKenna, Gutierrez, & Ungerleider, 2002; Pessoa, Kastner, & Ungerleider, 2002), so perhaps it is not solely preattentive processes that are affected by emotional stimuli. One way to look at this concept would be via tasks that require conscious detection of emotional stimuli, such as the visual search task. Ohman, Flykt & Esteves (2001) presented participants with visual arrays that included pictures of either "fear relevant" arousing stimuli such as snakes or spiders, or "fear irrelevant" nonarousing stimuli such as flowers or mushrooms. Reaction times were taken when participants detected an arousing or a nonarousing item among distracter items in the array. The results of this study suggested that participants were much quicker to detect arousing images amidst a matrix of nonarousing images. Other studies have found that this attentional prioritization of arousing items stands regardless of the valence of the item (Anderson, 2005; Calvo & Lang, 2004; Carretie et al., 2004; Juth, Lundvist, Karlsson & Ohman, 2005; Leclerc & Kensinger, 2008; Nummenmaa et al. 2006; Tipples, Young, Quinlan, Broks, & Ellis, 2002). Thus, it seems as though attention is directed more rapidly toward emotionally arousing information – at least in the visual search task. However, do these effects also apply to words as well as pictures? This question is especially important as words and pictures may be processed in different ways. Pictures may be processed faster than words (e.g., Friedman & Bourne, 1976; Kim, Yoon, & Park, 2004), and may elicit activation in emotion processing areas earlier than words (Giannotti et al., 2008; Schacht, 2008). Thus, the attentional direction towards words may or may not have the same prioritization as pictures.

A task that is often used to look at the processing of emotional words is the Rapid Serial Visual Processing (RSVP) task. In the RSVP task, participants view a series of words presented in rapid succession. They are asked to name the two target colored items (T1 and T2) in the stream of words that were presented in a different colored font from the surrounding distracters (See Figure 1). The typical response to the RSVP task is that the second target, if presented in close temporal succession to the first target, will go unnoticed, because the participant is still processing the first word. This effect has been referred to as an "attentional blink." However, Anderson & Phelps (2001) found that when the second target was an arousing word, people were more likely to detect this word than if the second word were a neutral word. Further, patients with damage to the amygdala did not have the same prioritization of processing for arousing information (e.g., attenuation of the attentional blink) that people with intact amygdalae exhibited. This finding suggests that attention may be directed toward emotional information more easily than it is directed toward neutral information and that the amygdala is necessary for this process. In other words, the appearance of an arousing word and the subsequent activation of the amygdala may override the attentional mechanisms used to process the first word, allowing for detection of the usually missed second word. Thus, in both the visual search and RSVP tasks, where participants are consciously aware of detecting emotional stimuli, arousing emotional information is the key determinant of what takes priority over nonarousing information.

This attentional priority given to emotional information seems to reflect an automatic or involuntary process as opposed to a contingent capture of attention that can be influenced by intentional or top-down processes. Evidence to support the automaticity of the effect has come from studies that have revealed a capture of attention by emotional information even in situations where that attentional capture is harmful to performance on the task. For example, studies have shown that attention towards task-irrelevant emotional information slows detection of nonemotional targets (Horstmann & Becker, 2008; Lipp & Waters, 2007). In addition, this "attentional rubbernecking" towards emotinal information occurs even when participants are highly incentivised (by providing a nienty dollar reward) to detect nonemotional targets (Most, Smith, Cooter, Levy & Zald, 2007). Thus, even when people are highly motivated to ignore emotional information they may be unable to override the automatic attentional priority that emotional information recieves.

Difficulty Disengaging from Emotional Information. Not only is attention directed toward emotional stimuli, it also may be sustained on emotional information longer than on nonemotional information due to difficulty in disengaging from emotional information. Some of this evidence has come from dot-probe experiments. In dot-probe experiments, an emotional and a nonemotional item are briefly presented in different locations on a screen. Then the pictures are removed to reveal a dot behind either the emotional item or the nonemotional item (See Figure 2). Participants are asked to indicate, as quickly as they can, on which side of the screen the dot appeared. Their speed of making this decision, referred to as their reaction time, is measured. A fast reaction time suggests that the participant's attention was directed towards the target that obscured the dot, while a slow reaction time indicates that the participant's attention was not on the target that obscured the dot.

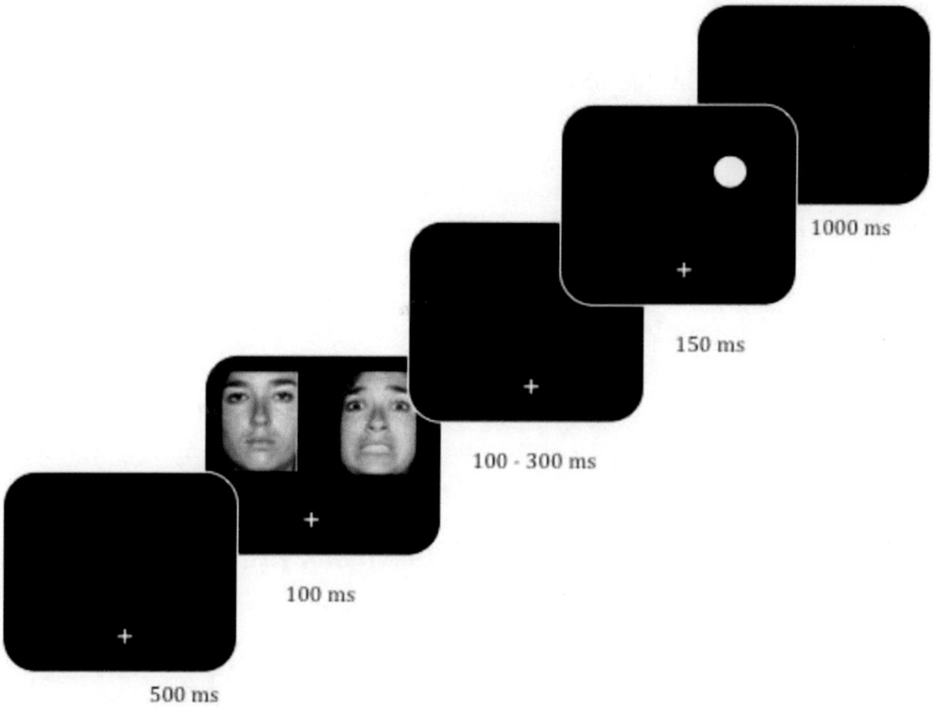

Figure 2. Dot Probe Paradigm. Participants are shown two stimuli side by side and are asked to press a button on the side where the dot appears. (Figure based on paradigm from Pourtois, Grandjean, Sander & Vuilleumer, 2004).

Many studies have shown that participants are faster to detect dots placed behind negative fear-related stimuli (Bradley et al., 1997; Derakshan, 2005; MacLeod, Mathews, & Tata, 1986; Mogg & Bradley, 1999; Pourtois, Grandjean, Sander & Vuilleumer, 2004). This may also be the case for some types of positive stimuli, at least if they are "nurturance relevant," or containing evolutionary significance (i.e., baby faces in Brosch, Sander, Pourtois & Scherer, 2008).

It has been recently suggested that the dot-probe effects may be partially attributed to difficulty in disengagement from an emotional stimuli, as opposed to vigilance for threatening information (Derryberry & Reed, 2002; Koster, Crombez, Verschuere & DeHouwer, 2003). This is because, when compared to a neutral baseline (two neutral pictures), the differences in reaction times were driven by incongruent threat trials as opposed to facilitation on congruent threat trials. In other words, people were slower to detect a dot behind a neutral target paired with a threatening target. However, they weren't any faster to detect a dot behind a threatening picture than they were to notice a dot behind a neutral picture paired with another neutral picture. This pattern of results suggests that the dot-probe task may actually demonstrate sustained attention in the form of a difficulty in disengaging from a threatening item (Koster, Crombez, Verschuere & DeHouwer, 2003). Thus, emotional information may not only direct people's attention, but also sustain it, leading to difficulty disengaging from the information.

This idea that individuals can have difficulties disengaging attention from emotional information is further supported by studies that traditionally have been used to study interference (in this case, the inability to attend to task relevant stimuli in the presence of an emotional stimulus). One task used to study emotional interference is the emotional Stroop paradigm (Stroop, 1935). In this paradigm, people are presented with emotional or neutral words that are written in different colors of font, and they are asked to name the color of font in which the words are written (See Figure 3). Participants tend to be slower to name the color of font in which threat words are written (McKenna & Sharma, 1995). Though there has been some indication that the emotional Stroop effect may be in part caused by the higher word frequency for non-emotional words (and the novelty of emotional words), this cannot fully explain the effects of valence (Kahan & Hely, 2008). Thus, negative arousing information appears to cause interference by commanding processing that may overpower top-down task-related goals (color naming). Both the dot probe task and the emotional Stroop task capture sustained attention due to difficulty in disengaging from emotional information.

Control	Traditional Stroop	Emotional Stroop *Emotional List*	Emotional Stroop *Neutral List*
XXXX	**RED**	**FAIL**	**CLOCK**
XXXX	**YELLOW**	**FEAR**	**GATE**
XXXX	**BLUE**	**CRASH**	**NOTE**
XXXX	**GREEN**	**GRIEF**	**THUMB**
XXXX	**BLUE**	**DEATH**	**FIELD**
XXXX	**RED**		
•	•	•	•
•	•	•	•
•	•	•	•

Figure 3. The Stroop Paradigm. Participants are asked to name the color of the text and reaction time is measured. Longer reaction times may indicate greater interference due to the meaning of the word. Words from the emotional stroop were taken from McKenna & Sharma (1995).

In summary, studies have shown that people without affective disorders attend to emotional information differently than non-emotional information. These differences arise from: 1) preattentive attentional orienting towards emotional information, 2) directed attention towards emotional information, and 3) the sustaining of attention on emotional information. These differences in the processing of emotional information may be caused by amygdalar-driven processes in the brain, separate from the attentional network used to process nonemotional information.

Attentional Processing in People with PTSD

Posttraumatic stress disorder is an anxiety disorder that develops in response to a traumatic event (Breslau, 2002). It is characterized by re-experiencing the trauma, avoiding the stimuli associated with the trauma, numbing of responsivity and affect, and hyperarousal (DSM-IV-TR). Changes in attention are key contributors to the disorder; people with PTSD tend to have difficulty concentrating or attending to neutral stimuli, while at the same time exhibiting hypervigilance, or increased sensitivity to detecting threat. People with PTSD also tend to have automatic re-experiencing of their trauma despite intentionally avoiding stimuli associated with the trauma. These symptoms seem to indicate differences in attentional processing towards stimuli associated with their trauma, and perhaps to emotional stimuli more generally.

Some studies have shown that patients with PTSD may attend to emotional information in a different way than people without an affective disorder. For example, attention to nonemotional information is not always allocated as efficiently in people with PTSD as in controls. People with PTSD often report "poor concentration," (Vasterling & Brewin, p.180) and they perform worse on attentional tasks in general – especially those requiring sustained attention or working memory (Gilbertson, Gurvits, Lasko, Orr & Pitman, 2001; Vasterling, Brailey, Constans, & Sutker, 1998). However, an important question is how PTSD affects attention allocation to emotional information. In other words, does PTSD result only in generalized attention deficits, or does it specifically affect the way in which attention is directed and sustained on emotional information?

Considerable debate has arisen as to whether people with PTSD have exaggerated 1) preattentive processing of emotional information, 2) conscious detection or directed attention towards emotional information, 3) sustained attention or the inability to disengage from emotional information, or 4) some combination of the three (see Buckley, Blanchard, & Neill, 2002 for review).

Preattentive Processes. As we know from the previous section, people without PTSD have differences in preattentive processes directed towards emotional information: even without conscious awareness, people are more likely to exhibit prioritization in processing of emotional information. Therefore, in order to determine if people with PTSD differ in preattentive processing of emotional information, they must be compared to groups without PTSD in order to make sure that any sort of facilitation surpasses that of a person without PTSD. In addition, it is important to compare the reaction to trauma-related stimuli as opposed to trauma-unrelated emotional stimuli, to see if these processes are trauma-specific or reflect a more generalized change in emotional processing.

Little research has been conducted to examine preattentive processing in PTSD, and those studies that have looked at this issue have revealed conflicting results. One paradigm that has been used to test preattentive processing in people with PTSD is a modified version of the Stroop task that uses the backwards-masking technique (see Buckley et al., 2002 for review and Figure 1 for a reminder of the backwards-masking approach). In this paradigm, emotional words are presented subliminally and are quickly replaced by a random string of letters that is equally as long as the emotional word.

One study found that PTSD patients showed an attentional advantage for negative words even though they were not consciously aware of the presence of the threat-related words (e.g., PTSD participants, but not trauma-matched controls, showed slower color naming of word strings that were masking threatening colored words as compared to neutral words; Harvey, Bryant, & Rapee, 1996). However, other studies have not found this to be the case when using this paradigm, perhaps indicating that this effect may be subject to habituation, or may not generalize across all task versions or subgroups of patients (Constans, 2005).

McNally, Amir, & Lipke (1996) found habituation effects when using this paradigm. This study did not find an overall Stroop effect for trauma words in people with PTSD as compared to trauma-matched controls. However, they did find an early attentional bias in the PTSD group: it took participants with PTSD, but not trauma-matched controls, longer to name the colors of masked trauma words on early trials, but this effect waned over the course of the experiment.

This study may also demonstrate that occurrence of comorbidity of depression along with PTSD may have lead to a lack of prioritization towards traumatic information. Most of the participants in McNally, Amir, & Lipke (1996) had depression as well as PTSD. As previous studies have shown that people with depression may not exhibit the emotional Stroop interference in the subliminal Stroop paradigm (Mogg, Bradley, Williams, & Mathews, 1993), the comorbid depression may be another reason why the overall Stroop effect may not have occurred. Therefore, the subliminal Stroop effect may not extend to people with PTSD who also have depression.

It also may not extend to people who have acute stress disorder (e.g., the duration of symptoms is less than three months). Paunovic, Lundh & Ost, (2002) found no preattentive advantage for subliminally presented trauma or positive words in the subliminal Stroop task for people with acute PSTD as compared to age-matched controls. Paunovic and colleagues suggested that this may have to do with the fact that their participants' had acute PTSD, and that the trauma network may become more generalized over time. Therefore, more research is necessary to tease out the effects of the subliminal Stroop, separate from potential differences in habituation and comorbidity.

As noted in the section discussing preattentive processing in healthy individuals, it can be a difficult phase of processing to isolate. Thus, research is beginning to move away from behavioral examinations of preattentive processing in PTSD and toward the use of neuroimaging methods to reveal whether PTSD patients show alterations in the neural processes engaged during the processing of stimuli that have not reached awareness. Studies have shown that when PTSD patients are presented with fear faces that are quickly masked with a neutral face, so that the participant is not consciously aware of seeing a fearful face, PTSD participants exhibit more amygdala activation to those masked stimuli than they exhibit to either explicitly perceived fear faces (Armony, Corbo, Clément, & Brunet, 2005) or to masked happy faces (Rauch, et al., 2000). However, these studies did not compare PTSD patients to a control group. Thus, the most convincing evidence for preattentive priortization of emotional information that reaches beyond that of the typical priortization of emotional information comes from one recent study which found increased amygdala as well as medial prefrontal cortex activity in people with PTSD for masked fear faces when compared to non-

PTSD controls (Bryant et al., 2008). Although few studies have focused specifically on preattentive processing in PTSD, it is possible that at least the preattentive processing of fearful faces may be exaggerated in people with PTSD. This may be an especially important finding because it suggests that even for stimuli that are not trauma-specific, there may be enhanced preattentive processing in people with PTSD.

In summary, the scarce research on preattentive processing of emotional stimuli has hinted at the idea that people with PTSD may have even more prioritized processing than people without PTSD. However, more work is needed, controlling for comorbidity and using control groups in order to firmly make this claim.

Directed Attention. The facilitation of attention towards emotional information in people with PTSD as compared to people without PTSD has been reported in few studies. However, one experiment that has looked at the emotional prioritization in PTSD using the visual search paradigm has found that people with PTSD do not exhibit an exaggerated facilitation of processing emotional stimuli as compared with people without PTSD. Pineles, Shiphert, Welch, and Yovel (2007) found no additional attentional facilitation for threat-related words for people with either high or low ratings of PTSD. Given only this one null result, it is hard to draw any conclusions about the effects of PTSD on directed attention. This area is ripe for further research, particularly because if preattentive processes are indeed affected by PTSD, then it seems likely that downstream attentional processes may be affected as well.

Neuroscience research may begin to help determine differences in directed attention for people with PTSD. When people with PTSD view a negative emotional item, they exhibit more amygdala activity than those who don't have PTSD (see Shin, Rauch, & Pitman, 2006). This amygdala over-activity may be related to under-activity in the anterior cingulate (part of the prefrontal cortex) and the hippocampus, regions which may be important in regulating the amygdalar activity (Yamasue et al., 2004). When someone without PTSD encounters something that appears to be threatening, the amygdala is activated. If this object turns out to be safe, areas in the prefrontal cortex such as the anterior cingulate as well as areas of the medial temporal lobe such as the hippocampus work to suppress the amygdalar activity. In people with PTSD, without the control of the prefrontal cortex and the hippocampus, the amygdala may become overactive and stay overactive - leading to an inability to disengage from emotional information (Shin et al., 2001). As activation of the prefrontal cortex is usually associated with conscious processes it is possible that the inactivity of this area may indicate that people with PTSD's attentional differences may function at a more subconscious level.

It has also been hypothesized that this dysfunction of the frontal-amygdalar network, as well as deficits in cortico-thalamic integration, may lead to generalized attentional and concentration problems in people with PTSD (Vasterling, Brailey, Constans & Sutker, 1998; Clark, et al., 2003). Future work focusing specifically on neural differences while doing attentional tasks are necessary to determine specific functional and anatomic brain differences that may lead to differences in attentional processing in people with PTSD.

Difficulty Disengaging from Emotional Information. Much more research has been done on whether PTSD patients have difficulty disengaging from emotional information. As noted in an earlier section, even individuals without PTSD find it difficult to disengage from emotional stimuli; however, these difficulties may be exaggerated in those with PTSD. In fact, the difficulties with disengagement may be so intense in people with PTSD that they may cause interference and be disruptive for further processing of task-relevant stimuli (Buckley et al., 2000).

One study has used traumatic distractors to explore disengagement from emotional information in people with PTSD. Participants were asked to complete a simple attention task while traumatic and non-traumatic pictures were presented in the background. People with PTSD were slower at responding when trauma-related distracters were used (Chemtob et al., 1999). Thus, it seems that the presence of traumatic pictures may cause interference effects on attention.

Much of the research on emotional disengagement has been studied by looking at interference using the emotional Stroop task. PTSD patients have repeatedly been shown to have exaggerated slowing as compared to people without PTSD when asked to name the color of trauma words rather than neutral words (see Vasterling & Brewin, 2005). This effect has been shown in people who developed PTSD after combat (Constans, McCloskey, Vasterling, Brailey & Mathews, 2004; Kaspi, McNally & Amir, 1995; McNally, Kaspi, Reinamm, & Zeitlin, 1990; Vrana, Roodman, & Beckman, 1995), violent crimes (Cassiday, McNally, & Zeitlin, 1992; Foa, Feske, Murdock, Kozak, & McCarthy, 1991), or accidents (Thrasher, Dalgleish & Yule, 1994; Bryant & Harvey, 1995; Buckley, Blanchard & Hickling, 2002). Most of these studies have shown the increased reaction times specifically for trauma-related words, though it may also extend to other negative words (Litz et. al, 1996; Thrasher, Dalgleish & Yule, 1994; Buckley, Blanchard & Hickling, 2002) or even to positive arousing words (Cassiday et al., 1992; Paunovic et al., 2002). In addition, Pineles, Shiphert, Welch, & Yovel (2007) found that people with high levels of PTSD, but not those with low levels, exhibited more interference. They suggested that this may mean that people with low levels of PTSD are better able to habituate to threat related words and therefore may allow them to be more responsive to exposure therapy. This finding suggests that there may be differences between individuals with PTSD that may lead to differences in attentional interference, underscoring the importance for future research to take an individual-differences approach when examining the effects of PTSD on attention toward emotional information.

In order to determine if volitional and motivational aspects may play a role in these Stroop effects, Buckley, Galovski, Blanchard, & Hickling (2004) trained professional actors to act like patients with PTSD, but they did not find the same slowing for threat words, as shown in PTSD. In addition, people with PTSD still exhibited the slowing effect for traumatic words, even when they were offered a financial reward for their success (Constans et al., 2004). These findings are significant because they indicate that these effects of emotion on disengagement may not be subject to volitional control.

However, one study found that the disengagement effect can be manipulated in other ways. Participants with PTSD did not show the emotional Stroop interference effect if they were told that they were going to encounter a stressful event such as watching a combat movie or giving a speech after the Stroop test (Constans et al., 2004). Thus, the attentional interference seems to not be under volitional control, but may be overridden by anticipatory anxiety. The authors suggest that this overriding may have occurred either because the inhibition effect may be awarded only to the most potent threat (e.g., the upcoming speech or movie), or because the stressor caused a narrowing of attention, which led to the ability to focus on the word color, ignoring the word meaning. These results are significant because they indicate that difficulty in disengagement can be overridden in people with PTSD.

It also has been suggested that whereas only high threat levels result in disengagement difficulties in people without PTSD, those people with PTSD may have trouble disengaging from even mild threats (Vasterling & Brewin, 2005). However, this claim stems mainly from research that was done on anxious individuals, not specifically those with PTSD (e.g., Mogg & Bradley, 1998), so future research will be required to elucidate whether the disengagement difficulties are more generalized in PTSD.

In summary, though the prioritization of emotional information in preattentive processing and directed attention may be enhanced only in certain situations, converging evidence suggests that people with PTSD often have more difficulty in disengaging from emotional stimuli than do people without PTSD. This interference may lead to differences in concentration and attending to nonemotional information as well as differences in encoding emotional information (Vasterling & Brewin, 2005). As we will later discuss, these difficulties may also have implications for the types of information that PTSD patients remember.

Emotional Memory

As discussed in the previous section, PTSD may affect the processes that are engaged while emotional items are encoded. These effects of PTSD on the processing of emotional information (in concert with influences on other factors such as consolidation and retrieval processes) may change the way that patients with PTSD remember emotional items. PTSD patients' emotional memories may have different subjective characteristics compared to the emotional memories of non-PTSD patients, and PTSD patients also may have altered access to their emotional memories. Some of these changes may be specific to information tied to their traumatic experience, whereas other changes may generalize to trauma-irrelevant emotional memories. In this section we will discuss how emotion affects the qualities of memories that are retrieved by individuals without PTSD, and then we will describe how PTSD may change the qualities most often associated with an emotional memory as well as the ways in which emotional memories are accessed. An underlying theme throughout these discussions will be whether the trauma memories of PTSD are supported by a special memory system or whether they arise via the same mechanisms that support other types of emotional memories.

Emotional Memory in People without PTSD

Even in individuals without PTSD, emotional memories differ from nonemotional ones in the quality with which they are remembered. Negative items, in particular, are remembered with subjectively rich detail. This subjective vividness has been shown in memory studies that ask people to indicate whether they vividly recollect emotional items or simply have a feeling of familiarity that lacks specific details. These studies have consistently shown that participants vividly recollect negative items more often than nonemotional items (Dewhurst & Parry, 2000; Kensinger & Corkin, 2003; Neisser & Harsch, 1992; Ochsner, 2000; Rubin & Kozin, 1984; Schmolck, Buffalo, & Squire, 2000; Sharot et al., 2004). It has also been found that the level of emotional arousal of an event is strongly correlated with subjective ratings of vividness that participants report (Reisberg, Heuer, McLean & O'Shaughnessy, 1988).

Corroborating evidence for the effect of emotion on memory for detail has come from objective assessments of memory for specific visual details. In one paradigm, participants were shown a series of emotional or nonemotional items. Then, at test, they were shown either the same item or a similar item. They were asked to distinguish between the two, requiring them to remember specific details of the studied item. Studies using this paradigm have found that people were more likely to distinguish "same" items from "similar" items if the items were negative as opposed to neutral, indicating that specific visual details may be retained more often for negative items (Kensinger, Garoff-Eaton, & Schacter, 2006, 2007a).

Richness in memory for other details has also been tested, revealing that for negative items, people may be more likely to remember the color of font in which a word was presented (D'Argembeau & Van der Linden, 2004; Doerksen & Shimamura, 2001; Kensinger & Corkin, 2003; MacKay et al., 2004), the location in which a word was presented on a computer screen (D'Argembeau & Van der Linden, 2004; MacKay & Ahmetzanov, 2005), or whether words or objects were visually presented or mentally imagined (Kensinger & Schacter, 2006). Therefore, there is increasing evidence that negative items are accompanied by an increased subjective and objective vividness. These qualitative differences may stem from differences at encoding: when one first views an emotional item. The attentional factors described in the previous section may be particularly important, because if an item is more likely to capture your attention at encoding, its details may be more likely to be remembered later.

There is some evidence to suggest that the enhanced vividness of an emotional memory may be specific to those events that elicit negative, rather than positive, emotions. Negative items can be more likely to be processed in a detailed manner and with a narrower focus of attention, while positive items often are processed in a more global or conceptual manner and are associated with a broadening of attention (Fredrickson & Branigan, 2005; Rowe, Hirsh & Anderson, 2007; Gasper & Clore, 2002). These attentional differences may lead to differences in later memory for emotional items. Specifically, while negative information is more likely to be remembered along with contextual details, positive information is often associated with a general sense of familiarity, lacking these specific details (e.g., LaBar & Phelps, 1998; Ochsner, 2000). In addition, areas of the brain associated with visual processing are more likely to be associated with the successful encoding of negative information, while areas associated with self-referential processing and episodic and semantic retrieval are more associated with for the successful encoding of positive items (Mickley & Kensinger, 2008; see also Mickley Steinmetz & Kensinger, 2009). Thus, the qualitative differences in the way that positive and negative information is remembered may be tied to encoding processes which differ based on valence.

Despite the evidence outlined above, it is not the case that all aspects of negative experiences are remembered well; this enhancement in vividness for negative items may come at a cost. While some aspects of a negative event may be more likely to be remembered, other aspects may actually be more likely to be forgotten. These effects have been called "memory trade-offs" in laboratory investigations (Kensinger, Garoff-Eaton, & Schacter, 2007b; Waring, Payne, Schacter, & Kensinger, 2010) or "tunnel memory" in the case of autobiographical memories (see Christianson & Safer, 1996; Safer, Christianson, Autry, & Osterlund, 1998). These terms refer to the fact that people can be less likely to remember information that surrounds an emotional item either spatially (one may be able to remember the emotional object within a scene, such as a snake, but not the background context; Christianson & Loftus, 1991; Kensinger, Piguet, Krendl, & Corkin, 2005; Waring, Payne, Schacter, & Kensinger, 2010) or temporally (you may be able to remember an emotional word, but not the word that followed it). Within investigations of eyewitness memory, this kind of phenomenon has also been described as the "weapon focus effect," referring to the fact that crime victims are more likely to remember the emotional object (the weapon) but not other important details such as their robber's face or clothing (Brown, 2003; Deffenbacher,1983; Pickel, French, & Betts, 2003; Shaw & Skolnick, 1994).

These memory trade-offs may be due to the narrowing of attention onto negative items (Easterbrook, 1959), leading to decreased encoding of surrounding information (see Reisberg & Heuer, 2004). Indeed, studies have found that when participants passively view a scene, they are more likely to exhibit memory trade-offs (Burke, Heuer & Reisberg, 1992; Kensinger, Garoff-Eaton, & Schacter, 2007b; Wessel, van der Kooy, & Merckelbach, 2000), while if they are directed to pay attention to specific details, the trade-off effect may be lessened or may be eliminated altogether (Kensinger et al., 2005; Kensinger et al., 2007b). These studies indicate that attentional mechanisms at encoding, when unconstrained, may serve to focus attention on negative information and may therefore be instrumental in leading to memory trade-offs. These studies emphasize that although negative emotion may increase the likelihood of encoding something vividly, negative emotion also may lead to the constriction of attention onto particular event details, lessening the likelihood that surrounding elements are incorporated into memory.

Emotional Memory in People with PTSD

People with PTSD often report general memory deficits when they are asked to recall nonemotional items (Vasterling & Brewin, 2005), suggesting that there are effects of PTSD on general memory mechanisms. However, it is less clear how PTSD affects the relationship between emotion and memory either in terms of the quality of a memory or in terms of the accessibility of a memory. For example, traumatic memories in people with PTSD are often associated with incredible vividness and a sense of reliving (Bremner, Krystal, Southwick, & Charney, 1995; Ehlers & Clark, 2000; Janet, 1904), but it is not clear if these characteristics reflect the same types of processes that lead to vivid memories in individuals without PTSD, or whether a distinct mechanism accounts for the vivid memories experienced by those with PTSD.

When considering the mechanisms that support traumatic memory in individuals with PTSD, one important distinction to make is whether it is a voluntary memory or an involuntary memory. Based on the different qualities of involuntary and voluntarily accessed memories, it has been proposed that distinct memory systems may underlie the formation or retrieval of these two types of memories. The Dual Representation Theory (see Brewin, Dalgleish & Joseph, 1996) posits that voluntarily accessed memories rely on the same system that supports autobiographical memory for non-traumatic memories. This system – postulated to be hippocampally-based - underlies "verbally accessible memories" which are remembered by deliberate retrieval. These are the memories that are tested in recall and recognition paradigms in the laboratory, when participants are asked to retrieve a memory and to assess that memory's qualities.

By contrast, involuntarily accessed memories, or "situationally accessible memories," may be triggered automatically by specific cues, leading to the flashbacks characteristic of PTSD. These situational memories may not rely on a hippocampal-based system, but may instead be cued by lower level perceptual processing of the traumatic information, leading to vivid recapitulation of visuo-spatial information without a higher-level narrative structure (Brewin, 2001). These memories are often triggered by internal or external cues that relate to some aspect of the traumatic event, and these cues elicit the recapitulation of the prior traumatic experience. This recapitulation can occur despite the presence of safety signals within environmental context. For example, a veteran with PTSD may experience an involuntary flashback from war in response to a car backfiring (which may sound like a gun-shot), despite the fact that the veteran is now in a safe environment and is not in a war zone. The hallmark of these intrusive memories is that the individual has no control over the retrieval of the memory, and once the memory is triggered, he cannot curtail the re-experiencing of the traumatic event.

Voluntary Memories. To study voluntary memories in PTSD, many researchers began by asking whether people with PTSD are more likely to remember items associated with their trauma than are people without PTSD. If the PTDS patients are more likely than controls to remember items associated with their trauma, this may indicate some difference in the memory processes engaged at encoding, consolidation, or retrieval. If the PTSD patients remember a similar proportion of items to the controls, this could suggest that similar memory processes may be at work whenever people have experienced trauma, regardless of whether they have PTSD. Alternatively, the same behavioral outcome could result from different neural processes in people with and without PTSD, thus neuroscience research is beginning to be used to provide further information about the memory mechanisms at work in people with and without PTSD.

The findings regarding the effect of PTSD on voluntary memory for trauma-related stimuli have been mixed. Some studies have found that when participants are asked to freely recall trauma-related and non-trauma-related words that were earlier embedded in an attentional task (such as the emotional Stroop task), people with PTSD remember proportionally more traumatic words than do non-patient controls (Chemtob et al., 1999; Paunovic, Lundh, & Ost, 2002; Vrana, Roodman, & Beckman, 1995). This finding goes along nicely with the previously discussed attention research, which has found that PTSD patients are more likely than control participants to process the meanings of these trauma words in the emotional Stroop task. Thus, this attention bias might lead to an enhancement in memory for trauma-related words in people with PTSD.

Other studies have indicated that this exaggerated memory enhancement for voluntarily accessed trauma items as compared to non-trauma items may be driven by the fact that PTSD patients have memory deficits for non-trauma related words and may not reflect a boost in their memory for trauma related words. In other words, people with PTSD may simply be *less impaired* in their memory for trauma-relevant stimuli than in their memory for trauma-irrelevant stimuli. For example, one study found that while crime victims with PTSD were equally as likely as people without PTSD to recognize faces that were perceived as threatening, they were less likely than people without PTSD to recognize non-hostile faces (Paunovic, Jundh & Ost, 2003). This finding suggests that people with PTSD may have less of a memory impairment for trauma related items than for trauma-irrelevant information. This conclusion is consistent with work indicating that recall of trauma words may be less impaired in PTSD than the recall of positive or neutral words (McNally, Metzger, Lasko, Clancy & Pitman, 1998). It also is compatible with a study of associative memory, revealing that Holocaust victims with PTSD were less likely to remember neutral word pairs than were those without PTSD, but that the individuals with PTSD showed an enhanced memory for word pairs associated with their traumatic experience (Golier, Yehuda, Lupien & Harvey, 2003).

Though these studies suggest that PTSD patients are more likely to be able to voluntarily access trauma-related information as compared to non-trauma-related information, some studies have found that when false alarms (times when participants incorrectly endorse items that were not presented) are controlled in a recognition memory task, there is no remaining difference in recognition accuracy between combat veterans with and without PTSD (Litz et al.,1996). This finding suggests that people with PTSD may have an enhanced response bias towards trauma-related stimuli: they may be more liberal in accepting that an item related to their trauma was presented, perhaps because it fits with their schema for what they saw (e.g., "I saw a series of pictures related to my trauma").

Together these studies suggest that although PTSD may be associated with global deficits in memory, those with PTSD may have less of an impaired memory for items related to their trauma. There is not much evidence that people with PTSD are more likely to remember items associated with their trauma than are people without PTSD. Rather, PTSD may lead to a larger discrepancy between memory for traumatic and non-traumatic items because individuals with PTSD retain the traumatic stimuli as well as the control group but are more likely to forget the stimuli that are not trauma-relevant.

Though the likelihood of voluntarily remembering a trauma-relevant item may be similar between people with and without PTSD, the *quality* of these memories may be very different in people with PTSD. Some research indicates that the voluntarily accessed trauma memories of PTSD patients are fragmented: i.e., disjointed and disorganized, with missing pieces of information (Foa, Molnar, & Cashman, 1995; Halligan, Michael, Ehlers & Clark, 2003; Nijenhuis & Van der Hart, 1999; Tromp, Koss, Figueredo & Tharan, 1995; van der Kolk and Fisler, 1995; van der Hart, Van der Kolk, & Boon, 1998; but see Controversies section for opposing view). It is not clear what types of deficits may lead to this disjointed recall. On the one hand, it is possible that this disjointed nature reflects a breakdown in the mnemonic retrieval processes engaged by PTSD patients. On the other hand, it is plausible that the disjointed memories reflect a more general deficit in verbal processing and that one consequence of this verbal deficit is a breakdown in memory retrieval. Although this issue continues to be debated, the fact that people with PTSD often report that their non-emotional memories are disjointed, and that they tend to have difficulty providing narratives of their past experiences, may suggest a more pervasive deficit that is not constrained to the retrieval of traumatic experiences (Hellawell & Brewin, 2002).

This "fragmentation," resulting in a memory that is missing pieces of information, may also be caused in part by memory trade-offs similar to those described for individuals without PTSD. Anecdotally, patients with PTSD often report "tunnel memory," or a detailed memory for the emotional element or gist of the scene without much memory for the surrounding elements or contextual details (LaBar, 2007). For example, someone with PTSD might have a vivid memory of a body in combat, but they may not remember the details of where the body was found. One recent study has found that people with higher anxiety levels and lower levels of cognitive control (e.g., lower ability to manage other cognitive processes, leading to poorer ability to plan, think abstractly, etc.) were more likely to show a trade-off; these individuals were particularly likely to remember the central emotional element at the cost of the background (Waring et al., 2010). Because those who develop PTSD tend to have higher levels of anxiety and lower levels of cognitive control than those who do not develop PTSD (see van der Kolk, 2004), it would make sense that people with PTSD may show more of a trade-off (or have more tunnel memory). However, the magnitude of the trade-off effect has not been systematically tested in a population with PTSD. Thus, it is unclear to what extent the voluntary memories that people with PTSD experience are supported by similar mechanisms to those that underlie extreme emotional memories in those without PTSD. More specifically, it is not clear whether the same mechanisms that lead to the trade-off effect in controls could also lead to the fragmented memories that PTSD patients voluntarily access.

Involuntary memory. In addition to differences in voluntarily recalled memory of trauma, people with PTSD also experience *involuntary* reliving experiences or flashbacks accompanied with vivid sensory and affective details (see Brewin, 1998; van der Kolk & Fisler, 1995; Hellawell & Brewin, 2004; Boals & Rubin, in press). These memories are usually visual in nature, but they may also include the re-experiencing of other sensations, including the smells, sounds, tastes and physiological reactions during the traumatic experience (Brewin et al., 1996; Ehlers & Clark, 2000; Ehlers & Steil, 1995; Ehlers, Hackmann, Steil, Clohessy, Wenninger & Winter, 2002; Foa & Rothbaum, 1998; Hackmann, Ehlers, Speckens & Clark, 2004). These involuntary memories are accompanied by a sense that the memory is happening in the present (Ehlers, Hackmann, & Michael, 2004; Michael, Ehlers, Halligan & Clark, 2004). In other words, these involuntary memories may lack temporal context (e.g. they may feel as though they are happening in the present) and spatial context (e.g. they may feel as though the trauma is happening at the current location). Thus, these memories feel phenomenologically as a "reliving" of the trauma as they are accompanied by an extremely vivid sensory experience, detached from temporal and spatial context.

One explanation for this lack of context may be a disruption of "contextual integration" at encoding (Steel & Holmes, 2007). When people without PTSD encode an experience, the hippocampus is thought to be important in binding the features of the information along with the spatial and temporal context (Eichenbaum, 1997; Squire, 1992). However, in PTSD this binding may be disrupted. During the trauma, the automatic processing of information via the direct path from the visual thalamus to the amygdala, discussed earlier, may be evoked allowing for a quick reaction to the stressful situation (LeDoux et al. 1988). This direct path may bypasses the hippocampus, thereby leading to a lack of the binding of the information with the spatial and temporal context. Ehlers & Clark (2000) have also suggested that during encoding of the trauma people may shift from "contextual processing" to "data driven" perceptual processing. The traumatic incident is processed in a deeply perceptual way, but without elaboration or integration of context. Thus, differences at encoding in processing and hippocampal activation may lead involuntary memories to be remembered in a vivid perceptual manner, lacking spatial and temporal context.

Though involuntary memories are most often discussed in reference to PTSD, people without PTSD also can have intrusive memories, both for negative and for extremely positive events (Berntsen, 2001; Brewin, 1996). However, in people with PTSD, intrusive memories occur more frequently, occur more often in a repetitive nature, and are more likely to be to be stressful (Berntsen, 1996; Brewin, 1998). Thus, these memories may be best characterized as a dysfunctional subclass of intrusive memories. Further, these memories may be self-perpetuating. This perpetuation may be set off by a number of factors. First, the negative nature of these memories may foster avoidance, but that very avoidance may require the patient to maintain awareness of the memory so as to be able to keep it out of mind (see Wegner, 1994 for discussion of this type of avoidance). Second, these intrusive memories may induce a negative mood in people with PTSD, which may make them more likely to experience negative intrusive memories as a function of mood-congruent recall (Berntsen, 1996). Third, people with PTSD may have a hard time accessing the content of their traumatic memory directly (see Brewin, 1998; van der Kolk and Fisler, 1995), and so this may make it more likely that the memory is cued involuntarily. Thus, even though involuntary recall of memories may occasionally occur in those without PTSD, those with PTSD may experience involuntary recalls much more often, and it may even serve as the core mode of access of traumatic memories for them (Brewin, 1998).

In summary, a hallmark of PTSD may be the tendency to remember past experiences both through voluntarily accessed memories and also through involuntarily accessed "flashbacks." It is still debated whether voluntary and involuntary memories reflect the operation of distinct memory systems, and it also is not clear whether the memory mechanisms at work are unique to PTSD or whether they generalize even to those without the disorder. What does seem clear is that the attentional effects described earlier in this chapter are likely to have downstream consequences both on the memories that are likely to be accessed involuntarily and also on the memories that are accessed voluntarily. Within the realm of involuntary memories, the attentional focus may explain why some cues can easily trigger a memory or why the memories often contain the particular sensory information that was being processed as the event initially unfolded. In addition, we propose that the fragmentation found in the voluntary memories of people with PTSD may be influenced by the way in which attention was focused at encoding, and may be another example of an emotion-induced memory trade-off (and see McNally, 2003 for further discussion). In other words, because attention is focused on an emotional element at encoding, the memory that is created may be less likely to contain information about the surrounding elements, resulting in the fragmented voluntary memories that so often occur with PTSD. Thus, both voluntary and involuntary memories may be influenced by biased attention at encoding.

Memory Controversy: Are Trauma Memories Unique?

One point that has been brought up repeatedly in this paper is the question of the uniqueness of trauma memories. Are the traumatic memories of people with PTSD processed and stored fundamentally differently from other emotional memories, or are they just an extreme version of emotional memory? The answer to this question continues to be debated in the current literature, and its resolution is vitally important both for the theoretical conceptualization of memory processes in PTSD and also for the treatment of this disorder.

One side of the argument states that the traumatic memories of PTSD patients are fundamentally unique from the emotional memories of individuals without PTSD. Quite a few different cognitive theories of PTSD conceptualize traumatic memories in this way. Though these theories differ from one another in some ways, they share two views in common. First, they state that traumatic stress is different than "routine" stress response, and thus that traumatic memories are encoded in a fundamentally different way than other memories in the duration of the biological and physiological stress response (van der Kolk, 2004). Second, and as discussed in detail earlier, these theories predict that traumatic memories are divided into two types: voluntary recollections and involuntary recollections.

According to this view, voluntary memories of trauma are unique from "typical" emotional memories in their fragmentation and their lack of a narrative structure. This "fragmentation hypothesis" in reference to voluntary recollections of trauma dates back to clinical references described by Pierre Janet and Sigmund Freud (Janet, 1919/1925; as cited in Hopper & van der Kolk, 2001; Breuer & Freud, 1893; as cited in Nemiah, 1998). However, it is also a fundamental component of modern theories.

The theories that characterize traumatic memories as unique have recently been labeled the "special mechanism view" (referring to a special mechanism for the encoding of traumatic memories as opposed to other memories, Berntsen, Rubin, & Bohni, 2008).

One of these theories, the Dual Representation Theory (described earlier), claims that both voluntary and involuntary memories are encoded and subsequently recalled in different ways from typical memories, recruiting different neural networks (see Brewin, Dalgleish & Joseph, 1996). Part of this difference may be due to the under-active hippocampi found in people with PTSD. These theories suggest specifically that voluntarily recalled memories are fragmented because they rely on a deficient hippocampally-based network (see Lamprecht & Sack, 2002; Peres, McFarlane, Nassello & Moores, 2008).

However, more recently, this view has been challenged. It has been suggested that instead of trauma memories being encoded and recalled in a unique way from other emotional memories, they just may be more extreme emotional memories (Berntsen, Rubin, & Bohni, 2008; McNally, 2003). By this view, neither voluntary nor involuntary memories of trauma are organized or integrated into the general autobiographical memory network in a fundamentally different way than any other emotional memories. This has been called the "basic mechanisms view," indicating that memories of trauma use the same mechanism of normal, extreme emotional memories.

One of the most logical ways to discover if people with PTSD's trauma memories are uniquely fragmented as compared to the memories of people without PTSD is to look at their narrative accounts of their trauma. Narrative studies have found that narrative fragmentation shortly after a trauma is associated with the development of chronic PTSD (Amir et al., 1998; Halligan et al., 2003; Murray, Ehlers, & Mayou, 2002). However, concerns about the anxiety caused by reporting one's trauma verbally, as well as the deficiency in verbal skills that is associated with PTSD, have lead to questioning about whether these results point to the fragmentation of traumatic narratives or to some more global deficit. To adjudicate between these alternatives, Gray & Lombardo (2001) compared the narratives of people with and without PTSD, controlling for variables such as verbal ability and writing skill. Only when these factors were controlled was there no difference in narrative fragmentation between the groups. These results suggest that differences in verbal skills may underlie the differences in the narrative reports of people with and without PTSD.

Because global deficits in verbal skills may influence the reporting of narratives, some studies have examined whether narrative ability may change over time while verbal skill may remain constant. The theoretical basis behind the fragmentation hypothesis indicates that although these trauma memories are unique, they can be integrated into a more typical memory system with treatment (see Brewin, Dalgleish & Joseph, 1996). Thus, one would expect that as people recover PTSD their narratives would become less fragmented. There are some studies that indicate that the fragmentation of trauma narratives may decrease with treatment (Foa, Molnar & Cashman, 1995). However, it may be that the narratives of those with PTSD become less fragmented due to practice in recounting their narrative rather than because of improvement in the symptoms of PTSD (van Minnen, Wessel, Dijkstra, & Roelofs, 2002). In other words, although verbal skills may remain constant through treatment, practice recounting the trauma narrative in therapy may increase the ability to communicate the trauma narrative, but may not be directly associated with the overall severity of the disorder. Thus, while there is evidence that fragmentation plays a role in the development of PTSD, it is not consistently associated with treatment of PTSD or direct comparisons between individuals with and without PTSD after they have developed the disorder. Though it may appear that the narratives of people with PTSD are more fragmented than people without PTSD and that the fragmentation may improve with treatment, this effect may actually be an artifact of factors such as verbal and writing skills and practice of trauma narratives.

Another explanation of the "the fragmentation hypothesis" is that people with PTSD may incorrectly perceive their memory of the traumatic event as fragmented (Kindt & van den Hout, 2003). According to this explanation, there is not a special mechanism for traumatic memory in PTSD; instead, traumatic memories may reflect a difference in metamemory, or the awareness of one's own memory. However, this idea has yet to be fully supported as the results of self-reports of fragmentation have been mixed. Some studies that have compared self-perception of traumatic memory in those with and without PTSD have found that people with PTSD report having more fragmented memories than people without PTSD who have also experienced trauma (Halligan, Michael, Clark & Ehlers, 2003; Koss, Figueredo, Bell, Tharan & Tromp, 1996; van der Kolk, Hopper, & Osterman, 2001); however, other studies have not found this difference in fragmentation (Berntsen, Willert & Rubin, 2003; Rubin, Feldman, & Beckham, 2004). In addition, some studies have found that people who reported having more fragmented memories immediately after their trauma had more severe PTSD symptoms later (Halligan et al., 2003; Murray et al., 2002). However initial self-report of fragmentation may not be a unique predictor of later developing PTSD. Thus, the verdict is still out on the possibility that there may be metamemory differences in people with PTSD.

Another factor that is important to consider is if these memories are unique to trauma memories or if all distressing memories are fragmented in people with PTSD. According to the fragmentation hypothesis, it is the trauma memory alone which is uniquely encoded and thus remembered in a fragmented nature. This would indicate that there would not be overall deficits in emotional memory in PTSD, but that it would be unique to the memory for the trauma. Though few studies have focused on this issue, there is some evidence that traumatic memories were reported as being more disorganized than other negative memories (van der Kolk & Fisler, 1995; Halligan et al., 2003). Some studies using non-clinical populations have found that trauma memories and memories for intense positive experiences both remembered very vividly (Porter & Birt, 2001; Byrne et al, 2001). However, though trauma memories were unique in that they differed in vantage point and number of details. Though this has yet to be studied in comparison to a population with PTSD, it may indicate that trauma memories themselves may be unique from other emotional memories.

The role of dissociation is also often reported as a unique feature in the encoding and memory for traumatic events. People with PTSD often describe dissociative features e.g., sensations like time slowing down, having an out of body experience, or a sense of unreality both at the encoding as well as the recall of the traumatic event. Dissociation at the time of the trauma seems to be linked with PTSD. Specifically, reports of dissociation are correlated with the development of PTSD (Holen, 1991; Koopman, Classen & Spiegel, 1994; Marmar et al., 1999; Shalev, Peri, Canetti & Schreiber, 1996; but see Freedman, Brandes, Peri & Shalev, 1999). Thus, dissociation is cited as a factor that may make the encoding and subsequent recall of traumatic memories unique. However, dissociation may occur in the absence of trauma, such as in novice skydivers before their first jump (Sterlini & Bryant, 2002). So, dissociation may be one factor that influences the development of PTSD symptoms, but it may not be unique to individuals with PTSD.

Another explanation that has been proposed in dispute of the fragmentation hypothesis is that perhaps the memories of people with PTSD appear to be fragmented because they are exhibiting a traditional memory trade-off (see McNally, 2003). In other words, if the attention of people with PTSD is more readily caught by a central emotional element, they may be unable to attend to or encode other pieces of the trauma experience. This may lead to a fragmented or disjointed memory, lacking critical pieces of information. This idea has been yet to be empirically tested, though the counter argument has pointed to case studies in which people may not be able to remember something that one would think would be the central emotional element, such as a gun (Ehlers, Hackmann, & Michael, 2004). Further, these memory trade-offs may play the largest role in single episode traumas, as it may be the case that with repeated episodes of trauma people learn to shift their attention to something else, allowing decreased encoding of the central emotional component. For example, in a case of repeated abuse, an individual may shift the focus of their attention from the perpetrator and to a seemingly neutral detail in the environment, such as the wallpaper (see Speigel, 2006 for a discussion of this type of dissociation). Thus, more research is needed to see if people with PTSD do exhibit more of a memory-trade off for their traumatic memory than for other memories, and if so, whether the memory trade-off may be associated with the fragmentation of their memory.

As this section highlights, the question if trauma memories are unique in PTSD is still left unanswered. There have been many issues that have confused the research on this topic. First, there is often not a consistent definition of fragmentation (Zoellner & Bittenger, 2004). Studies have defined fragmentation in a variety of different ways, from confusion, to muddled thoughts, to disorganization, to repetitions in narratives, to missing pieces of information. Second, it is important to make sure that differences in narrative fragmentation are not confounded by global differences in verbal intelligence or speaking or writing abilities (Gray & Lombardo, 2001). Third, studies must be careful not to mix the measure of fragmentation in voluntary memory with that in involuntary memory; instead, studies must specifically test the theory that these two kinds of memories are different (Zoellner & Bittenger, 2004). Lastly, carefully matched control groups are necessary in order to determine to what extent the differences are specific to PTSD and to what extent they may generalize to traumatic memory more generally.

GENERAL CONCLUSIONS

In summary, emotion biases attention at multiple levels of processing. These attentional biases (along with potential differences at consolidation and retrieval, which have not been reviewed here) lead to a more vivid, detailed memory for experiences that elicit emotion. However, while some elements of these experiences are remembered well, the attentional focus may come at a cost for the memory of surrounding items. Although these effects exist even in people without PTSD, people with PTSD may exhibit exaggerated attentional biases with enhanced prioritization of emotional information and an increased difficulty disengaging attention from emotional information. These attentional biases may influence the memories that are retrieved either voluntarily or involuntarily in individuals with PTSD. Focusing attention on the emotional details of a traumatic experience may lead to a vivid memory for that event, and may lead the memory to be likely to be cued even by inappropriate contextual triggers. On the other hand, although it has yet to be specifically tested in a PTSD population, we suggest that this attentional focus may also lead to a lack of processing of other elements of the trauma. This may lead to a vivid memory for traumatic elements, along with poorer memory for the context. It may be this deficient memory for context that potentially could lead to the triggering of the memory in contextually inappropriate situations.

REFERENCES

Adams, R. B. & Kleck, R. E. (2003). Perceived gaze direction and the processing of facial displays of emotion. *Psychological Science*, *14*, 644-47.

Amir, N., Stafford, J., Freshman, M. S. & Foa, E. B. (1998). Relationship between trauma narratives and trauma pathology. *Journal of Traumatic Stress*, *11*, 385-392.

Anderson, A. K. (2005). Affective influences on the attentional dynamics supporting awareness. *Journal of Experimental Psychology: General*, *134*, 258-261.

Anderson, A. K. & Phelps, E. A. (2001). Lesions of the human amygdala impair enhanced perception of emotionally salient events. *Nature*, *411*, 305-309.

Armony, J. L., Corbo, V., Clement, M. H. & Brunet, A. (2005). Amygdala response in patients with acute PTSD to masked and unmasked emotional facial expressions. *American Journal of Psychiatry*, *162*, 1961-1963.

Berntsen, D. (2001). Involuntary memories of emotional events. Do memories of traumas and extremely happy events differ? *Applied Cognitive Psychology*, *15*, 135-158.

Berntsen, D. (1996). Involuntary autobiographical memory. *Applied Cognitive Psychology*, *10*, 435-454.

Berntsen, D., Rubin, D. C. & Bohni, M. K. (2008). Contrasting models of posttraumatic stress disorder: Reply to Monroe and Mineka (2008). *Psychological Review*, *115*, 1099-1107.

Berntsen, D., Willert, M. & Rubin, D. (2003). Splintered memories or vivid landmarks? Qualities and organization of traumatic memories with and without PTSD. *Applied Cognitive Psychology*, *17*, 675-693.

Boals, A. & Rubin, D. (in press). The integration of emotions in traumatic memories: Cognitive-emotional distinctiveness and posttraumatic stress disorder. *Applied Cognitive Psychology*.

Bradley, B. P., Mogg, K., Millar, N., Bonham-Carter, C., Fergusson, E., Jenkins, J. & Parr, M. (1997). Attentional biases for emotional faces. *Cognition and Emotion*, *11*, 25-42.

Bremner, J. D., Krystal, J. H., Southwick, S. M. & Charney, D. S. (1995). Functional neuroanatomical correlates of the effects of stress on memory. *Journal of Traumatic Stress*, *8*, 527-553.

Brewin, C. R. (2001). A cognitive neuroscience account of posttraumatic stress disorder and its treatment. *Behaviour Research and Therapy*, *39*, 373-393.

Brewin, C. R. (1998). Intrusive autobiographical memories in depression and post-traumatic stress disorder. *Applied Cognitive Psychology*, *12*, 359-370.

Brewin, C. R., Dalgleish, T. & Joseph, S. (1996). A dual representation theory of posttraumatic stress disorder. *Psychological Review*, *4*, 670-686.

Breslau, N. (2002). Epidemiologic studies of trauma, posttraumatic stress disorder, and other psychiatric disorders, *Canadian Journal of Psychiatry*, *47*, 923-9.

Brosch, T., Sander, D., Pourtois, G. & Scherere, K. R. (2008). Beyond fear. *Psychological Science*, *19*, 362-370.

Brown, J. M. (2003). Eyewitness memory for arousing events: Putting things into context. *Applied Cognitive Psychology*, *17*, 93-106.

Bryant, R. A. & Harvey, A. G. (1995). Processing of threatening information in posttraumatic stress disorder. *Journal of Abnormal Psychology*, *104*, 537-541.

Bryant, R. A., Kemp, A. H., Felmingham, K. L. Lidell, B., Olivieri, G. Peduto, A., Gordon, E. & Williams, L. M. (2007). Enhanced amygdala and medial prefrontal activation during nonconscious processing of fear in posttraumatic stress disorder: An fMRI study. *Human Brain Mapping*, *29*, 517-523.

Buckley, T. C., Blanchard, E. B. & Neill, T. W. (2000). Information processing and PTSD: A review of the empirical literature. *Clinical Psychology Review*, *28*, 1041-1065.

Buckley, T. C., Blanchard, E. B. & Hickling, E. J. (2002). Automatic and strategic processing of threat stimuli: A comparison between PTSD, panic disorder, and nonanxiety controls. *Cognitive Therapy and Research*, *26*, 97-115.

Buckley, T. C., Galovski, T., Blanchard, E. B. & Hickling, E. J. (2003). Is the emotional Stroop paradigm sensitive to malingering? A between-groups study with professional actors and actual trauma survivors. *Journal of Traumatic Stress*, *16*, 59-66.

Burke, A., Heuer, F. & Reisberg, D. (1992). Remembering emotional events. *Memory and Cognition*, *20*, 277-290.

Byrne, C. A., Hyman, I. E. & Scott, K. L. (2001). Comparison of memories for traumatic events and other experiences. *Applied Cognitive Psychology*, *15*, S119-S133.

Calvo, M. G. & Lang, P. J. (2004). Gaze patterns when looking at emotional pictures: Motivationally biased attention. *Motivation and Emotion*, *28*, 221-243.

Carretie, L., Hinojosa, J. A., Martin-Loeches, M., Mercado, F. & Tapia, M. (2004). Automatic attention to emotional stimuli: Neural correlates. *Human Brain Mapping*, *22*, 290-299.

Cassiday, K. L., McNally, R. J. & Zeitlin, S. B. (1992). Cognitive processing of trauma cues in rape victims with post-traumatic stress disorder. *Cognitive Therapy and Research*, *16*, 283-295.

Christianson, S. A. & Loftus, E. F. (1991). Remembering emotional events: The fate of detailed information, *Cognition and Emotion*, *5*, 81-108.

Christianson, S. A. & Safer, M. A. (1996). Emotional events and emotions in autobiographical memories. In D., Rubin, (Eds.), *Remembering our past: Studies in autobiographical memory*. (218-243). New York: Cambridge University Press.

Clark, C. R., McFarlane, A. C., Morris, P., Weber, D. L., Sonkkilla, C., Shaw, M., et al. (2003). Cerebral function in posttraumatic stress disorder during verbal working memory updating: a positron emission tomography study. *Biological Psychiatry, 53*, 81-474.

Chemtob, C. M., Roitblat, H. L., Hamada, R. S., Muraoka, M. Y., Carlson, J. G. & Bauer, G. B. (1999). Compelled attention: the effects of viewing trauma-related stimuli on concurrent task performance in posttraumatic stress disorder. *Journal of Traumatic Stress, 12*, 309-26.

Constans, J. I. (2005). Information-processing biases in PTSD. In: J. J., Vasterling, C. R. Brewin, (Eds.), *Neuropsychology of PTSD: Biological cognitive, and clinical perspectives*. (105-130). New York: The Guilford Press.

Constans, J. I., McCloskey, M., Vasterling, J. J., Brailey, K. & Mathews, A. (2004). Suppression of attentional bias in PTSD. *Journal of Abnormal Psychology, 113*, 315-323.

Cohen, A. (2005). Selective attention. In L. Nadel (Ed.) *Encyclopedia of Cognitive Science*. (1033-1037). Nature Publishing Group (Macmillan).

D'Argembeau, A. & Van der Linden, M. (2004). Influence of affective meaning on memory for contextual information. *Emotion, 4*, 173-188.

Deffenbacher, K. A. (1983). The influence of arousal on reliability of testimony. In: S. M. A., Lloyd-Bostock, B. R., Clifford, (Eds.), *Evaluating Witness Evidence: Recent Psychological Research and New Perspectives*, 235-251. Chichester: Wiley.

Derakshan, N. & Lipp, O. V. (2005). Attentional bias to pictures of fear-relevant animals in a dot probe task. *Emotion, 5*, 365-69.

Derryberry, D. & Reed, M. A. (2002). Anxiety-related attentional biases and their regulation by attentional control. *Journal of Abnormal Psychology, 111*, 225-236.

Dewhurst, S. A. & Parry, L. A. (2000). Emotionality, distinctiveness, and recollective experience. *European Journal of Cognitive Psychology, 12*, 541-551.

Doerksen, S. & Shimamura, A. (2001). Source memory enhancement for emotional words. *Emotion, 1*, 5-11.

Driver, J. & Vuilleumier, P. (2001). Perceptual awareness and its loss in unilateral neglect and extinction. *Cognition, 79*, 39-88.

Easterbrook, J. A. (1959). The effect of emotion on cue utilization and the organization of behavior. *Psychological Review, 66*, 183-201.

Egeth, H. E. (1997). Visual attention: control, representation, and time course. *Annual review of psychology, 48*, 269-97.

Ehlers, A. & Clark, D. (2000). A cognitive model of posttraumatic stress disorder. *Behaviour Research and Therapy, 38*, 319-345.

Ehlers, A. & Steil, R. (1995). Maintenance of intrusive memories in posttraumatic stress disorder: A cognitive approach. *Behavioural and Cognitive Psychotherapy, 23*, 217- 249.

Ehlers, A., Hackmann, A. & Michael, T. (2004). Intrusive re-experiencing in post-traumatic stress disorder: Phenomenology, theory, and therapy. *Memory, 12*, 403-415.

Ehlers, A., Hackmann, A., Steil, R., Clohessy, S. & Wenninger, K. (2002). The nature of intrusive memories after trauma: The warning signal hypothesis. *Behaviour Research and Therapy, 40*, 995-1002.

Eichenbaum, H. (1997). Declarative memory: Insights from cognitive neurobiology. *Annual Review of Psychology, 48*, 547-572.

Foa, E. B., Feske, U., Murdock, T. B., Kozak, M. J. & McCarthy, P. R. (1991). Processing of threat-related information in rape victims. *Journal of Abnormal Psychology, 100*, 156-162.

Foa, E. B., Molnar, C. & Cahsman, L. (1995). Change in rape narratives during exposure therapy for posttraumatic stress disorder. *Journal of Traumatic Stress, 8*, 675-690.

Foa, E. B. & Rothbaum, B. O. (1998). *Treating the trauma of rape*. New York Guilford Press.

Fredrickson, B. L. & Branigan, C. (2005). Positive emotions broaden the scope of attention and thought-action repertoires. *Cognition and Emotion, 19*, 313-332.

Freedman, S. A., Brandes, D., Peri, T. & Shalev, A. (1999). Predictors of chronic posttraumatic stress disorder: A prospective study. *British Journal of Psychiatry, 174*, 353-359.

Friedman, A. & Bourne, L. (1976). Encoding the levels of information in pictures and words, *Journal of Experimental Psychology: General, 105*, 169-90.

Gasper, K. & Clore, G. L. (2002). Attending to the big picture: Mood and global versus local processing of visual information. *Psychological Science, 13*, 34-40.

Gianotti, L. R., Faber, P. L., Schuler, M., Pascual-Margui, R. D., Kochi, K. & Lehmann, D. (2008). First valence, then arousal: the temporal dynamics of brain electric activity evoked by emotional stimuli. *Brain Topography, 20*, 143-156.

Gilbertson, M. W., Gurvits, T. V., Lasko, N. B., Orr, S. P. & Pitman, R. K. (2001). Multivariate assessment of explicit memory function in combat veterans with posttraumatic stress disorder. *Journal of Traumatic Stress. 2*, 1573-6598.

Golier, J. A., Yehuda, R., Lupien, S. J. & Harvey, P. D. (2003). Memory for trauma-related information in Holocaust survivors with PTSD. *Psychiatry Research, 121*, 133-143.

Gray, M. J. & Lombardo, T. W. (2001). Complexity of trauma narratives as an index of fragmented memory in PTSD: A critical analysis. *Applied Cognitive Psychology, 15*, S171-S186.

Hackmann, A., Ehlers, A., Speckens, A. & Clark, D. M. (2004). Characteristics and content of intrusive memories in PTSD and their changes with treatment. *Journal of Traumatic Stress, 17*, 231-240.

Halligan, S. A., Michael, T., Clark, D. M. & Ehlers, A. (2003). Posttraumatic stress disorder following assault: The role of cognitive processing, trauma memory, and appraisals. *Journal of Consulting and Clinical Psychology, 71*, 419-431.

Harvey, A. G., Bryant, R. A. & Rapee, R. M. (1996). Preconscious processing of threat in posttraumatic stress disorder. *Cognitive Therapy and Research, 20*, 613-623.

Hellawell, S. J. & Brewin, C. R. (2004). A comparison of flashbacks and ordinary autobiographical memories of trauma: Content and language. *Behaviour research and therapy, 42*, 1-12.

Holen, A. (1991). A longitudinal study of the occurrence and persistence of post-traumatic health problems in disaster survivors. *Stress Medicine, 7*, 11-17.

Hopper, J. W. & van der Kolk, B. A. (2001). Retrieving, assessing, and classifying traumatic memories: A preliminary report on three case studies of a new standardized method. *Journal of Aggression, Maltreatment, and Trauma, 4*, 33-71.

Horstmann, G. & Becker, S. I. (2008). Attentional effects of negative faces: Top-down contingent or involuntary? *Perception & Psychophysics, 70*, 1416-1434.

Janet, P. (1904). L'amnesie et la dissociation des souvenirs par l'emotion. *Journal de Psychologie*, *1*, 417-453.

Juth P., Lundqvist, D., Karlsson, A. & Ohman, A. (2005). Looking for foes and friends: Perceptual and emotional factors when finding a face in the crowd. *Emotion*, *5*, 379-395.

Kahan, T. A. & Hely, C. D. (2008). The role of valence and frequency in the emotional Stroop task. *Psychonomic Bulletin & Review*, *15*, 956-60.

Kaspi, S. P., McNally, R. J. & Amir, N. (1995). Cognitive processing of emotional information in posttraumatic stress disorder. *Cognitive Therapy and Research*, *19*, 433-444.

Keane, T. M., Kolb, L. C., Kaloupek, D. G., Orr, S. P., Blanchard, E. B., et al. (1998). Utility of psychophysiological measurement in the diagnosis of posttraumatic stress disorder: results from a Department of Veterans Affairs Cooperative Study. *Journal of Consulting and Clinical Psychology*, *66*, 914-23.

Kensinger, E. A. & Corkin, S. (2003). Effect of divided attention on the memory benefit for negative as compared to neutral words. *Brain and Cognition*, *51*, 223-225.

Kensinger, E. A, Garoff-Eaton, R. J. & Schacter, D. L. (2007a). Effects of emotion on memory specificity in young and older adults. *Journal of Gerontology: Psychological Science*, *62*, 208-215.

Kensinger, E. A., Garoff-Eaton, R. J. & Schacter, D. L. (2007b). Effects of emotion on memory specificity: Memory trade-offs elicited by negative visually arousing stimuli. *Journal of Memory and Language*, *56*, 575-591.

Kensinger, E. A., Garoff-Eaton, R. J. & Schacter, D. L. (2006). Memory for specific visual details can be enhanced by negative arousing content. *Journal of Memory and Language*, *54*, 99-112.

Kensinger, E. A., Piguet, O., Krendl, A. C. & Corkin, S. (2005). Memory for contextual details: Effects of emotion and aging. *Psychology and Aging*, *20*, 241-250.

Kensinger, E. A. & Schacter, D. L. (2006). Reality monitoring and memory distortion: Effects of negative, arousing content. *Memory and Cognition*, *34*, 251-260.

Kim, K. H., Yoon, H. W. & Park, H. W. (2004). Spatiotemporal brain activation pattern during word/picture perception by native Koreans. *NeuroReport*, *15*, 1099-1103.

Kindt, M. & van den Hout, M. (2003). Dissociation and memory fragmentation: Experimental effects on metamemory but not on actual memory performance. *Behaviour Research and Therapy*, *41*, 167-178.

Koopman, C., Classen, C. & Spiegel, D. (1994). Predictors of posttraumatic stress symptoms among survivors of the Oakland/Berkeley, California, Firestorm. *American Journal of Psychiatry*, *151*, 888-894.

Koss, M. P., Figueredo, A. J. Bell, I. Tharan, M. & Tromp, S. (1996). Traumatic memory characteristics: A cross-validated mediation model of response to rape among employed women. *Journal of Abnormal Psychology*, *105*, 421-432.

Koster, E. H. W., Crombez, G., Verschuere, B. & De Houwer, J. (2004). Selective attention to threat in the dot probe paradigm: differentiating vigilance and difficulty to disengage. *Behaviour Research and Therapy*, *42*, 1183-1192.

LaBar, K. S. (2007). Beyond Fear: Emotional memory mechanisms in the human brain. *Current Directions in Psychological Science*, *16*, 173-177.

LaBar, K. S. & Phelps, E. A. (1998). Arousal-mediated memory consolidation: Role of the medial temporal lobe in humans. *Psychological Science*, *9*, 490-493.

Leclerc, C. M. & Kensinger, E. A. (2008). Effects of age on detection of emotional information. *Psychology and Aging*, *23*, 209-215.

Lamprecht, F. & Sack, M. (2002). Posttraumatic stress disorder revisited. *Psychosomatic Medicine*, *64*, 222 237.

LeDoux, J. E. (1996). *The Emotional Brain*. New York: New York Magazine.

LeDoux, J. E. (2000). Emotion circuits in the brain. *Annual Review of Neuroscience*, *23*, 155-184.

LeDoux, J. E., Iwata, J., Cicchetti, P. & Reis, D. J. (1988). Different projections of the central amygdaloid nucleus mediate autonomic and behavioral correlates of conditioned fear. *Journal of Neuropsychiatry and Clinical Neurosciences*, *14*, 254-261.

Lipp, O. V. & Waters, A. M. (2007). When danger lurks in the background: Attentional capture by animal fear-relevant distractors is specific and selectively enhanced by animal fear. *Emotion*, *7*, 192-200.

Litz, B. T., Weathers, F. W., Monaco, V., Herman, D. S., Wulfoshn, M., Marx, B. & Keane, T. M. (1996). Attention, arousal, and memory in posttraumatic stress disorder. *Journal of Traumatic Stress*, *9*, 497-519.

MacKay, D. G. & Ahmetzanov, M. V. (2005). An experimental analogue of flashbulb memories. *Psychological Science*, *16*, 25-32.

MacKay, D. G., Shafto, M., Taylor, J. K., Marian, D. E., Abrams, L. & Dyer, J. (2004). Relations between emotion, memory and attention: Evidence from taboo Stroop, lexical decision, and immediate memory tasks. *Memory & Cognition*, *32*, 474-488.

MacLeod, C., Mathews, A. & Tata, P. (1986). Attentional bias in emotional disorders. *Journal of Abnormal Psychology*, *95*, 15-20.

Marmar, C. R., Weiss, D. S., Metzler, T. J., Delucci, K. L. Best, S. R. & Wentworth, K. A. (1999). Longitudinal course and predictors of continuing distress following critical incident exposure in emergency services personnel. *Journal of Nervous and Mental Disease*, *187*, 15-22.

McKenna, F. P. & Sharma, D. (1995). Intrusive cognitions: An investigation of the emotional Stroop task. *Journal of experimental psychology*, *21*, 1595-1607.

McNally, R. J. (2003). Psychological mechanisms in acute response to trauma. *Biological Psychiatry*, *53*, 779-788.

McNally, R. J., Amir, N. & Lipke, H. J. (1996). Subliminal processing of threat cues in posttraumatic stress disorder? *Journal of Anxiety Disorders*, *10*, 115-28.

McNally, R. J., Kaspi, S. P., Riemann, B. C. & Zeitlin, S. B. (1990). Selective processing of threat cues in posttraumatic stress disorder. *Journal of Abnormal Psychology*, *99*, 398-402.

McNally, R. J., Metzger, L. J., Lasko, N. B., Clancy, S. A. & Pitman, R. K. (1998). Directed forgetting of trauma cues in adult survivors of childhood sexual abuse with and without posttraumatic stress disorder. *Journal of Abnormal psychology*, *107*, 596-601.

Michael, T., Ehlers, A., Halligan, S. L. & Clark, D. M. (2005). Unwanted memories of assault: what intrusion characteristics are associated with PTSD? *Bahaviour research and therapy*, *43*, 613-628.

Mickley, K. R. & Kensinger, E. A. (2008). Emotional Valence Influences the Neural Correlates Associated with Remembering and Knowing. *Cognitive, Affective, and Behavioral Neuroscience*, *8*, 143-152.

Mickley Steinmetz, K.R. & Kensinger, E.A. (2009). The effects of valence and arousal on the neural activity leading to subsequent memory. *Psychophysiology, 46,* 1190-99.

Mogg, K. & Bradley, B. P. (1998). A cognitive-motivational analysis of anxiety. *Behaviour Research and Therapy, 36,* 809-48.

Mogg, K., Bradley, B. P., Williams, R. & Mathews, A. (1993). Subliminal processing of emotional information in anxiety and depression. *Journal of Abnormal Psychology, 102,* 304-11.

Morris, J. S., DeGelder, B., Weiskrantz, L. & Dolan, R. J. (2001). Differential extrageniculostriate and amygdala responses to presentation of emotional faces in a cortically blind field, *Brain, 124,* 1241.

Most, S. B., Smith, S. D., Cooter, A. B., Levy, B. N. & Zald, D. H. (2007). The naked truth: Positive, arousing distractors impair rapid target perception. *Cognition and Emotion, 21,* 964-981.

Murray, J., Ehlers, A. & Mayou, R. A. (2002). Dissociation and post-traumatic stress disorder: Two prospective studies of road traffic accident survivors. *British Journal of Psychiatry, 180,* 363-368.

Neisser, U. & Harsch, N. (1992). Phantom flashbulbs: False recollections of hearing the news about Challenger. In E., Winograd, & U., Neisser, (Eds.), *Affect and accuracy in recall: **Studies of 'flashbulb' memories*** (9-31). Cambridge: Cambridge University Press.

Nemiah, J. C. (1998). Early concepts of trauma, dissociation, and the unconsciousL Their history and current implications. In: J. D., Bremner, & C. R., Marmar, (Eds.) *Trauma, memory and dissociation* (1-26). Washington, DC: American Psychiatric Press.

Nijenhuis, E. R. S. & van der Hart, O. (1999). Forgetting and reexperiencing trauma. In J. Goodwin & R. Cittias (Eds.), *Splintered reflections: Images of the body in the trauma,* (39-65). New York: Basic Books.

Nummenmaa, L. & Hyönä, J. & Calvo, M. G. (2006). Eye movement assessment of selective attentional capture by emotional pictures. *Emotion, 6,* 257-268.

Ochsner, K. N. (2000). Are affective events richly "remembered" or simply familiar? The experience and process of recognizing feelings past. *Journal of Experimental Psychology: General, 129,* 242-261.

Ohman, A., Flykt, A. & Esteves, F. (2001). Emotion drives attention: Detecting the snake in the grass. *Journal of Experimental Psychology: General, 130,* 466-478.

Orr, S. P., Pitman, R. K., Lasko, N. B. & Herz, L. R. (1993). Phychophysiological assessment of posttraumatic stress disorder imagery in World War II and Korean combat veterans. *Journal of Abnormal Psychology. 102,* 152-159.

Paunovic, N., Lundh, L. G. & Ost, L. G. (2002). Attentional and memory bias for emotional information in crime victims with acute posttraumatic stress disorder. *Journal of Anxiety Disorders, 16,* 675-692.

Parkhurst, D., Kilnton, L. & Ernst, N. (2002). Modeling the role of salience in the allocation of overt visual attention. *Vision research, 42,* 107-23.

Peres, J. F. P., McFarlane, A., Nasello, A. G. & Moores, K. A. (2008). Traumatic memories: bridging the gap between functional neuroimaging and psychotherapy. *Australian and New Zealand Journal of Psychiatry, 42,* 478-488.

Pessoa, L., Kastner, S. & Underleider, L. G. (2003). Neuroimaging studies of attention: From modulation of sensory processing to top-down control. *Journal of Neuroscience, 23,* 3990-3998.

Pessoa, L., McKenna, M., Gutierrez, E. & Ungerleider, L. G. (2002). Neural processing of emotional faces requires attention. *PNAS*, *99*, 11458-63.

Pickel, K. L., French, T. A. & Betts, J. M. (2003). A crossmodal weapon focus effect: the influence of a weapon's presence on memory for auditory information. *Memory*, *11*, 277-292.

Pineles, S. L., Shipherd, J. C., Welch, L. P. & Yovel, I. (2007). The role of attentional biases in PTSD: Is it interference or facilitation? *Behaviour research and therapy*, *45*, 1903-1913.

Pitman, R. K., Orr, S. P., Forgue, D. F., Altman, B., de Jong, J. B. & Herz, L. R. (1990). Psychophysiologic responses to combat imagery of Vietnam veterans with posttraumatic stress disorder versus other anxiety disorders. *Journal of Abnormal Psychology*, *99*, 49-54.

Pitman, R. K., Orr, S. P., Forgue, D. F., DeJong, J. B. & Claiborn, J. M. (1987). Psychophysiologic assessment of posttraumatic stress disorder imagery in Vietnam combat veterans. *Archives of general psychiatry*, *44*, 970-975.

Porter, S. & Birt, A. R. (2001). Is traumatic memory special? A comparison of traumatic memory characteristics with memory for other emotional life experiences. *Applied Cognitive Psychology*, *15*, S101-S117.

Pourtois, G., Grandjean, D., Sander, D. & Vuilleumier, P. (2004). Electrophysiological correlates of rapid spatial orienting towards fearful faces. *Cerebral Cortex*, *14*, 619-633.

Rauch, S. L., Whalen, P. J., Shin, L. M., McInerney, S. C., Macklin, M. L., Lasko, N. B., Orr, S. P. & Pitman, R. K. (2000). Exaggerated amygdala response to masked facial stimuli in posttraumatic stress disorder: a functional MRI study. *Biological psychiatry*, *47(9)*, 769-76.

Reisberg, D. & Heuer, F. (2004). Remembering emotional events. In D., Reisberg, P., Hertel, (Eds.), *Memory and emotion*, (3-41). New York: Oxford University Press.

Reisberg, D., Heuer, F., McLean, J. & O'Shaughnessy, M. (1988). The quantity, not the quality, of affect predicts memory vividness. *Bulletin of the Psychonomic Society*, *26*, 100-103.

Rensink, R. A. (2005). Visual attention. In: L., Nadel, (Ed.) *Encyclopedia of Cognitive Science*. (509 - 515). Nature Publishing Group (Macmillan).

Rowe, G., Hirsh, J. B. & Anderson, A. K. (2007). Positive affect increases the breadth of attentional selection. *Proceedings of the National Academy of Sciences of the United State of America*, *104(1)*, 383-8.

Rubin, D. C., Feldman, M. E. & Beckham, J. C. (2004). Reliving, emotions and fragmentation in the autobiographical memories of veterans diagnosed with PTSD. *Applied Cognitive Psychology*, *18*, 17-35.

Rubin, D. C. & Kozin, M. (1984). Vivid memories. *Cognition*, *16*, 63-80.

Russell, J. A. (1980). A circumplex model of affect. *Journal of Personality and social Psychology*, *39*, 1161-1178.

Safer, M. A., Christianson, S. A., Autry, M. W. & Osterlund, K. (1998). Tunnel memory for traumatic events. *Applied Cognitive Psychology*, *12*, 99-117.

Sarter, M., Givens, B. & Bruno, J. P. (2001). *Brain Research Reviews*, *35(2)*, 146-60.

Schact, A. & Sommer, W. (2008). Emotions in word and face processing: Early and late cortical responses. *Brain and Cognition*, *69*, 538-550.

Schmolck, H., Buffalo, E. A. & Squire, L. R. (2000). Memory distortions develop over time: Recollections of the O. J., Simpson trial verdict after 15 and 32 months. *Psychological Science*, *11*, 39-45.

Shalev, A. Y., Peri, T., Canetti, L. & Schreiber, S. (1996). Predictors of PTSD in injured trauma survivors: A prospective study. *American Journal of Psychiatry*, *153*, 219-225.

Shalev, A. Y., Orr, S. P. & Pitman, R. K. (1993). Psychophysiologic assessment of traumatic imagery in Israeli civilian patients with posttraumatic stress disorder. *American Journal of Psychiatry*, *150*, 620-624.

Sharot, T., Delgado, M. R. & Phelps, E. A. (2004). How emotion enhances the feeling of remembering. *Nature Neuroscience*, *7*, 1376-1380.

Shaw, J. I. & Skolnick, P. (1994). Sex differences, weapon focus, and eyewitness reliability. *Journal of Social Psychology*, *134*, 413-420.

Shin, L. M., Rauch, S. L. & Pitman, R. K. (2005). Structural and functional anatomy of PTSD. In: J. J., Vasterling, & C. R., Brewin, (Eds). *Neuropsychology of PTSD: Biological, Clinical, and Cognitive Perspectives*. New York: Guilford Press.

Shin, L. M., Whalen, P. J., Pitman, R. K., Bush, G., Macklin, M. L., Lasko, N. B., Orr, S. P., McInerney, S. C. & Rauch, S. L. (2001). An fMRI study of anterior cingulate function in posttraumatic stress disorder. *Biological Psychiatry*, *50*, 932-942.

Speigel, D. (2006). Trauma, dissociation, and memory. *Annals of the New York Academy of Sciences*, *821*, 225-237.

Squire, L. (1992). Memory and the hippocampus: A synthesis from findings with rats, monkeys and humans. *Psychological Review*, *99*, 195-231.

Steel, C. & Holmes, E. A. (2007). Involuntary memories in posttraumatic disorder and psychosis. In: J. H., Mace, (Eds.), *New Perspectives in Cognitive Psychology: Involuntary Memory*. Malden, MA: Blackwell.

Sterlini, G. L. & Bryant, R. A. (2002). Hyperarousal and dissociation: A study of novice skydivers. *Behaviour research and therapy*, *40*, 431-437.

Stroop, J. R. (1935). Studies of interference in serial verbal reactions. *Journal of Experimental Psychology*, *18*, 643-662.

Thrasher, S. M., Dalgleish, T. & Yule, W. (1994). Information processing in post-traumatic stress disorder. *Behaviour Research and Therapy*, *32*, 247-254.

Tipples, J., Young, A. W., Quinlan, P., Broks, P. & Ellis, A. W. (2002). Searching for threat. *The Quarterly journal of experimental psychology. A, Human experimental psychology*, *55*, 1007-26.

Tromp, S., Koss, M. P., Figueredo, A. J. & Tharan, M. (1995). Are rape memories different? A comparison of rape and other unpleasant, and pleasant memories among employed women. *Journal of Traumatic Stress*, *8*, 607-627.

van der Hart, O., Van der Kolk, B. A. & Boon, S. (1998). The treatment of dissociative disorders. In: J. D., Bremner, C. A., Marmar, (Eds.) *Trauma, memory, and dissociation*. (253-283) Washington, DC: American Psychiatric Press, 1998.

van der Kolk, B. A. (2004). Psychobiology of posttraumatic stress disorder. In J. Pankesepp (Ed.) Textbook of Biological Psychiatry. New Jersey: Wiley-Liss, Inc.

van der Kolk, B. A. & Fisler, R. (1995). Dissociation and the fragmentary nature of traumatic memories: Overview and exploratory study. *Journal of Traumatic Stress*, *8*, 505-525.

van der Kolk, B. A., Hopper, J. W. & Osterman, J. E. (2001). Exploring the nature of traumatic memory: Combining clinical knowledge with laboratory methods. *Journal of Aggression, Maltreatment, and Trauma*, *4*, 9-31.

van Minnen, A., Wessel, I., Dijkstra, T. & Roelofs, K. (2002). Changes in PTSD patients' narratives during prolonged exposure therapy: A replication and extension. *Journal of Traumatic Stress*, *15*, 255-258.

Vasterling, J. J. & Brewin, C. R. (2005). *Neuropsychology of PTSD: Biological cognitive, and clinical perspectives*. New York: The Guilford Press.

Vasterling, J. J., Brailey, K., Constans, J. I. & Sutker, P. B. (1998). Attention and memory dysfunction in posttraumatic stress disorder. *Neuropsychology*, *12*, 125-133.

Vrana, S. R., Roodman, A. & Beckman, J. C. (1995). Selective processing of trauma-relevant words in posttraumatic stress disorder. *Journal of Anxiety Disorders*, *9*, 515-530.

Vuilleumier, P. & Schwartz, S. (2001). Beware and be aware: Capture of spatial attention by fear-related stimuli in neglect. *NeuroReport*, *12*, 1119-1122.

Waring, J. D., Payne, J. D., Schacter, D. L., & Kensinger, E. A. (2010). Impact of individual differences upon emotion-induced memory trade-offs. *Cognition and Emotion, 24,* 150-167.

Wegner, D. M. (1994). *White bears and other unwanted thoughts: Suppression, obsession, and the psychology of mental control*. New York. The Guilford Press.

Wessel, I., van der Kooy, P. & Merckelbach, H. (2000). Differential recall of central and peripheral details of emotional slides is not a stable phenomenon. *Memory*, *8*, 95-109.

Whalen, P. J., Kagen, J., Cook, R. G., Davis, F. C., Hackjin, K., Polis, S. McLaren, D. G., Somerville, L. H., McLean, A. A., Maxwell, J. S. & Johnstone, T. (2004). Human amygdala responsivity to masked fearful eye whites. *Science*, *306*, 2061.

Yamasue, H., Kasai, K., Iwanami, A., Ohtani, T., Yamada, H., Abe, O., Kuroki, N., Fukuda, R., Tochigi, M., Furukawa, S., Sadamatsu, M., Sasaki, T., Aoki, S., Ohtomo, K., Asukai, N. & Kato, N. (2003). Voxel-based analysis of MRI reveals anterior cingulate gray-matter volume reduction in posttraumatic stress disorder due to terrorism. *PNAS U S A*, *100*, 9039 -9043.

Yantis, S. (1998). Goal-directed and stimulus-driven determinants of attentional control. In Monsell, S. & Driver, J. (Eds.) *Control of Cognitive Processes*. Boston: MIT Press.

Zoellner, L. A. & Bittenger, J. N. (2004). On the uniqueness of trauma memories in PTSD. In G. M. Rosen (Ed.) *Posttraumatic stress disorder: Issues and controversies*. (147-162). West Sussex: Wiley.

In: Learning and Memory Developments...
Editors: L. C. Eklund, A. S. Nyman, pp. 33-70
ISBN: 978-1-60876-397-9

Chapter 2

LIFE SKILLS INSTRUCTION IN A TIME OF ACCOUNTABILITY

Beth Ackerman and Katherine Quigley
Liberty University, School of Education, Lynchburg, VA, USA.

ABSTRACT

The current legislation, *No Child Left Behind,* mandates that students with intellectual disabilities have access to core curriculum courses. This action research investigates a comprehensive life skills program, Life Centered Career Education (LCCE), being integrated into the curriculum of high school students with intellectual disabilities. The LCCE program was utilized to educate students on Personal-Social Skills, Daily Life skills, and Occupational lessons with an academic emphasis.

INTRODUCTION

Currently the *No Child Left Behind* (NCLB, 2002) federal legislation mandates that students with disabilities receive instruction in the core curriculum classes of English, math, science, and social studies, and that Adequate Yearly Progress in these courses be maintained by all schools. In addition, public schools are responsible for assessing students with special needs at the same intervals as their regular education peers. "Alternate assessments are relatively new in most states, developed for students who were not included in most large-scale assessments until Federal law mandated their participation" (National Center on Educational Outcomes, 2005, p. 1). As a result, students with intellectual disabilities must be assessed in the four core curriculum areas. The implementation of these alternate assessments provides the government with accurate statistics regarding the success of students. As a result, this academic curriculum does not always reflect the social needs of students with intellectual disabilities. According to Agran, Alper, & Wehmeyer (2002):

> There is an intentional narrowing of the curriculum. When the narrowing is combined with high-stakes testing procedures established to ensure accountability, the result too often is that the 'general curriculum' focuses only on core academic content areas, to the exclusion of other areas that might be just as (or more) important to students with significant disabilities (p. 124).

It has become increasingly evident that students with severe cognitive delays require a curriculum that incorporates functional academics, daily living, occupational, and social skills training. "Special education must resist the constant push for an academic curriculum emphasis rather than the more important career/life skills approach that their students will need for successful community living and working" (Brolin, 1997, p. 7). A life skills curriculum supported by academics allows for students with intellectual disabilities to learn how to utilize skills that enable them to live and work as independently as possible, as well as remain in compliance with federal legislation.

Background of the Study

The manner in which students with disabilities have been educated has varied greatly throughout history. This was evident when reviewing the history of special education, pertinent legislation, the manner in which students with intellectual disabilities are educated, and the need for specific curriculum and social skills training. Throughout the 1800s and the turn of the 20th century, children with disabilities were placed in institutions from an early age. This was where they resided throughout their lifetime, receiving little instruction. This trend began to change in the 1880s and 1890s with the beginnings of deinstitutionalization of those people with mild handicaps (Lawrence, 1999).

Legislation

In 1954 with *Brown v. Topeka Board of Education*, the law stated that education was an equal right to all students. The debate of integration culminated with the passage of federal legislation in 1974 titled the *Education for All Handicapped Children Act*, which is now titled the *Individuals with Disabilities Education Act* (IDEA). The act mandated that "students with disabilities be provided an appropriate education designed to meet their need in the least restrictive environment (LRE)" (Kavale, 2000, p. 4). In addition, the concept of mainstreaming was introduced with Public Law 94-142 as schools were now required to place children with disabilities with their nondisabled peers to the maximum extent possible. "Depending upon a student's functioning level and the structure of the school system, the student may either be in an integrated setting with non-disabled peers or a segregated environment with other disabled students" (DeWeaver & Kropf, 1992, p. 38).

Another key legislative action was Section 504 of the *Rehabilitation Act of 1973* (Section 504). This civil rights law served as a protection of rights entitled to students with disabilities. "Section 504 requires entities receiving federal funds (e.g., schools, colleges) to make 'reasonable accommodations to known physical or mental limitations of an otherwise qualified handicapped (person)'" (Shriner, 2000, p. 232).

The *Americans with Disabilities Act of 1990* (ADA) only served as a reinforcement of the principles found within Section 504. The ADA reiterated that the primary focus should remain on making individual decisions regarding reasonable modifications on policies, procedures, and practices. *Goals 2000: Educate America Act of 1994* (Goals 2000) and the *Improving America's Schools Act of 1994* (IASA) provided a framework for the requirement of setting performance goals and standards.

Current legislation entitled *No Child Left Behind* "continues the legacy of the *Brown v. Topeka Board of Education* decision by creating an educational system that is more inclusive, responsive, and fair" (Paige, 2004, p. 13). This has had a tremendous impact on the education of students with intellectual disabilities. Historically, legislation has worked to provide accommodations as well as access to general education classes and the curriculum. The 1997 amendments to IDEA specify that "students with disabilities have access to and progress in the general education curriculum" (Wehmeyer et al, 2002, p. 157).

Social Skills

The curriculum for students with disabilities can easily be divided into the areas of academic and nonacademic skills. Social skills instruction would be considered nonacademic sklls. "Traditionally, the emphasis on social skills has been overshadowed by academics. However, many educators acknowledge the need for an increased emphasis on social skills development to promote greater social competency for students with high-incidence disabilities" (Kolb & Hanley-Maxwell, 2003, p. 163).

Similar to other skills, social skills instruction must be deliberate and skills must be learned and practiced within the various natural settings and the environments that they will occur (St. Peter, Ayres, Meyer, Park-Lee, 1989). Students with intellectual disabilities can learn to get along with others and adjust to various social situations when taught these social skills. According to the American Association for Intellectual Disabilities (AAID), "impairments in adaptive behavior can seriously limit an individual's opportunities in work situations, living arrangements, and leisure activities" (Thomas, 1996, p. 349).

Education of Students with Disabilities

There are two concepts that are essential to understanding the education of students with intellectual disabilities: intelligence and adaptive behavior. The construct of intelligence refers to the general mental capabilities. According to the 9th edition of Mental Retardation: Definition, Classification, and Systems of Supports, significantly sub-average intellectual functioning was "defined as an IQ of approximately 70 to 75 or below" (Cuskelly, 2004, p. 118).

The second essential concept to be aware of is adaptive behavior. "It now consists of three areas, as resulting from factor analytical research studies" (de Bildt, Serra, Luteijn, Kraijer, Sytema, & Minderaa, 2005, p. 318). These areas are conceptual, social, and practical skills that enable students to function independently. These conceptual skills include reading and expressive language, reading and writing, money concepts, and self-directions.

Furthermore, social skills included interpersonal relationships, responsibility, self-esteem, and following rules and laws. Finally, the practical skills are defined as personal hygiene and grooming, daily living activities, and occupational skills (AAMR, 2002).

The awareness of these two concepts enabled an educator to have a thorough understanding of intellectual disabilities. In order to meet the needs of the students in special education, specific skills in these deficit areas must be taught. Due to recent changes in legislation, research-based curriculum specifically designed for students with intellectual disabilities is emerging. As a result, nonacademic skills such as daily living, social, and occupational skills are not receiving enough attention (Brolin, 1997).

This study sought to analyze this relationship by determining if students participating in a curriculum focusing on personal-social skills achieved significantly higher scores on the Knowledge Battery and Competency Rating Scale (CRS) than students who did not participate in the program.

Statement of the Problem

According to Ford, Schnorr, Meyer, Davern, Black, & Dempsey (1989): We know that many of the curricular offerings in today's schools (e.g., language arts, math, science, social studies, physical education, and fine arts) can accommodate these new students when adaptations are planned and instructional supports are made available. But further examination reveals that the existing scope of schools' curricula is not broad enough to encompass all the activities or areas of competence that may be appropriate for a given student (p. 3).

It is essential to expose students with intellectual disabilities to personal or social skills. The development of independence, self-confidence, socially acceptable behavior, and maintenance of friendships were among the essential social skills necessary for students to learn in order to function within their community (Brolin, 1997).

Hypothesis

Students in classes that utilized the Life Centered Career Education's (LCCE) Personal-Social Skills program achieved significantly higher scores on the Knowledge Battery (KB) and Competency Rating Scale (CRS) than students who did not participate in the program.

LITERATURE REVIEW

It was important to recognize the need for students with intellectual disabilities to be exposed to a curriculum that was both academic and functional in order for students to learn essential social skills. This was accomplished by reviewing the historical developments, legislative progress, and curriculum developments.

Historical Review

A chronological review indicated that the manner in which students with disabilities have been viewed and educated had varied greatly. According to *Mental Retardation* (Payne & Patton, 1981), the historical perspectives regarding the attitudes and treatment of individuals with intellectual disabilities can be divided into nine distinct periods. The first era, prior to 1700, was considered a state of confusion. Since there was a limited knowledge base, the attitudes about and the treatment and perceptions of people with mental deficiencies varied greatly. There was no consensus among Western societies as to who should be treated and why and how they should be treated. As a result, different patterns of treatment developed reflecting a time of confusion. If any service was provided, it would typically be nourishment and housing.

Following this era was the Awakening, from 1700 to 1800, which created two key concepts that impacted people with intellectual disabilities. The first was a new social attitude; "it held that all 'men'- even those who were exceptional – had rights" (Payne & Patton, 1981, p. 6). As a result of this attitude, the second implication would be that the attitudes and time were conducive for idealistic people to develop their philosophies of Humanism.

According to Payne & Patton (1981) the era of "Early Optimism" occurred from 1800 to 1860 and was illustrated through the enthusiasm towards working with people with disabilities. In addition, the birth of special education occurred in Europe with the work of John Marc Itard (1774-1838). He developed five major objectives to help overcome metal problems. However, this optimism and belief that people with intellectual disabilities could be cured were later replaced by the pessimism in the fourth period of Disillusionment occurring between 1860 and 1890. People with intellectual disabilities was now being perceived as incurable.

This period of disillusionment led to the "Sounding the Alarm" period. Between 1890 and 1930 the institutions that were originally designed to train individuals with intellectual disabilities were now assuming the role of caregiver. More dramatically, the change in social attitudes toward the population of people with intellectual disabilities was detrimental. In 1964 Kanner wrote, "The mental defectives were viewed as a menace to civilization, incorrigible at home, burdens to the school, sexually promiscuous, breeders of feebleminded offspring, victims and spreaders of poverty, degeneracy, crime, and disease. Consequently, there was a cry for the segregation of all mental defectives, with the aim of purifying society, of erecting a solid wall between it and its contaminators" (Payne & Patton, 1981, p.13).

Following this era, the progress in the treatment was simply put "On Hold" between 1930 and 1950. However, views were slowly changing with the realization of several key concepts regarding the scientific research on the causes of intellectual disabilities. These changes in views in the causes of intellectual disabilities led to the time referred to as "A Turning Point" occurring between 1950 and 1960 (Payne & Patton, 1981). This quiet revolution was marked by the formation of the National Association for Retarded Children (NARC) in 1950. This organization served as lobbyist, service provider, and advocate for research for people with intellectual disabilities. In addition to the establishment of the NARC, social and political views were shifting from fear and repulsion to tolerance and compassion.

From 1960 to 1970 special education began to take "Center Stage." National attention was placed on people with intellectual disabilities as President Kennedy had a sister with intellectual disabilities. He established a President's Panel to serve as a guide and source for national policy which led to the establishment of what is now the Office for Special Education and Rehabilitative Services. Consequently, the Civil Rights Movement was extended to people with disabilities (Payne & Patton, 1981).

Finally, the era "From Action to Introspection" occurred from 1970 to the 1980s, when it was established that people with intellectual disabilities have personal and civil rights, guaranteeing services and protection which must be extended to the educational setting. The historical changes in this time period were a result of the numerous legal rulings that occurred.

Throughout history the terminology of special education has undergone continuous changes. The vocabulary most often chosen to describe people with cognitive limitations has been historically "mental retardation"and more recently "intellectual disabilities" is the term that is being used. *IDEA* used the term "disability" which is "probably an unfortunate choice of terms because it conflicts with current philosophy in special education and with the intent of the *IDEA* by focusing on a person's lack of ability" (Thomas, 1996, p. 5). This term has slowly begun to be viewed as unacceptable just as its predecessors: mental deficient, idiot, imbecile, and moron. The National Association for Retarded Children chose to change its name to "the Arc" eliminating any reference to retardation by eliminating the acronym. Likewise, in 2002 the Council for Exceptional Children's Division on Mental retardation voted to change the name to The Division on Developmental Disabilities (Hourcade, 2002).

Legislation

Beginning in 1954 with *Brown v. Topeka Board of Education*, the law stated that education was an equal right to all students. Following this groundbreaking case, two key pieces of civil rights legislation have had an impact on education: Section 504 of the Rehabilitation Act of 1973 and the Americans with Disabilities Act (ADA). Since these two pieces of legislation were civil rights acts, it was mandatory for schools to adhere to these laws.

The first of these legislative actions was Section 504 of the *Rehabilitation Act of 1973*. Section 504 prohibited the discrimination against individuals who meet the definitions of a disability. According to Wegner (1988), Congress's primary objective was to "honor the requirements of 'simple justice' by ensuring that federal funds not be expended in a discriminatory fashion" (Smith, 2001, p. 336). This civil rights law served as a protection of rights entitled to students with disabilities. "Section 504 requires entities receiving federal funds (e.g., schools, colleges) to make 'reasonable accommodations to known physical or mental limitations of an otherwise qualified handicapped (person)'" (Shriner, 2000, p. 234).

Section 504 strived to provide students with disabilities an equal opportunity to gain the same benefits from school and to reach the same level of achievement as their nondisabled peers. It is important to note that Section 504 applies only to entities that obtain federal subsidies. On the other hand, the *Americans with Disabilities Act of 1990* (ADA) applies to most entities, regardless of whether they receive federal funds. The ADA served as a reinforcement of the principles found within Section 504 and reiterated that the primary focus should remain on making individual decisions regarding reasonable modifications on policies, procedures, and practices. "The ADA was intended as companion legislation to the *IDEA* and Section 504 of the Rehabilitation Act of 1973. The most comprehensive civil rights legislation enacted since the 1960s, the ADA expands the prohibition of discrimination against people with disabilities to the area of employment, transportation, communications, and public accommodations and reinforces rights guaranteed in earlier pieces of legislation" (Rea & Davis-Dorsey, 2004, p. 66).

The ADA contained several titles which corresponded to various aspects of discrimination for people with disabilities. Title I focused on discrimination within the work place. Title II dealt with state and local governmental entities such as prohibiting discrimination within schools. Finally, Title III focused on public accommodations such as within stores, hotels, and restaurants. According to the ADA, all entities were required to make reasonable accommodations and modifications to guarantee that people with disabilities had access to goods and services. In the educational setting, the ADA had produced numerous positive results such as "a more diverse workforce; increased accessibility of opportunities, activities, and facilities; increased labor resources; a refreshing call for innovation, creativity, and flexibility; and a new recognition and appreciation of the strengths, contributions, and abilities of people with disabilities" (Rea & Davis-Dorsey, 2004, p. 69).

The definition of a disability under Section 504 and the ADA contained three main criteria (Rehabilitation Act & sec; 706[8]):

1. has a physical or mental impairment that substantially limits one or more of such person's major life activities,
2. has a record of such impairment, or
3. is regarded as having such impairment (Smith, 2001, p. 338).

There were two requirements detailed in Section 504 and the ADA which affected students: nondiscrimination and free, appropriate public education (FAPE). The nondiscrimination policy referred to the concept that the students with disabilities should be allowed to participate in activities that were available for all students. This would include the same academic curriculum, nonacademic extracurricular activities, health services, recreational activities, athletics, student employment, clubs, specific courses, and field trips. It is essential to understand that students must meet the "otherwise qualified" criterion as stated in IDEA. "This means that a person with a disability must be qualified to do something before the presence of a disability can be a factor in discrimination" (Smith, 2001, p. 340).

In addition to nondiscrimination, Section 504 and ADA required that schools provided students with disabilities with a FAPE. This would include the provisions that were designed to meet the individual educational needs of students with disabilities comparable to that of the needs of the nondisabled students. A FAPE must be provided regardless of the nature and severity of the disability. Students must have nondiscriminatory evaluations and placement. Furthermore, procedural safeguards enables parents to contribute significantly in decisions concerning the evaluation and placement of their students. Finally, students must be integrated with their nondisabled peers to the maximum scope possible, a trend referred to as mainstreaming.

In addition to Section 504 and ADA, the concept of mainstreaming was enforced with Public Law 94-142 as schools were now required to place children with disabilities with their nondisabled peers to the maximum extent possible. "Depending upon a student's functioning level and the structure of the school system, the student may be in either an integrated setting with nondisabled peers or a segregated environment with other disabled students" (DeWeaver & Kropf, 1992, p. 38).

The debate of integration culminated with the passage of federal legislation in 1974 entitled the *Education for All Handicapped Children Act.* This law was revised and reauthorized as the *Individuals with Disabilities Education Act (IDEA)* of 1997. *IDEA* mandated that students with disabilities be provided an education planned to meet their needs in the least restrictive environment. The placement of students with disabilities is one of the most important decisions agreed upon by the IEP team. Likewise, it can be a controversial area resulting in many due process hearings (Yell & Katsiyannis, 2004, p. 29).

The two essential principles of *IDEA* were the FAPE and providing these services within the students' LRE. This legislation details that support for special education and related services to children be provided in a variety of settings such as child care, preschool, elementary, middle, and high school. According to *IDEA* this is accomplished through the development of Individual Education Programs (IEPs) that provide students with disabilities with a free, appropriate education in a minimally-restrictive environment. This must be provided for students, age three to 21, who have been found eligible for services. This document was considered the cornerstone of the *IDEA* as a means of providing students with a FAPE (Gartin & Murdick, 2005).

IDEA was a federal programmatic mandate that governed all special education services and therefore provided funding for students identified as eligible. On the other hand, Section 504 was a civil rights statute; therefore, no funding was provided to assist in compliance. The criteria for determining identification, eligibility, appropriate education, least restrictive environment, and due process were all different between *IDEA* and *Section 504.*

The major differences center on the flexibility of the procedures. There were less specific criteria for students found eligible under Section 504. Therefore, schools may offer less assistance and monitoring. Students found eligible for services under *IDEA* must meet specific criteria as well as the degree of regulation was more specific with regards to timeframes, parental participation, and paperwork requirements. Furthermore, *IDEA* made provisions for students with disabilities from ages 3 to 21, while Section 504 covered people with disabilities throughout their lifespan. In addition, *IDEA* focused on the educational needs of people with disabilities, while Section 504 covered a variety of aspects of people's lives such as employment, public access, transportation, as well as their educational needs (deBettencourt, 2002).

The 2004 *IDEA* reauthorization (*IDEA 2004*) made provision for many positive changes. According to the Council for Exceptional Children (2006), the most important of these changes include:

- Guaranteed that students with disabilities participate in accountability systems.
- Reduced the paperwork burden.
- Established methods to decrease the number of students from culturally and linguistically diverse backgrounds inappropriately placed in special education.
- Ensured the discipline provisions for students with disabilities continue to protect the rights of students to a free, appropriate public education.
- Provided funding for professional development for special educators.

The most current legislation entitled *No Child Left Behind* is "the 21st century iteration of this first major foray into education policy" (Paige, 2004, p. 13). This has had a tremendous impact on the education of students with intellectual disabilities. Previously, legislation had worked to provide accommodations as well as access to general education classes and the curriculum. The 1997 amendments to *IDEA* specify that "students with disabilities have access to and progress in the general education curriculum" (Wehmeyer et al, 2002, p. 158).

It is also important to review the legislation specific to working with students who are mentally retarded. The first landmark case was *Diana v. State Board of Education* (1970) which required the state of California to correct assessment procedures. Three important results of this case were that students must be tested in their primary language, culturally unfair items must be eliminated from test and assessments, and intelligence tests must be developed to reflect Mexican-American culture (NASET, 2006).

Later in 1984 *Larry P v. Riles* similar results indicated California was discriminating against students who were mentally retarded by using IQ tests as the assessment measure for eligibility. *Wyatt v Stickney* (1972) directed that children with intellectual disabilities in state institutions had the right to treatment. *PARC v Commonwealth of PA* (1972) would play a fundamental role in future federal special education laws. This legislation assured that schools could not exclude students with intellectual disabilities and that these students must be provided with a free public education. Furthermore, it called for deinstitutionalization due to inhumane conditions (Black & Salas, 2001). Similarly, *Mills v Board of Education of DC* (1972) provided guidelines for a free public education and due process. In addition, it was mandated that special education services must be provided despite the school's financial capability (NASET, 2006).

Curriculum

Historically, curriculum planning began with the passage of PL 94-142 when schools became responsible for the education of students with intellectual disabilities and IEPs drove the curriculum. Barnes and Barnes (1989) described guidelines for the development of a curriculum specifically designed for students with intellectual disabilities. The major goal was to identify what needed to be taught, by moving them toward independence in adulthood. Goals and objectives should be developed in the areas of academic, recreational, prevocational and vocational, social and emotional, and life skills. The key is to strike a balance between students being left in academic classes and functional life skills (Sutton, 1993).

The curriculum for students with intellectual disabilities should be driven by the specific needs of individual students, rather than their label, current issues, or the general education curriculum (Thomas, 1996). However, recent changes in legislation have created shifts in philosophical views and have directly impacted curriculum planning. "As societal perspectives change, so does the focus of school curriculum. One of the strongest current influences on curriculum is the school accountability movement" (Ahlgrim-Delzell, Algozzine, Browder, Flowers, Karvonen, & Spooner, 2004, p. 1).

Instruction for students with intellectual disabilities was at one time characterized by a developmental approach to teaching. Students with disabilities were often asked to complete repeated drill and practice on isolated skills that were not easily transferable to the general community. Since students with disabilities typically take a longer time to acquire a skill, they were often focusing on similar skills throughout their education without progressing. As a result, educators found that students were completing their education with the skills associated with younger children rather than adults made ready to enter the community (Ford, 2001). Therefore, specific instruction should be provided in functional academic skills that will be used in everyday life. "As these individuals move to secondary education settings, the curriculum should take on a stronger career preparation and life skills emphasis" (Hourcade, 2002, p. 4).

Current educational trends and legislation allows for students with intellectual disabilities to receive special education services in an environment which provided access to the general education curriculum. "The State shall have such academic standards for all public elementary school and secondary school children, including children served under this part, in subjects determined by the State, but including mathematics, reading or language arts, and (beginning in 2005-2006 school year) science, which shall include the same knowledge, skills, and levels of achievement expected of all children" (CEC, 2003, p. 7). This mandated that students with disabilities take part in a curriculum appropriate for their age and grade level.

In addition to participating in the general education curriculum, students must demonstrate that they have made progress in this curriculum. Adequate yearly progress (AYP) is a controlling measurement to determine accountability towards each student's achievement (CEC, 2001). Since schools are now mandated to maintain AYP in the areas of mathematics, reading or language arts, and science, students with intellectual disabilities must be exposed to a curriculum that contained these subjects.

"Over the past 30 years there has been a significant shift in the focus of the curriculum for students with significant cognitive disabilities. As a field we have moved from a developmental model to a functional life skills model to one that promotes access to the general education curriculum" (VDOE, 2006-2007, p.7). However, as students with cognitive disabilities progress through school, a focus should be placed on the maturation of functional academic skills. Educators must find a balance between providing the students access to the general education curriculum and providing instruction in a functional curriculum. As students advanced to secondary education settings, a career preparatory and life skills emphasis is placed on curriculum and instructional matters (Hourcade, 2002).

Finding a curriculum that allows students with mental disabilities to be exposed to the general education curriculum, while receiving instruction in these vital areas continues to be of utmost importance. *IDEA* mandated that the curricula used within special education classes be research-based and peer-reviewed (Cernosia, 2005). In addition, "In education, national policies such as No Child Left Behind (NCLB) require that teachers use scientifically proven practice in their classrooms" (Odom, Brantlinger, Gersten, Horner, Thompson, & Harris, 2005, p. 137). NCLB requires that all students be assessed in reading, math, social studies, and science, which was contradictory to the functional approach typical of how skills were acquired for students with disabilities (Browder & Cooper-Duffy, 2003).

The concept of a life skills curriculum has been increasing in awareness and practice. According to the 1989 text *Best Practices in Mild Mental Retardation* (Robinson, et. al.) curriculum options were discussed and, "although there are a number of curricular options, we believe that the one best suited for a vast majority of students with mild intellectual disabilities is one based on the principles inherent in the life skills/adult outcomes approach" (p. 25). In 1994, Smith and Hilton determined that the curriculum should be driven by the needs of the students rather than by clinical labels, philosophical issues, or the initiatives occurring with regular education (Thomas, 1997).

Syracuse Community-Referenced Curriculum Guide

Within the field of disabilities two leading life and vocational curriculums are the Syracuse Community-Referenced Curriculum Guide for Students with Moderate and Severe Disabilities and the Life Centered Career Education program. Both of these curriculums tie assessment and lesson planning together (Moon, 2000). The Syracuse Curriculum Guide was based on the premise that, "every student, no matter how severe his or her disabilities, is capable of living, working, and recreating in the community" (Ford, Schnorr, Meyer, Davern, Black, & Dempsey, 1989, p. 3).

The Community-Referenced Curriculum Guide focused on the community living domains of self-management/home living, vocational, recreational/leisure, and community functioning. In addition functional academic skills like reading, writing, money handling, and time management were addressed. Furthermore, the embedded social, communication, and motor skills were concentrated on throughout instruction in all of the content areas. This would include interacting positively with peers, using vocalizations and symbol systems, and moving about in the environment effectively. All of these areas were targeted as they would allow students to function in the real world.

The Syracuse Community-Referenced Curriculum Guide addressed the concern for educators of how to integrate life skills into an academic curriculum. It is proposed that this curriculum be used as one part of the numerous other course offerings available. If the content areas cannot be met in regular education classes, an alternate method would be to incorporate the content area into informal parts of the day, natural learning times, or recess and free time.

The community living domains of self-management/home living, vocational, recreational/leisure, and community functioning were all areas where students must receive this consistent deliberate instruction. The self management/home living realm encompasses skills that were essential to everyday functioning. "These types of skills are common in people's daily lives and present frequent opportunities to make personal choices (e.g., what to eat, when to do something). By not teaching students to participate in such common and regular daily routines, we may seriously restrict their opportunities to influence decisions about their personal lives (Ford, Schnorr, Meyer, Davern, Black, & Dempsey, 1989). The six major goal areas include eating and food preparation, grooming and dressing, hygiene and toileting, safety and health, assisting and taking care of others, and budgeting and planning/scheduling.

According to the Syracuse Guide, vocational skills were essential in helping to establish a positive self-image, gain the respect of others, and make contributions to the community. The vocational domain covered three major goal areas: classroom/school jobs, neighborhood jobs, and actual community jobs. These settings represent a variety of integrated environments and build the students' vocational resumes (Ford, Schnorr, Meyer, Davern, Black, & Dempsey, 1989).

The recreational/leisure skills domain was centered on increasing the life skills of a person with disabilities. This would include five major goals areas: school and extracurricular, activities to do alone, activities to do with family and friends at home, activities to do with friends in the community, and activities that increase one's physical fitness (Ford, Schnorr, Meyer, Davern, Black, & Dempsey, 1989).

Finally, general community functioning was based on the fact that learning can take place in various settings. "Meaningful instruction is not limited to school settings; it can also take place in the surrounding community where students can learn and practice skills in real-life settings" (Ford, Schnorr, Meyer, Davern, Black, & Dempsey, 1989, p. 77). One cannot assume that students with intellectual disabilities will acquire these skills based on exposure alone. Educators must provide instruction in order for students to receive consistent and repeated opportunities to develop these skills.

In addition to the community living domains, The Syracuse Community-Referenced Curriculum Guide stressed the instruction of embedded skills. These skills included communication, motor, and social skills. These skills were reinforced throughout all aspects of instruction in a variety of content areas. With regard to social skills, there are 11 social skill functions identified. "No cookbook approach to social skills instruction could meet the widely varied needs of students with moderate and severe disabilities. Rather, we have provided some guidelines for thinking about social skills in general as well as for planning specific social skills programs." (Ford, Schnorr, Meyer, Davern, Black, & Dempsey, 1989, p. 184).

Life Centered Career Education

The LCCE curriculum was based on the premise that career education is more than just a part of an educational program--it should be the major focus of a program. Career education began in the early 1970s as educators became aware of the need to refocus their instruction on specific skills that benefited students in their adult life. The concept of career education focused on the facilitation of growth and development for all roles in life, settings, and events. These roles were defined as "a productive and independent family member, citizen, employee, and participant in a variety of avocational/leisure activities such as recreational pursuits and hobbies" (Brolin, 1997, p.17). Furthermore, emphasis is made that educational experiences should be community-based to provide students with events in a variety of settings.

"Research during the past three decades clearly revealed that students must learn four major categories of skills: academic, daily living, personal-social, and occupational" (Brolin, 1997, p. 9). The LCCE placed its emphasis on three domains: daily living skills, occupational skills, and personal-social skills. "This is not to imply that career education is the only education students should receive, but it should be a significant and pervasive part of what is taught" (Brolin, 1997, p. 9).

LCCE was chosen as the curriculum for the purposes of this study due to the integration of academics with life skills training as well as the assessment instruments available. The LCCE curriculum contained a set of curriculum-based assessment instruments designed to measure the Daily Living Skills, Personal-Social Skills, and Occupational Guidance and

Preparation. This curriculum focused on career education for regular and special education students. These competencies were identified as targeted areas based upon research, input from previous studies, and professional opinions (Brolin, 1997). Each competency was then classified under one of the three major curriculum areas referred to as domains.

The Daily Living Skills domain contained competencies that were essential goals for students in special education to reach their most independent level possible. These targeted competencies included managing personal finances, selecting and managing a household, caring for personal needs, raising children and meeting marriage responsibilities, buying, preparing, and consuming food, buying and caring for clothing, exhibiting responsible citizenship, using recreational facilities and leisure time, and getting around the community (mobility).

An additional domain targeted would be that of Occupational Guidance and Preparation. In an effort to help students attain their highest potential, students must be exposed to a variety of aspects related to vocational awareness. Addressing students' need to become aware of the diverse job possibilities available to them accomplishes this objective. In addition, students were helped to develop the necessary skills, participate in a variety of work experiences, and learn to make logical and viable job choices. The competencies that were designated to address occupational curriculum are knowing and exploring occupational possibilities, selecting and planning occupational choices, exhibiting appropriate work habits and behaviors, seeking, securing, and maintaining employment, exhibiting sufficient physical-manual skills, and obtaining a specific occupational skill.

The third domain was the Personal-Social competency area and served as the curriculum utilized within this study. The Personal-Social competency focused on the independence, self-confidence, socially acceptable behavior, and maintenance of friendships for the students with intellectual disabilities participating within the study. The primary competencies that were included in instruction were achieving self-awareness, acquiring self-confidence, achieving socially responsible behavior, maintaining good interpersonal skills, achieving independence, achieving problem-solving skills, and communicating with others. The following are LCCEs Domains.

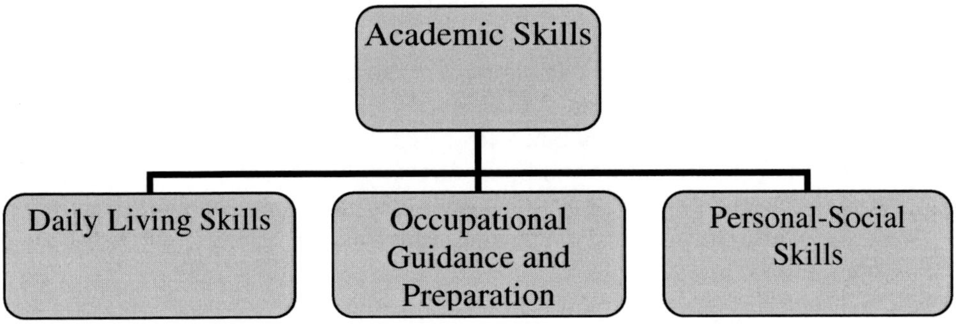

Chart 1. LCCE Curriculum Domains (Brolin, 1997, p. 13).

LCCE's personal-social domain

Achieving Self-Awareness

1. Identify Physical and Physiological Needs

    List basic physical needs
    Identify ways to meet physical needs
    List basic psychological needs
    Identify ways to meet psychological needs

2. Identify Interests and Abilities

    Identify abilities common to most people
    Identify interests common to most people
    Demonstrate goal setting in relation to pursing an interest or ability and show how goals are attained

3. Identify Emotions

    Identify common emotions (fear, love, hate, sadness)
    List ways in which one's emotions affect the behavior of self and others
    Identify ways in which one may cope with emotions
    Differentiate particular emotions in self and others

4. Demonstrate Knowledge of Physical Self

    Identify major systems of the body
    List personal physical characteristics
    Describe physical characteristics and dimensions
    Identify major parts of the body

5. Acquiring Self-Confidence

    1. Express Feelings of Self-Worth
        List positive physical and psychological attributes
        Express ways in which positive attributes make him/her feel good
        List the characteristics necessary to feel good about oneself
        Describe ways in which the actions of others affect one's feelings of self-worth
    2. Describe Others' Perception of Self
        List potential reactions of others to oneself
        Construct a personal view of how others see oneself
        Describe the relationship between one's own behaviors and others' reactions
        Demonstrate awareness of individual differences in others
    3. Accept and Give Praise
        Identify statements of praise in everyday activities
        List appropriate and inappropriate responses to praise
        Respond to praise statements by others
        List the effects of praise on oneself
    4. Accept and give criticism
        Identify critical and/or rejecting types of statements

List appropriate ways to respond to criticism and/or rejection
Respond appropriately to critical statements
List positive and negative effects of criticism

5. Develop confidence in oneself
   Identify and describe positive characteristics of oneself in a variety of areas
   List appropriate ways to express confidence in oneself
   Make positive statements about oneself
   Identify potential reactions of others to expressions of self-confidence

6. Achieving Socially Responsible Behavior

   1. Demonstrate respect for the rights and properties of others
      Identify personal and property rights of others
      Identify reasons for respecting the rights and properties of others
      Demonstrate respect for others and their property
      List appropriate situations and procedures for borrowing the property of others
   2. Recognize authority and follow instructions
      Identify common authority roles
      Identify aspects of following instructions
      Identify situation in which the individual has the right to disregard instructions from authorities
   3. Demonstrate appropriate behavior in public places
      Identify appropriate behavior in public places
      Identify and demonstrate appropriate behaviors when using transportation facilities
      Identify and demonstrate appropriate behaviors when using eating facilities
      Identify and demonstrate appropriate behaviors when using recreational facilities
   4. Know important character traits
      Identify own acceptable character traits
      Identify acceptable character traits in others
      List character traits necessary for acceptance in group activities
      List character traits that inhibit acceptance
   5. Recognize personal roles
      Identify current roles
      Identify possible future roles
      List roles of significant others
      Describe the rights and obligations in personal roles as they interact with the roles of others

7. Maintaining Good Interpersonal Skills

   1. Demonstrate listening and responding skills
      Identify proper listening and responding techniques
      Identify positive outcomes of listening and responding appropriately
      Identify negative aspects of listening and responding inappropriately
   2. Establish and maintain close relationships
      Identify qualities of an individual who would be desirable in the dating process
      Identify and demonstrate appropriate procedures for making a date
      List activities that are appropriate for a date

Identify characteristics of close relationships
List different types of close relationships
Recognize and respond to intimate feelings of others
Identify persons with whom one could establish a close relationship

3. Make and maintain friendships
Identify necessary components for a friendship
List personal considerations in choosing a friend
List rights and responsibilities important in personal friendships
List activities that can be shared with friends

8. Achieving Independence

1. Strive towards self-actualization
Identify important characteristics for personal growth
List elements necessary for a satisfactory personal life
Identify sources for continued educational/psychological growth
2. Demonstrate self-organization
Develop plan of daily activities
Identify areas of responsibility in personal life
Identify reasons for organizing one's responsibilities/activities
Develop ways in which personal organization relates to greater independence
3. Demonstrate awareness of how one's behavior affects others
List ways in which behavior affects others around us
List appropriate behaviors for a variety of situations
List different cues elicited by others that behavior is inappropriate
List ways to correct inappropriate behavior

9. Making Adequate Decisions

1. Locate and utilize sources of assistance
Identify situations in which one would need advice
List available resources for resolving problems
Given particular situations, describe the procedures for contacting persons for assistance
List potential outcomes of seeking advice
2. Anticipate consequences
Describe consequences or outcomes of decision-making
List and demonstrate knowledge of ways in which personal behavior produces consequences
Describe the concept of maximum gain for minimum risk
3. Develop and evaluate alternatives
Define the meaning of alternatives
List possible alternatives with respect to a personal goal
Describe a compromise with respect to a personal goal
List resources for information that develops alternatives
4. Recognize nature of a problem
Given a list of situations with positive/negative aspects of personal ideas, examine each as a positive or negative

Identify why ideas, values, and plans have both potentially positive and negative implications
Identify a situation which requires examination of positive/negative aspects
5. Develop goal-seeking behavior
Identify ways that goals affect one's life
List outcomes to be considered in goal setting
List examples of individuals who have set and attained their goals
Set one goal for school, home, recreation
Set short-term and long-term personal goals
Identify characteristics of realistic goals
Identify appropriate persons for obtaining assistance with setting and achieving goals
Identify potential barriers to goals
Set model personal goals

10. Communicating with Others
1. Recognize and respond to emergency situations
Identify sights and sounds of emergency situations
Identify appropriate authorities to contact in emergency situations
Describe personal communication indicating emergency situations
List personal responsibilities in emergency situations
2. Communicate with understanding
Demonstrate a variety of verbal expressions related to communication
Identify and demonstrate methods of speaking appropriately in a social conversation
Demonstrate proper use of telephone
Demonstrate appropriate volume and intensity in conversation
3. Know subtleties of communication
Identify nonverbal elements of communication
Identify verbal expressions that correspond to feelings
Identify verbal expressions that are consistent with feelings
Demonstrate verbal and nonverbal elements of communication
(Brolin, 1997, pp. 69-104).

Social Skills

Social skills training was typically an integral aspect of programs for people with intellectual disabilities. It was essential that students initiate and maintain positive social relationships with their family, peers, teachers, and people within their community. "Social skills are often defined as a complex set of skills that include communication, problem-solving and decision-making, assertion, peer and group interactions, and self-management" (Kolb & Hanley-Maxwell, 2003, p. 163).

Social skills are both observable and measurable behaviors that promoted independence, acceptability, and a good quality of life. "These skills are crucial to adjustments and normal functioning, and deficits have been closely linked to psychopathology and behavior problems" (Matson, Mayville, Lott, Bielecki, & Logan, 2003, p. 58). The research on intellectual disabilities indicated that social skills were of utmost importance in the quality of life and adjustment of people with intellectual disabilities into their community and vocation. "Numerous studies have proven that the lack of appropriate social skills is a major factor contributing to the failure of persons with intellectual disabilities in community placements" (Paraschiv & Oiley, 1999, p.3).

According to Barnes and Barnes (1989) educators have four major goals when teaching social skills. The first is to support students in learning how to read social cues and develop suitable responding behaviors. Secondly, it is essential to provide opportunities to socialize and practice these skills. Next educators must take on the role of educating others regarding the unique social needs of students with intellectual disabilities. Finally, it is essential to provide direct instruction on these specific social skills (Sutton, 1993). Similarly, Bertone, Boyle, Mitchel, & Smith (1999) stated that social skills goals can be met by incorporating direct instruction, structuring a positive classroom environment, and implementing cooperative learning strategies and activities.

In a historical review of special education, social deficits were identified early as detrimental to the development of students with intellectual disabilities. However, there were few instances of social skills training. In the 1950s authorities on disabilities indicated that social competency was most affected by the experiences within school. As students were integrated into regular education classrooms, poor social skills contributed to the fact that students with disabilities were frustrated with failure. This resulted in students being placed in separate classes to create a non-threatening classroom environment. "The less threatening academic atmosphere would ensure success experiences resulting in enhanced self-concept and decreases in showing off, teasing, and stealing other children's things that were believed to be part of the youngsters' with mild mental retardation behavioral repertories" (Robinson et al, 1989, p.271).

One of the earliest social skills training programs was the Social Learning Curriculum (Goldstein, 1974) developed by the Curriculum Research and Development Center in Mental Retardation at Yeshiva University. This was a social education curriculum directly geared toward addressing social interaction skills and providing information to students regarding their community and the daily living environment. Since the development of that curriculum, special education service delivery models changed focus and attempted to program for students with disabilities in the least restrictive environment (Robinson et al, 1989).

According to Taylor & Larson (1999) specific social skills training during adolescence can be effective in positively influencing students' behavior (Kolb & Hanley-Maxwell, 2003). Despite this research, there was little consensus within current curricula regarding what the content of social skills training should include. "Social incompetence can lead to failure cycles and eventual poor school and adult outcomes" (Cartledge & Kiarie, 2001, p. 40). Despite this fact, there was little evidence that social skills were being systematically taught.

Ethical Considerations in Special Education Research

In 1969 the AAMR(America Association of Mental Retardation) adopted ten general principles when performing research on students with intellectual disabilities. The first principle centered on the fact that all research must conform to the same scientific, legal, and moral principles which justify all research. Secondly, all research with human subjects must be performed by qualified individuals. Furthermore, the research can only be carried out if the benefits of the objective outweighed the potential risk to the participants. The fourth principle reflected the fact that caution should not be limited to physical harm but should preclude psychological damage to the subjects as well as to their families (AAMR, 2006).

The fifth ethical principle to be implemented was that coercion of students is prohibited. In addition, compensation must be provided for any unusual inconvenience resulting from the study. It is also important to understand that all ethical aspects in the experimentation with people who were mentally retarded is clearly stated and that consent must be obtained if there is any risk or if one's identity may be revealed. The ninth principle centered on the premise that experimentation should be planned in a manner in which pain, suffering, and inconvenience was avoided. Finally, it was the researcher's responsibility to report the findings to the scientific community (AAMR, 2006).

Since qualitative research was empirical, it relied on factual information as well as observations and direct experiences. When completing the LCCE's Competency Rating Scale (CRS) forms, it was essential to be aware of the ethical standards that related to qualitative research. It was essential to recognize standards of high-quality work and to avoid or expose unethical behavior. "Qualitative field research, like all behavior, must follow the four cardinal virtues of antiquity: prudence, justice, wisdom, and courage" (Bruckerhoff, 1996, p. 2).

It was suggested that qualitative research was about human relationships. In order to establish an appropriate relationship between the researcher and the persons being studied, the researcher must have an interest in the people being studied, listen well, show respect, keep accurate records, be honest regarding intentions of the study, exercise caution, do no harm, and report the limitations of the study (Bruckerhoff, 1996).

Theoretical Review

Typically social skills are defined as the ability to get along with others and the exhibition of character traits. The concept of social skill acquisition relates to the theory of Emotional Intelligence described by Daniel Goleman (1997). "Emotional intelligence is the ability to access and interpret a given situation accurately and to manage oneself to relate effectively with others" (Kolb & Hanley-Maxwell, 2003, p.170). The five distinct dimensions found within emotional intelligence were self-awareness, managing emotions or self-control, motivation, recognizing emotions in others, and handling relationships. Research indicated that a person's emotional intelligence was more predictive of achievement within school and the workplace than IQ. "Children need to learn to manage their feelings appropriately, interact effectively with others, and motivate themselves if they are to be productive students and or workers" (Menta, 2006, p.1).

In addition, Albert Bandura's Social Leaning theory can be applied to the social skills development of students with intellectual disabilities. Social learning emphasized the importance of the observation and subsequent modeling of behaviors, attitudes, and emotional reactions of others. This theory was based on the premise that social interactions play a fundamental role in the development of cognition. "Bandura's social cognitive theory posits that behavior change is a function of setting goals based on outcome expectations associated with the behavior change, the tasks required to achieve those goals, and self-efficacy expectations for achieving the goals" (Heller & Rimmer, 2006, p. 1).

The Social Learning theory can easily be applied to the education of students with intellectual disabilities. "Social learning theory explains human behavior in terms of continuous reciprocal interaction between cognitive, behavioral, and environmental influences" (Kearsley, 2006, p.1). Bandura's theory also sets the theoretical framework for behavior modification techniques. These techniques were frequently used within special education classrooms to help achieve desired behaviors. As the social learning theory dictated, the LCCE curriculum focused on blending academics, daily living, personal-social, and occupational skills through social interactions within a variety of instructional settings (Brolin, 1997).

METHODOLOGY

No Child Left Behind mandates that students with intellectual disabilities have access to core curriculum courses. The life skills program, Life Centered Career Education (LCCE), was integrated into the curriculum of high school students with intellectual disabilities. The LCCE program was chosen as it integrated essential academic instruction along with Personal-Social skills, Daily Living skills, and Occupational Knowledge lessons.

The study determined improvements made in the social skills of students pre- and posttest scores of the LCCE Knowledge Battery and Competency Rating Scale (CRS). Observations in the differences between the control group and an experimental group were made. Therefore, the hypothesis was that students in classes that utilized the LCCE's Personal-Social Skills program achieved significantly higher scores on the Knowledge Battery and Competency Rating Scale (CRS) than students who did not participate in the program.

Procedures

The study began with the four educators participating being trained on the administration of the Knowledge Battery (Form A) and CRS. This was accomplished by each educator being provided with the introductory material that described the instrument and gave guidelines for test administration, detailed instructions to students, and scoring information along with templates for scoring and student recording forms. All educators began by administering the pretest evaluation. The LCCE Knowledge Battery determined the initial level of each student's Personal-Social skills.

The two special education teachers participating in the experimental instruction of the 39 subjects were trained on the LCCE program. The LCCE curriculum was administered to the selected 19 subjects over the course of seven weeks. Each week focused on one competency of the LCCE's Personal-Social curriculum:

- Week 1: Competency 10: Achieving Self-Awareness
- Week 2: Competency 11: Acquiring Self-Confidence

- Week 3: Competency 12: Achieving Socially Responsible Behavior
- Week 4: Competency 13: Maintaining Good Interpersonal Skills
- Week 5: Competency 14: Achieving Independence
- Week 6: Competency 15: : Making Adequate Decisions
- Week 7: Competency 16: Communicating with Others

The competencies addressed each week contained three specific sections for educators to apply. These sections included objectives, activities or strategies, and the role of adults in helping students achieve the identified goals. The teachers were provided with identical lesson plans and materials. Following the completion of the LCCE program, all four of the educators administered the equivalent, Form B, of the Knowledge Battery and reevaluated the students using the CRS, to determine the effectiveness of the intervention. Finally, a LCCE survey was administered to the educators involved in the study in order to provide additional information regarding any improvements that occurred in the study.

This experiment was classified as a nonequivalent control group, pretest/posttest design. This can be illustrated as administering a pretest to determine the dependent variable (Y_1) to the experimental and control group, applying the experimental treatment or independent variable (X), and the administration of a posttest to both groups that once again measured the dependent variable (Y_2). This was classified as nonequivalent since the student selection was based upon the students school.

Sample

The students were placed either into the LCCE class for seven weeks or continued to receive instruction from the current curriculum. The schools selected for the study had previously not participated in any of the LCCE programs. The LCCE classes were taught in seven weeks by the students' special education teachers. Students in the non-LCCE classes continued to receive instruction according to the Augusta County curriculum for high school students with intellectual disabilities.

The 39 subjects participating resided in Augusta County, Virginia, a rural community. The students all have been found eligible for services under the category of intellectual disabilities. The participants fell between 14 and 22 years of age. The control group consisted of 20 students from two separate high schools and the experimental group was composed of 19 students from two separate high schools.

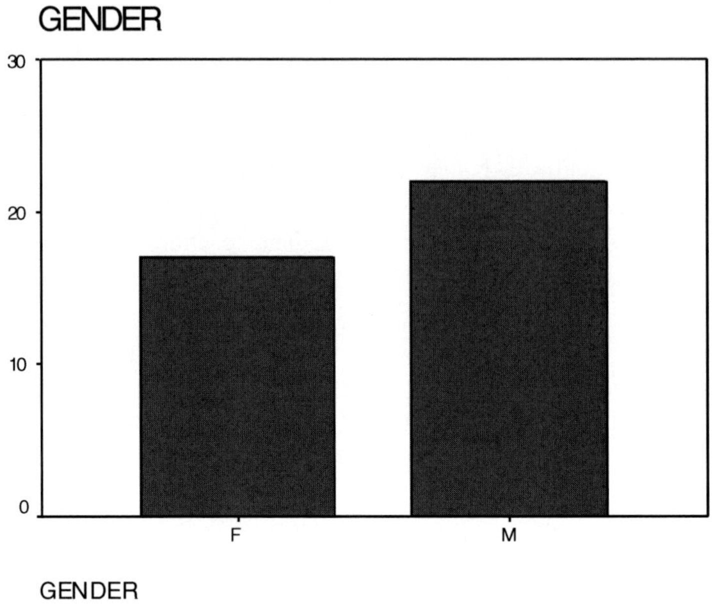

Graph 1. Frequency of Gender.

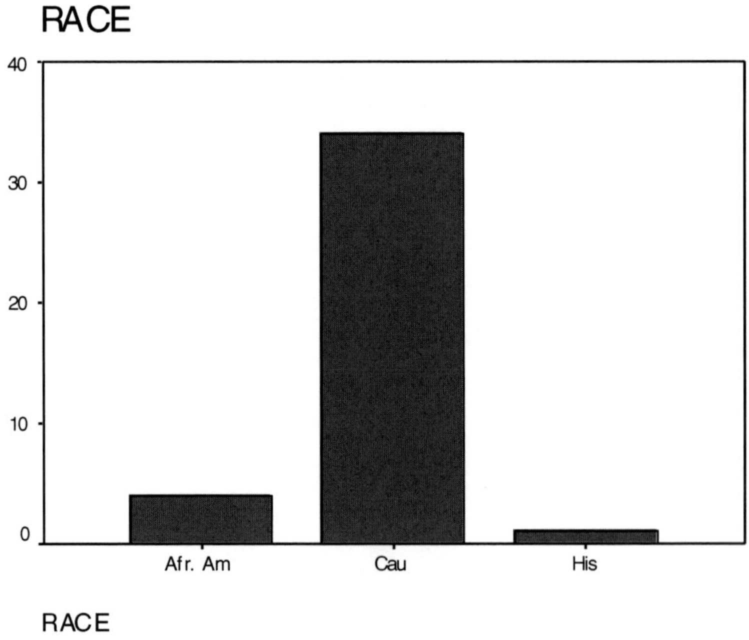

Graph 2. Frequency of Race.

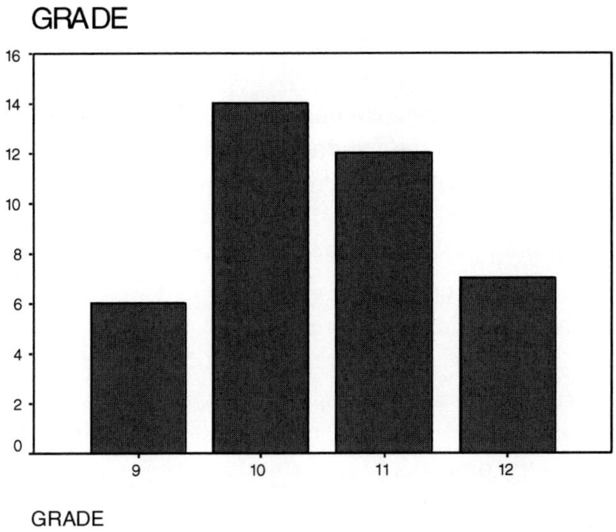

Graph 3. Frequency of Grade.

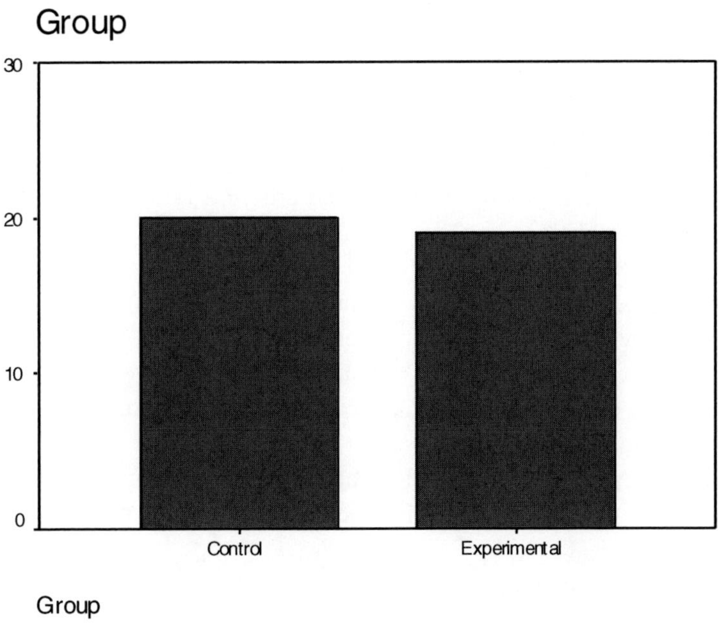

Graph 4. Frequency of Control and Experimental groups.

Descriptive Statistics on Frequency

The descriptive statistics regarding gender indicated there were 17 females (43.6%) and 22 males (56.4%) who participated in the study.

The ethnicity of the participants demonstrated that 87.2% of the subjects were Caucasian. This is significantly higher than the national overall population average of 61% (Education Thrust, 2004). Furthermore, the African-American population was represented by 10.3% of the subjects, compared to the national overall population average of 17%. The frequency of Hispanics within the study represented was 2.6%, well below the national overall population average of 16% (Education Thrust, 2004).

An analysis of the grade level data represented within the study demonstrated that 9th graders represented 15.4%, 10th graders represented 35.9%, 11th graders represented 30.8% and 12th graders represented 17.9%.

The following descriptive statistics correspond to the frequency of subjects within acontrol group and the experimental, LCCE group.

Instruments

The LCCE Battery of assessment tested the students' general knowledge of the 21 competencies as well as their ability to demonstrate the desired competencies. The Knowledge Battery was broken into the three LCCE domains: Daily Living, Occupational Knowledge, and Personal-Social. In order to assess student improvement, educators administered the LCCE's Knowledge Battery specifically related to the Personal-Social competencies.

The Knowledge Battery was a standardized criterion-referenced instrument consisting of 200 multiple choice questions covering all of the curriculum domains, 21 competencies, and 97 sub-competencies. The Personal-Social portion contained questions for each of the targeted competencies with a total of 70 questions.

The Knowledge Battery's main purpose was to assess the knowledge important to functioning as a family member, an employee, a productive citizen, and in meaningful vocational activities (Brolin, 1997). This curriculum-based instrument field tested specifically for students with mild intellectual disabilities. In addition to the Knowledge Battery, the LCCE's Competency Rating Scale (CRS) also sought to identify strengths and weaknesses and determine the effectiveness of instructional strategies within the special education classroom.

Statistical analysis indicated the Kuder Richardson formula (KR 20) was utilized to determine reliability of each test, domain, and the total battery. Results indicated that the reference group scored one standard deviation below the mastery level, which was 17 out of 20 items. This translated into the fact that this battery was useful in the identification of student instructional needs and that there was not any test that was either too easy or too difficult. In addition, the KR 20s ranged between .55 and .82 with a median score of .72. The total battery on the KR 20 was .98, indicating that "the stability of the tests and total battery were also found to be good" (Brolin, 1997, p. 126). For the domain of Personal-Social skills, the Pre KR 20 score was .95, Post KR score was .96, and Test/Retest was .90, all indicating that the items have a high correlation to the domain they represent. Final measures of reliability, determined using the Pearson product moment correlations, ranged from .58 to.83 with a median of .745; for the total battery the correlation was .94. This indicated that the items correlate strongly with their respective domains (Brolin, 1997).

The LCCE Knowledge Battery demonstrated construct, content, and criterion-related validity. The construct validity was discerned on the basis of several projects from the Office of Special Education Programs through the US Department of Education and a federal special education project called the Competency Assessment Inventory Project (CAI). This allowed the LCCE curriculum to be developed with the input of special education teachers, as well as other educators. "The result was a competency-based curriculum which purported to cover all critical career/life skills that needed to be taught to mildly handicapped students (K-12)" (Brolin, 1997, p.119).

The content validity of the LCCE was addressed in numerous ways. This was accomplished through item writers developing questions that spanned the range of instructional objectives. Next, the administrators of tests evaluated test items through the utilization of field tests and agreed upon the appropriateness and status of items within the test. Finally, nine experts were given a field test with the task of analyzing each item to determine what competency they believed the questions addressed. Results indicated that the Personal-Social domain questions most often fell outside their domain. It was determined that "many of the items were written using a daily living or vocational example" (Brolin, 1997, p.127).

Criterion-related validity was performed in field tests as well as teacher judgments of the mastery, partial mastery, or non-mastery for each competency. This was completed in order to provide an external criterion against which the student was compared. Correlations between the actual scores and the teacher ratings were also made with a "Pearson product moment correlations revealed significant correlations at the .05 level for 17 out of 20 competencies" (Brolin, 1997, p.128).

The Personal-Social skills correlations score of .80 indicated a high level of correlation between the two Personal-Social skill tests. "Equivalency correlations between Form A and Form B are approximately equal when comparing pretest and retest" (Brolin, 1997, p. 130).

In addition to these quantitative methods, the use was utilized through an observational scale and educator survey. The LCCE's Competency Rating Scale (CRS) was completed along with the pretests and posttests. The CRS was a means of "providing educators with a systematic means of assessing student mastery of the subcompetencies" (Brolin, 1997, p. 151). Furthermore, the CRS can be employed to determine individual strengths and weaknesses, evaluation and development, and curriculum planning.

Since the CRS required subjective judgments to be made, it was essential that raters used the same criteria when completing the assessment. The CRS provided four ratings for student performance based upon the educators' observations, personal records or notes, and written or verbal reports from other personnel. Students were considered: Not Competent, Partially Competent, Competent, or Not Rated.

The educators completed the CRS for the Personal-Social domain. Following the completion of each CRS, the student's total actual score (TAS), which was the sum of all ratings, was determined. The actual score (AS) per item was then calculated by dividing the TAS by the number of items rated (N). The AS was then employed to evaluate progress made between pretests and posttests.

In addition, the educators completed the Communication Styles Checklist and the Curriculum Content Checklist developed by the CEC (Council for Exceptional Children) to be used in conjunction with the LCCE. These checklists were utilized to provide additional information regarding the rationale behind the results. The checklists were originally designed to help educators promote awareness of individual differences. "The checklists give teachers a tool to determine areas in which individual and cultural differences can be promoted, as well as areas that can be improved" (Brolin, 1995, p. ix).

Data Analysis

The means of the experimental and control groups were compared utilizing the statistical technique of Analysis of Covariance (ANCOVA). The ANCOVA procedure examined the inequalities among group means, taking into account the influence of a covariate. By comparing the means for the two groups, experimental and control, the linear associations between the posttest and pretest were given.

RESULTS OF THE STUDY

It has become increasingly apparent that students with severe cognitive delays required a curriculum that integrated functional academics, daily living, occupational, and social skills training. A functional curriculum supported by academics allows for students with intellectual disabilities to utilize functional skills that enabled them to live and work within their community. However, the current trend is for students to be exposed to the general education curriculum, preventing students from receiving essential instruction in nonacademic areas such as personal-social skills. The Life Centered Career Education (LCCE) curriculum was a viable option for educating students with cognitive delays in an integrated life skills and academic curriculum.

Data Organization

The descriptive statistics were compared with respect to each student's scores on the LCCE Knowledge Battery and CRS pretests and posttests. By utilizing the standard scores on the Knowledge Battery and CRS, the mean and standard deviation were determined and utilized for comparison.

Statistical Procedures

To examine the efficacy of the Personal-Social Skills program, two groups of students (experimental and control) were compared on the two dependent measures, which were KB scores and CRS scores. For both the KB and CRS variables, the Analysis of Covariance (ANCOVA) was used to test the above-described hypothesis.

Knowledge Battery (KB) Assessment

The Knowledge Battery was a standardized criterion-referenced instrument covering the three curriculum domains of Daily Living, Occupational Knowledge, and Personal-Social Skills. The Personal-Social skills segment contained questions for each of the targeted competencies with a total of 70 questions. Since the Knowledge Battery was a curriculum-based instrument, it is specifically designed to measure the instruction provided with the Personal-Social skills lessons. The results of the assessment were represented as a percentage.

Table 1. KB Descriptive Statistics.

Descriptive Statistics

Dependent Variable: KB Posttest

Group	Mean	Std. Deviation	N
Control	57.55	21.717	20
Experimental	60.26	15.231	19
Total	58.87	18.644	39

Competency Rating Scale (CRS)

The CRS required subjective judgments to be made on each of the Personal-Social skills subcompetencies. Students were rated on performance based upon the educator's observations, personal records or notes, and written or verbal reports from other personnel. Students were considered Not Competent (0), Partially Competent (1), Competent (2), or Not Rated.

Analyses of Data

Analyses of Knowledge Battery (KB) Assessment

The Analysis of Covariance (ANCOVA) statistical procedure examined the inequalities between the group means while taking into account the influence of a covariate. By comparing the means for the two groups, experimental and control, the linear associations between the posttest and pretest were given.

The effect of the covariate was significant, $F(1, 36) = 33.257$, $p < .0005$, indicating that the KB posttest and KB pretest were significantly correlated. However, the effect between groups was not significant F(1, 36) 1.535, p=.223. For this analysis, the equality-of-variances assumption was met, $F(1, 37) = 0.439$, $p = .512$ (Table 6). Furthermore, Graph 5 depicts the relationship between the KB posttest and KB pretest. The two variables had a positive relationship. However, no clear separation was seen between the two groups. In summary, the

ANCOVA tells us that the two groups' means were not significantly different and the LCCE treatment did not have an effect.

Table 2. CRS Descriptive Statistics.

Descriptive Statistics

Dependent Variable: CRS Postest

Group	Mean	Std. Deviation	N
Control	1.3530	.53183	20
Experimental	1.2674	.39353	19
Total	1.3113	.46547	39

Table 3. Pretest, Posttest, and Adjusted Means for Treatment Groups: Knowledge Battery.

Group	Pretest	Posttest	Adjusted Posttest
Experimental	51.58	60.20	61.691
Control	55.15	57.55	56.193

Analyses of Competency Rating Scale (CRS)

The CRS pretest data shows that the means of CRS scores for the experimental and control groups were 0.851 and 1.356, respectively. For the CRS posttest, the means for the two groups were 1.267 and 1.353, respectively. Numerically, therefore, it appears that there was a sizable increase in the CRS score for the experimental group of students. However, the Analysis of Covariance statistical test reflected a more accurate analysis.

Table 4. Pretest, Posttest, and Adjusted Means for Treatment Groups: Competency Rating Scale.

Group	Pretest	Posttest	Adjusted Posttest
Experimental	.851	1.267	1.515
Control	1.356	1.353	1.118

Table 5. KB ANCOVA: Analysis of Covariance Summary: Knowledge Battery.

Source	Type III Sum of Squares	df	Mean Square	F	Sig.
Covariate (Pretest)	6308.163	1	6308.163	33.257	.000
Effect (Study)	291.065	1	291.065	1.535	.223
Error	6828.471	36	189.680		
Total	148378.000	39			
Corrected Total	13208.359	38			

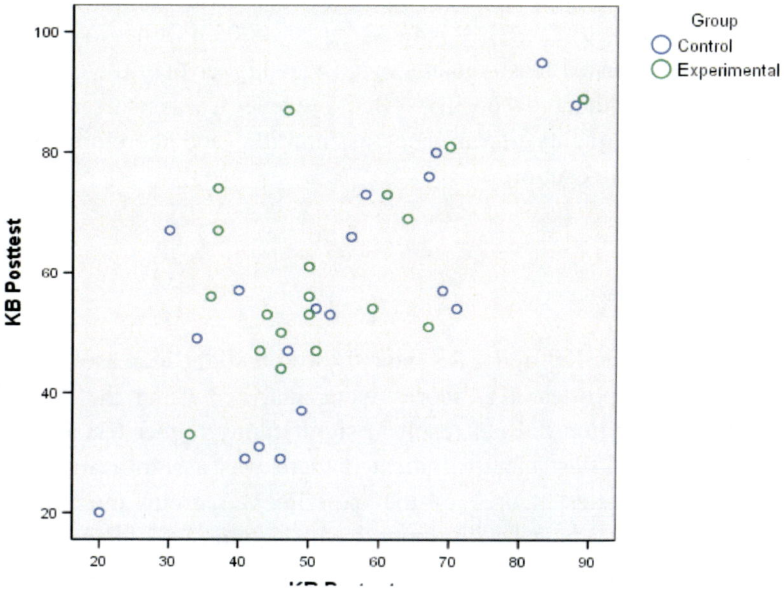

Graph 5: KB Pre and Posttest Results.

Table 6. CRS Equality of Variances.

Levene's Test of Equality of Error Variances[a]

Dependent Variable: CRS Postest

F	df1	df2	Sig.
44.342	1	37	.000

Tests the null hypothesis that the error variance of the dependent variable is equal across groups.

a. Design: Intercept+crspre+study

Table 7. CRS ANCOVA: Analysis of Covariance Summary: Competency Rating Scale.

Source	Type III Sum of Squares	df	Mean Square	F	Sig.
Covariate (Pretest)	6.922	1	6.922	200.971	.000
Effect (Study)	1.158	1	1.158	33.611	.000
Error	1.240	36	.034		
Total	75.292	39			
Corrected Total	8.233	38			

The effect of covariate was significant, $F(1, 36) = 200.971$, $p = .0005$. This indicated that the CRS posttest (response variable) and CRS pretest (covariate) were significantly correlated. The effect between groups was also significant, $F(1, 36) = 33.611$, $p < .0005$. The adjusted least-squares mean for the experimental group was higher ($M = 1.515$) than it was for the control group ($M = 1.118$). For this analysis, however, the equality-of-variances assumption was violated, $F(1, 37) = 44.342$, $p < .0005$ (Table 8). In conclusion, the experimental group's adjusted least-squares mean was higher than the control group's. This means that the treatment did have a positive effect however it was necessary to understand the ANCOVA violated the equality-of-variances assumption, and therefore interpretation as a positive result must be with caution.

Summary

In conclusion, both the KB and CRS data showed a slight increase in scores. However, when both the pre and posttest KB scores were analyzed using the ANCOVA, the test indicated that the intervention did not result in significantly higher test scores. On the other hand, the CRS ANCOVA test clearly indicated there was a significant increase in scores between the pre and posttest scores of the experimental group over the control group. Nevertheless, these results must be interpreted with caution due to the CRS violating the equality of variance assumption. Therefore, the hypothesis was rejected as the students in the experimental group, LCCE's Personal-Social Skills program, did not achieve significantly higher scores on the Knowledge Battery (KB) and Competency Rating Scale (CRS) than students in the control group, who did not participate in the program.

Educator Survey

The educators completed the Communication Styles Checklist and the Curriculum Content Checklist which provided additional information regarding the rationale behind the results. Both educators agreed that any of the students' improvements were a result of the direct extensive instruction spent on the personal-social skills lessons and the immediacy in which the tests were given following the instructional intervention. Both educators expressed the belief that repetitive instruction on any subject would likely yield similar results. In addition, concern over whether or not students would retain information over time was addressed by both educators involved.

Summary and Discussion

The hypothesis stated that students in classes that utilize the LCCE's Personal-Social Skills program achieved significantly higher scores on the Knowledge Battery and Competency Rating Scale (CRS) than students who did not participate in the program. The results of the KB suggested that the means of the experimental group of students were not significantly different that the means of the control group. On the other hand, it was determined that the CRS variable for the experiment and control mean scores demonstrated some increase, while those of the control group showed nearly no change. It could be assumed that the LCCE program was successful in increasing the personal–social skills scores. However, it is essential to be cautious while interpreting this data as the ANCOVA test did violate the equality-of-variances assumption.

In conclusion, the results indicated that the research hypothesis was rejected; students participating in the experimental group did not show a greater increase in scores on the Knowledge Battery and Competency Rating Scale than the students who belonged to the control group. Furthermore, interviews with the participating instructors indicated that the experimental group would potentially demonstrate significantly higher scores if the personal-social skills curriculum was continued over an extended period of time and continuously reinforced.

However, the slight increase in scores suggested that with direct intervention, students with disabilities can exhibit improvement in specific areas. By reviewing the degree of change between the experimental and control group (posttest minus pretest) it was clear that there was a greater increase in scores within the experimental group. For the KB, the mean change scores for the control group were 2.40, compared to the mean change score of 8.68 for the experimental group. Similarly, on the CRS, the mean change score were 0.416 for the experimental group and -0.003 for the change group. These change scores clearly illustrated that although minimal, the intervention was successful in increasing the scores of the experimental group.

As a result of this slight increase in change scores within the experimental group, it can be assumed that over time a personal-social skills curriculum can have positive effects. Consequently, a functional curriculum supported by academics allows for students with intellectual disabilities to utilize functional skills that enabled them to live and work within their community. Nevertheless, the current trend is for students to be exposed to the general education curriculum, preventing students from receiving essential instruction in nonacademic areas such as personal-social skills. According to VDOE (2006-2007):

Recognition that students with significant cognitive disabilities have instructional needs that are beyond the regular standards adopted by the general population is an accepted fact by researchers in the field of severe disabilities. However, NCLB and IDEA require that general grade level state standards be accessible for all students, including those with the most significant cognitive disabilities (p. 5).

Therefore, the curriculum utilized in the education of students with cognitive delays must include integrated life skills as well as an academic curriculum. One such vital life skill essential for students with intellectual disabilities to be exposed to was personal or social skills. The implementation of a specific personal or social skills program, such as LCCE, was essential in the development of social skills necessary for students to learn in order to function within their community.

Similar Studies

Current studies within the field of special education that relate to this study center on students' participation and progress within the general education curriculum (Hager and Slocum, 2002). Many educators were seeking to determine if the standards-based reform was creating a curriculum for students with intellectual disabilities that was more academic, resulting in less time being spent on functional skills (Agran, Alper, and Wehmeyer, 2002).

Similar studies have been completed with regard to the LCCE curriculum and social skill integration with students with intellectual disabilities. The LCCE curriculum can be employed to increase the self-determination needs in youth with mild cognitive disabilities. This study focused on the four specific goals within the LCCE domains that specifically addressed self-determination: self-awareness, self-confidence, choice and decision-making skills, and goal attainment behaviors. "The LCCE offers today's educators a comprehensive and effective means for fulfilling their critical role in facilitating the development of self-determination in students with and without disabilities" (Wehmeyer, 1995, p. 165).

Similar studies utilizing the LCCE program compared the Occupational Guidance and Preparation domains' competencies and subcompetencies with specific data found on IEPs of high school students with learning disabilities (Schlegel, 1998). In another study, (O'Leary, 1991) the LCCE curriculum was employed as the curriculum framework to measure educational outcomes. The purpose of this study was to measure the most important educational outcomes perceived by parents, special educators, regular educators, and employers of students with intellectual disabilities. Results indicated that the "validation for the major curricular areas (domains) and competencies in the LCCE model is provided by parents, regular educators, and employers" (O'Leary, 1991, p. 1).

In addition to studies utilizing the LCCE curriculum, similar studies have been completed with the integration of social skills training with students who are mentally retarded. Defalco (1989) incorporated real-life probes to show that three specific social skills were acquired by three students with intellectual disabilities. This instruction reported that students were able to successfully generalize social skills into real-life situations through the use of both interventions: stimulus-control and response-consequences.

An additional study conducted by Quintana (2004) in social skills with students with intellectual disabilities involved a single subject study utilizing an A-B-A-B design and the implementation of a social skills training program addressing negative behaviors. Results indicated that there was a positive effect between the social skills training and the subject's behavior.

According to the Office on Special Education Rehabilitation Services (OSERS), current related research focused on the use of alternate assessments and their relationship with the general education curriculum and social skills training. Research conducted by Agran, Alper, & Wehmeyer (2002) focused on the federal mandates to assure access for all students and that it might not be beneficial for students with severe disabilities.

We maintain that the ultimate goal of access to the general education curriculum for students with disabilities is successful and meaningful outcomes. We also agree with McDonnell, Thorson, and McQuivey's (2000) call for more research focused on how to embed a variety of social, functional academics, and transition skills within the ongoing activities and curriculum in the general education classroom (p. 130).

In addition, the researchers had teachers rank the importance of nine skill areas essential for facilitating access for students to the general education curriculum. Results indicated that social skills and communication skills were scored as the two most important skill areas. These results further indicated the need for a functional curriculum with social skills instruction.

Applications

For students with intellectual disabilities, a functional curriculum supported by academics allows them to utilize functional skills that enabled them to live and work within their community. However, the current trend is for students to be exposed to the general education curriculum, preventing students from receiving essential instruction in nonacademic areas such as personal-social skills. The increase in scores of the Personal-Social skills curriculum indicated that long-term extensive instruction could be beneficial to continue to incorporate necessary functional life skills into the curriculum of students with intellectual disabilities.

In addition, a curriculum that addressed academics and life skills, such as the LCCE program, could be utilized to address other vital issues within the special education field. Current trends in special education reflect several issues: integration, participation in an outcomes-based assessment process, self-determination, functional life skills, and transitional services (Brolin, 1997). The LCCE curriculum contained considerable elements that relate to each of these movements. The utilization of LCCE's curriculum can have an influence on all of these issues.

The first trend of integration stems from the concept of normalization. "Normalization dictates that both the means and the ends of education for people with disabilities should be as normal as possible" (Hallahan & Kauffman, 2000, p. 44). The drive towards integration has been instigated by the deinstitutionalization movement and the push for full inclusion. During the 1960s people with disabilities were slowly moved out of institutional settings into community placements. Likewise, inclusion advocates fought for the rights for students with disabilities to attend their neighborhood schools, placing the responsibility of education on the local educational systems. The utilization of the LCCE curriculum would assist in increasing students' social skills. As a result, students were more successful when integrated into regular education classes.

The second trend that the LCCE curriculum addressed was the use of outcomes-based education (OBE). OBE was based on the tenets that education should equip all students with the knowledge, skills, and competencies needed for mastery. OBE also established the conditions with schools that maximize the achievement and success for all students. The LCCE curriculum was an outcomes-based education system. "Many schools implementing LCCE have recognized this fact and have designated LCCE as their outcomes-based response to their state's and/or school district's mandate to implement the OBE approach" (Brolin, 1997, p. 3).

The third trend in special education was striving for students to learn to become self-determined. Self-determination was characterized by the attitudes within people that allow them to set goals for themselves and then take the initiative to meet these goals. The LCCE curriculum contained numerous strategies that work to increase students' self-determination. "The LCCE provides a comprehensive foundation upon which student instruction in self-determination can be accomplished and through which students can become more self-determined and involved in their educational process" (Brolin, 1997, p. 3).

In addition, there is a movement towards the utilization of functional skills and the need to blend academics with functional skills instruction within the school, home, and community settings. The functional skills addressed within the LCCE curriculum consist of independent living, social, communication, and vocational skills. Since the LCCE curriculum focused on 22 major functional skills, it provided a comprehensive background for delivering functional skills that will allow students with disabilities to function as productive members of their communities and as employees.

Finally, the mandate for transitional services has spurred a new movement. These services included postsecondary education, vocational training, integrated employment, continuing and adult education, adult services, independent living, and community participation. These services were mandates to be incorporated into the IEP with an emphasis on both employment and issues pertaining to the enhancement of students with disabilities' quality of life. This trend directly related to the need to have a vocational and life skills curriculum for students with intellectual disabilities. Transition is now mandated by IDEA to begin no later than age 16 and to be addressed within the IEP. The LCCE helps students to "learn and develop the critical skills they will need to be productive and successful upon making the transition from school to community life and work" (Brolin, 1997, p. 2).

Implications for Practice

One essential provision of *IDEA* was the mandate that every student found eligible for special education be provided with transition services. The LCCE enabled educators to fulfill this requirement through curriculum-based assessments and IEP documentation forms. As a result, the social skills of students with disabilities can easily be addressed and linked to students' Individualized Education Plan (IEP) goals and objectives. The CRS can be used in the development of IEPs as well as evaluations. "The cumulative average score resulting from a complete CRS rating can be used as one general index" (Brolin, 1997, p. 151). Furthermore, results of the LCCE Knowledge Battery can be an excellent source for documentation on the Present Level of Performance section of Eligibilities or annual IEPs.

The LCCE program has developed forms that allows for ease of integrating the curriculum into an IEP (See Appendix F). The LCCE Individualized Education Plan Forms allow educators to develop present levels of performance, goals, and objectives from the results of the CRS. "The LCCE IEP form could be used as the transition component and attached to the regular IEP form used by the school district" (Brolin, 1997, p.139).

Significance of the Study

By successfully incorporating a Personal-Social skills curriculum into a special education program for students with intellectual disabilities, other subpopulations could benefit. The concept would involve incorporating a social skills training into other populations such as students with learning disabilities, students with emotional disturbances, students in Alternative schools, students in General Education Degree (GED) programs, or even students who participate in English as a Second Language (ESL) programs.

In addition, general education teachers could become motivated to integrate universal life skill lessons, from LCCE, into core curriculum classes. An additional application of the LCCE curriculum would be to emphasize the incorporation of social skills training into other subgroups found within school settings. This would be an excellent opportunity to provide this form of instruction to students who are learning disabled or emotionally disturbed.

Furthermore, social skills integration can be an excellent opportunity to incorporate state standards into lessons. The use of a program which incorporates social skills instruction with functional academics can provide instruction for a high school student which is practical, age appropriate, and easily linked to state specified Standards of Learning.

Finally, by determining the effectiveness of a social skills program for students with special needs, educators will be able to better serve students who are cognitively disabled. By implementing a successful program, school systems can address the personal and social needs. When students with special educational needs receive specific instruction on social skills, potential behavioral problems can also be reduced.

Limitations of the Study

It was critical to understand the limits of the study being completed. These limits centered on the subjects as well as the time. First, the nature of working with students with mental disabilities was often inconsistent. It was often difficult to ascertain progress of students with intellectual disabilities as they frequently progress at slower rates and required additional time and instruction to grasp essential concepts. "Special education research, because of its complexity, may be the hardest of the hardest-to-do sciences. One feature of special education research that makes it more complex is the variability of the participants" (Odom et al, 2005, p. 139).

Furthermore, the demographics represented were limited with regard to race and ethnicity. Augusta County Schools are located in a rural community with less than one percent of the students being African-American and Hispanic. This limitation made it difficult to generalize the findings of the study to the general population. In addition, the small sample size could be viewed as a potential limitation. Since there were only 39 students participating in the study, results of the findings could be difficult to relate to the population of special education students.

Along the same lines as the limitations that the population might impose, the time constraints of the study could also be an indicator affecting the outcomes. The study occurred over the course of seven weeks. The LCCE curriculum was a comprehensive curriculum that could be utilized over the middle or high school careers of students with intellectual disabilities. The Personal-Social domain should be incorporated into instruction repeatedly before students could show progress. As a result, the degree of improvement found within a seven week study was minimal.

Recommendations for Further Research

This study created numerous opportunities for further research. First, this study could be expanded to include a larger population of students participating.

Furthermore, it would be beneficial to complete a longitudinal study to determine the degree of students' improvements over the course of middle and high school as instruction is provided throughout their education. Finally, further studies resulting from this research could revolve around incorporating any portion of the LCCE curriculum into various populations such as students with learning disabilities or emotional disabilities.

REFERENCES

American Association on Mental Retardation. (2002). *The definition of mental retardation.* Available online from: http://www.aamr.org.

Agran, M., Alper, S. & Wehmeyer, M. (2002). Access to the general curriculum for students with significant disabilities: What it means to teachers. *Education and Training in Mental Retardation and Developmental Disabilities, 37(2)*, 123-133.

Ahlgrim-Delzell, L., Algozzine, R., Browder, D., Flowers, C., Karvonen, M. & Spooner, F. (2004). The alignment of alternate assessment content with academic and functional curricula. *Journal of Special Education, 37.*

Bertone, L., Boyle, J., Mitchel, J. & Smith, J. (1999). Improving pro-social behavior through social skills instruction. *U.S. Department of Education.*

Black, R. & Salas, B. (2001). Forty years of progress: Where have we been? Where are we now? *Annual Meeting of the American Association on Mental Retardation.*

Brolin, D. (1997). *Life centered career education.* The Council for Exceptional Children.

Browder, D. M. & Cooper-Duffy, K. (2003).Evidence-based practices for students with severe disabilities and the requirement for accountability **in "No Child Left Behind".** *The Journal of Special Education, 37*, 3, 157-163.

Bruckerhoff, C. (1996). Who knows what? *Curriculum research and evaluation.*

Cartledge, G. & Kiarie, M. (2001). Learning social skills through literature for children and adolescents. *Teaching Exceptional Children, 34*, 2, 40-47.

Cernosia, A. (2005). The reauthorization of IDEA and significant judicial decisions. *California Department of Education Sponsored Training.*

Council for Exceptional Children (CEC). (2003). No Child Left Behind Act of 2001: implications for special education policy and practice. *Council for Exceptional Children.*

Cuskelly, M. (2004). The evolving construct of intellectual disability: is everything old new again? *International Journal of Disability, Development and Education, 51*, 1.

deBettencourt, L. (2002). Understanding the differences between Section 504 and ADA. *Teaching Exceptional Children, 34*, 3, 16-23.

de Bildt, A., Serra, M., Luteijn, E., Kraijer, D., Sytema, S. & Minderaa, R. (2005). Social skills in children with intellectual disabilities with and without autism. *Journal of Intellectual Disability Research, 49*, 5, 317-328.

Defalco, G. A., (1989).Generalized use of social skills in natural settings by people with mental retardation. Available: *DAI, 51,* no. 04B (1989). 2057.

DeWeaver, K. & Kropf, N. (1992). Persons with mental retardation: A forgotten minority in education. *Journal of Social Work Education, 28*, 1, 36-47.

Ford, A., Schnorr, R., Meyer, L., Davern, L., Black, J. & Dempsey, P. (1989). *The Syracuse community referenced curriculum guide: for students with moderate and severe disabilities.* Baltimore, MD: Brookes Publishing:

Gartin, B. & Murdick, N. (2004). IDEA 2004: The IEP. *Remedial and Special Education, 26*, 6, 327-331.

Hallahan, D. & Kauffman, J. (2000). *Exceptional learners: introduction to special education.* Boston: Allyn & Bacon.

Kearsley, G. (2006). Social Learning Theory (A. Bandura). *Exploration in Learning & Instruction: The theory into practice database.* Available online from:http://tip.psychology.org/bandura.html

Kolb, S. & Hanley-Maxwell, C. (2003). Critical social skills for adolescents with high incidence disabilities: parental perspectives. *Council for Exceptional Children, 69*, 2, 163-179.

Matson, J., Mayville, E., Lott, J., Bielecki, J. & Logan, R. (2003). A comparison of social and adaptive functioning in persons with psychosis, autism, and severe or profound mental retardation. *Journal of Developmental and Physical Disabilities, 15*, 1.

Menta Group. (2006). *Clinical services model. Special Education Services.* Available online: www.mentagroup.com.

NASET. (2006). Landmark cases in special education. *National Association of Special Education Teachers.* www.naset.org/landmarkcases.0.html

National Center on Educational Outcomes. (2005). Available online: *http://education.umn.edu/NCEO*

Odom, S., Brantlinger, E., Gersten, R., Horner, R., Thompson, B. & Harris, K. (2005). Research in special education: Scientific methods and evidence-based practices. *Council for Exceptional Children, 71*, 2, 137-148.

O'Leary, E. E., (1991). Consensual validation of educational outcomes for high school students with mild disabilities. Available: *DAI, 52,* no. 07A, 2503.

Paige, R. (2004) A guide to education and *No Child Left Behind. U.S. Department of Education.* Available online: www.ed.gov.

Paraschiv, I. & Oiley, G. (1999). Generalization of social skills: Strategies and results of a training program in problem solving skills. *U.S. Department of Education*

Payne, J. & Patton, J. (1981). *Mental Retardation.* Charles E. Merrill Publishing Co. Columbus.

Quintana, A. (2004). Efficacy of a social skills training procedure used on a child having moderate mental retardation. Available: *MAI, 43, no. 03,* 663.

Rea, P. & Davis-Dorsey, J. (2004). ADA in the public school setting. *Journal of Disability Policy Studies, 15, 2*, 66-69.

Robinson, et al. (1989). *Best practices in mild mental disabilities.* The Division on Mental Retardation of the Council for Exceptional Children.

Schlegel, B. J. (1998). A comparison of the life-centered career education model to the individual transition plans of high school students with learning disabilities. Available: *MAI, 37, no. 01*, 0051.

Shriner, J. G. (2000). Legal perspectives on school outcome assessment for students with disabilities. *Journal of Special Education, 33, 4*, 232-240.

Smith, T. (2001). Section 504, the ADA, and Public Schools. *Remedial & Special Education.*, *6*, 335-344.

Sutton, J. (1993). *Special education: A biblical approach* South Carolina:Hidden Treasure.

Thomas, G. (1996). *Teaching students with metal retardation: a life goal curriculum approach.* Prentice-Hall, Inc.: New Jersey.

VDOE (2006-2007). *Virginia Alternate Assessment Program (VAAP) Instructional Manual: A teacher resource for the aligned standards of learning*. Division of Special Education Instructional Services.

Wehmeyer, M. (1995). A career education approach: self-determination for youth with mild cognitive disabilities. *Intervention in School & Clinic, 30, 3*, 157-164.

Wehmeyer, M., Lance, G. & Bashinski, S. (2002). Promoting access to the general education curriculum for students with mental retardation: A multi-level model. *Education and Training in Mental Retardation and Developmental Disabilities, 37*, 3, 223-234.

Yell, M. & Katsiyannis, A. (2004). Placing students with disabilities in inclusive settings: Legal guardians and preferred practices. *Preventing School Failure*, Fall

In: Learning and Memory Developments...
Editors: L. C. Eklund, A. S. Nyman, pp. 71-101
ISBN: 978-1-60876-397-9

Chapter 3

PRO-INFLAMMATORY CYTOKINES IN LEARNING AND MEMORY

Amaicha Mara Depino
Consejo Nacional de Investigaciones Cientificas y Tecnologicas, Conicet—Faculty of Exact and Natural Sciences, University of Buenos Aires, Buenos Aires, Argentina

ABSTRACT

In animals and in humans, cytokines are typically immune system molecules that help orchestrate the host responses to infection. Pro-inflammatory cytokines coordinate immune, physiological, metabolic and behavioral responses that are collectively termed the acute phase reaction. In addition to their role in immunoregulation of inflammatory processes, pro-inflammatory cytokines represent the major communication link between peripheral immunity and the central nervous system. Cytokines are known to play a role in the physiological and behavioral adjustments that occur during sickness, leading to "sickness behavior". One of the most salient symptoms of the sickness behavior syndrome is alteration in learning and memory processes. Studies in animals have demonstrated that acute activation of pro-inflammatory cytokine signaling in the brain in response to peripheral immune activation is associated with deficits in hippocampal-dependent memory.

Recent studies suggest that brain cytokines may also have some physiological roles in neural, neuroendocrine, and behavioral regulation in non-pathological situations. Cytokine-induced modulation of memory processes is a complex phenomenon, including both detrimental and beneficial effects, depending on the specific pro-inflammatory cytokine, its levels (particularly within the brain), and the particular condition that elicits the cytokine secretion. Some cytokines, e.g., Interleukin (IL)-1, have been shown to significantly influence memory consolidation. IL-1, IL-6 and tumor necrosis factor (TNF)-α are the main cytokines involved in learning and memory modulation. These behavioral data are consistent with the impairing effect of enhanced cytokine signaling on hippocampal long-term potentiation.

We will review the literature, including our own contribution, on human and animal model studies of the role of cytokines in learning and memory.

Introduction

The interactions between the immune and the central nervous systems have been described many years ago. One of the main discoveries was that peripheral interleukin (IL)-1 activates the hypothalamus-pituitary-adrenal (HPA) system [1]. The number of cytokines involved in brain-immune system interactions is now known to be huge [2, 3], and includes both pro-inflammatory and anti-inflammatory molecules. In recent years, the discovery of multiple functions of cytokines within the central nervous system (CNS) suggests that cytokines play a central role in the CNS function, independent of their role as messengers from the immune system to the brain.

Cytokines are a class of polypeptides that are expressed at low levels in healthy tissue but can be induced rapidly in response to tissue trauma or immune challenges to serve a variety of immune signaling and functions. More than 40 different cytokines have been identified to date, as well as numerous cytokine receptor types and subtypes. The knowledge of the functional role of cytokines has broadened since the characterization of the first cytokine, IL-1. Several authors have proposed the division of cytokines into "families" on the basis of functional or molecular characteristics.

Across classificatory schemes, members of each proposed cytokine family is either constitutively expressed or inducible in brain cells. The primary cellular sources of cytokines in the CNS are activated microglia and to a lesser extent astrocytes. Cytokines can also be synthesized in neurons, and small amounts may enter the brain from peripheral circulation. The brain-derived cytokines constitute the majority of the CNS cytokine pool and have predominantly paracrine and autocrine actions. They function as nerve growth factors crucial to embryogenesis and tissue repair and remodeling, as chemotactic factors, as mediators of phagocytosis, and as mediators of a variety of immunoregulatory functions in both the periphery and in the CNS.

The over-expression of cytokines has been associated with numerous pathological states (both within the CNS and in the peripheral nervous system), such as infection (viral, bacterial and fungal), autoimmune diseases (e.g., multiple sclerosis and systemic lupus erythematosus), stroke, trauma, neurodegenerative diseases (e.g., Alzheimer´s, Parkinson´s and prion diseases) and in neuropsychiatric disorders, such as depression and schizophrenia [4, 5]. More specifically, some cytokines such as interleukin-1β (IL-1β), interleukin-6 (IL-6) and tumor necrosis factor alpha (TNF-α) have been associated with cognitive decline and dementia in several cross-sectional and prospective population studies.

It is now believed that cytokine-mediated pathophysiological processes underlie the cognitive impairments associated with several neuropsychiatric diseases, making cytokines ideal targets for therapeutic interventions. Despite these pathological implications, cytokines have also been shown to exert physiological and even neuroprotective functions. The role of cytokines in modulating learning and memory, however, has been barely studied. Evidence from peripheral and central inflammation suggest that at least some pro-inflammatory cytokines can affect learning and memory formation. A few studies have evaluated the role of endogenous, normally expressed cytokines in these processes.

SOURCES OF CYTOKINES IN THE BRAIN

Brain immunity is mediated predominantly by glial cells, particularly astrocytes (approximately 85% of the glial cell population) and microglia (approximately 10% of glial cells). Immune activated glial cells produce a host of immune signaling and effector molecules, including pro-inflammatory and anti-inflammatory cytokines, chemotactic and cell adhesion molecules, complement proteins, and cytotoxic free radicals. Neurons, too, have been demonstrated to produce some cytokines.

Astrocytes are cells from ectodermic origin that actively support normal physiological processes of neurons (e.g., in GABA and glutamate synthesis). Astrocytes can be activated (a process called "gliosis") in response to cytokines or other soluble molecules released during tissue injury, triggering astrocyte proliferation and increased synthesis and secretion of a range of immune effector molecules. Cytokines produced by astrocytes affect, in turn, the physiology of neighboring neurons and glial cells.

Microglia cells are endodermic cells that invade the developing brain and stay through life as resident macrophages in the CNS. Microglia are activated when surface receptors are engaged by mitogens, such as bacterial endotoxin or circulating immune factors including certain cytokines, prostanoids, and complement proteins. Activation can result in increased synthesis and secretion of soluble factors including cytokines, nitric oxide, reactive oxygen and nitrogen species, complement proteins, amino acid neurotransmitters and prostanoids.

Transmission of immune signals between the periphery and CNS may be a necessary event in the development of inflammatory brain damage in certain neurological disorders, including AIDS dementia, Multiple Sclerosis, and Alzheimer´s disease. A pathogen entering the body elicits a rapid immune response mediated by macrophages. Recognition of lypopolysaccharide (LPS), a component of the cell wall of Gram-negative bacteria, by the Toll-like receptor 4 (TLR4), or the Gram-positive bacteria by TLR2, activates macrophages [6]. This activation results in the production of the pro-inflammatory cytokine IL-1, which is then able to induce its own synthesis and the synthesis of other cytokines that potentiate its effect (e.g., TNF-α and IL-6).

Immune cells and molecules in circulation can enter the brain directly through the blood-brain barrier [7, 8]. Cytokines are relatively large proteins, ranging in molecular weight from 8 to 40 kDa, and are hydrophilic, so they would not readily cross the blood-brain barrier. However, '**activation**' of brain endothelial cells by immune signals such as LPS or certain cytokines promotes interaction between circulating proteins and vascular endothelial cells by inducing expression of membrane adhesion molecules on endothelial cells [7-11]. Immune-activated brain endothelial cells can undergo changes in morphology, causing gaps to form in the wall of the blood-brain barrier [7, 10] and leakage of immune mediators into the brain.

Cytokines also enter the brain parenchyma at circumventricular organs—areas of the brain vasculature which lack tight cellular junctions—and modulation of neuroendocrine parameters at the organum vasculosum lamina terminalis (OVLT), a circumventricular organ adjacent to the hypothalamus, has been attributed to the actions of circulating cytokines [12]. Finally, saturable, active transport of the cytokines IL-1α, IL-1β, IL-6 and TNF-α across the blood-brain barrier has been demonstrated in rodents [9, 13], although the active transport occurs at too low a level to account for the concentration of cytokines in the brain after peripheral administration of immune stimulants [2].

Although monocytes can produce pro-inflammatory cytokines that circulate in the blood and can reach far distant targets, most cytokines act locally in a paracrine manner. Neural afferents, such as the vagus nerves, can be the target of these cytokines. Sensory neurons of the vagus nerves express receptors for IL-1, and IL-1 stimulates vagal sensory activity [14]. Dantzer [15] and others [16, 17] have shown that vagus nerve afferents, stimulated by peripheral cytokines, can carry a neural code capable of triggering an inflammatory cascade in the brain. Sub-diaphragmatic lesion of the vagus nerve in rats attenuates brain cytokine production, corticosterone release and behavioral effects after i.v. IL-1 administration [18, 19]. Vagotomy also blocks behavioral effects of intraperitoneal IL-1 [20, 21], and the induction of cytokines in the brain [22, 23]. Intraperitoneal IL-1, however, was efficient in inducing fever in vagotomized mice [24]. This evidence suggests that there are different mechanisms to communicate peripheral inflammation that result in different central responses.

Low levels of circulating cytokines could trigger cytokine production by glial cells in some cases of brain inflammation. However, numerous studies indicate that the neurotoxic consequences of brain inflammation are mostly attributable to brain-derived, not peripheral, immune factors [3, 25, 26]. Cytokines and their receptors are expressed by brain cells, both glia and neurons [2, 27]. These endogenous molecules not only serve as communicators of immune signals into the brain and modulators of glial response, but they also appear to contribute to brain function.

CYTOKINES IN DISEASE

Sickness Behavior

Animals and humans experiencing viral or bacterial infections usually exhibit various changes in behavior commonly referred as **'sickness behavior'** [28]. This behavior comprises malaise, weakness, listlessness, inability to concentrate, depression, lethargy, little interest in the surroundings, reduced appetite, numbness, reduced sexual activity and fatigue. These psychological and behavioral components of sickness represent, together with the fever response and the associated neuroendocrine changes, a highly organized strategy of the organism to fight infection [29]. The necessary synchrony between metabolic, physiological, and behavioral components of the systemic response to infection is dependent on the same molecular signals as those that are already responsible for the local inflammatory response. These signals are pro-inflammatory cytokines, such as interleukin-1 (IL-1), interleukin-6 (IL-6), tumor necrosis factor-α (TNF-α), and interferons (IFNs).

Cytokine-induced sickness behavior has had different interpretations since its first observation in the late 1980s [30]. In 1989 Dantzer and Kelley [31] proposed that the sickness-inducing properties of cytokines were not an artifact but reflected the genuine action of these proteins in the brain. They proposed that the immune system would require communication ways with the brain to regulate the host response to pathogens, and that the brain would in time require communicating to the immune system. Hart [32] similarly saw sickness behavior as an adaptive response to reduce energy consumption at a time of increased energy demand that is necessary to maintain fever and to fight infection. However, it was later shown that IL-1-induced sickness behavior is independent of the febrile response [33]. A different view proposed that cytokines are responsible for the hyperalgesia that occurs during inflammation [34] and that the sickness response to cytokines is just an avatar of this necessity to deal with pain [35].

The current view of sickness behavior as the expression of a motivational state came only later [28]. This view took Hans Selye proposal that infectious agents are stressors that trigger a counter regulatory response aiming at re-establishing homeostasis. This way of defining cytokine-induced sickness behavior as a motivational state implies that it belongs in the realm of physiology, just as fear, hunger or thirst. As a consequence, sickness behavior needs to be studied independently of other phenomena such as fever.

Decreased social exploration of juvenile conspecifics has been used as a convenient way to assess sickness behavior in laboratory rodents. It offers the advantage of being reproducible and quantifiable. Systemic administration of LPS, IL-1β and TNF-α to adult rats or mice consistently decreases the time spent in exploration of juveniles [36-38].

Systemic administration of IL-1β and TNF-α also consistently suppresses feeding. This effect has been observed using various measurements of food intake under *ad libitum* as well as deprived conditions [39-41]. In contrast to the decrease in social exploration that takes about 2 hours to develop, the suppression of food intake occurs within 1 hour following treatment.

Exploiting a natural rodent behavior, the burrowing test has proved to be very useful in detecting sickness behavior even when fever is not observed [42]. Mice and rats spontaneously empty a tube filled with food pellets, gravel or other substances. This test is extremely sensitive to cytokines in rats, and LPS in mice and rats.

The pathways of cytokine-induced sickness behavior in the brain are still under investigation. Several studies have demonstrated that peripheral cytokines induce the synthesis and release of cytokines in the brain. Intraperitoneal injection of LPS, for instance, induces the expression of IL-1α, IL-1β, and TNF-α, followed by that of IL-6 in many regions of the brain, including the hippocampus, the striatum and the thalamus [25, 43-45]. In this case, the main cellular sources of IL-1 are microglial cells and perivascular and meningeal macrophages [46].

Intraperitoneal challenge with the synthetic double-stranded RNA poly inosinic:poly cytidylic acid (poly I:C) results in alterations in core-body temperature, loss of body weight, reduced locomotor activity and reduced engagement in a species-typical behavior, namely burrowing [4]. These changes are accompanied by synthesis of IL-1β, IL-6, TNF-α and IFN-β in the hippocampus and the hypothalamus.

By administrating the IL-1 receptor antagonist (IL-1ra) into the lateral ventricle of the brain, it was shown that blocking brain IL-1 receptors abrogated the depressing effect of peripherally administered IL-1 on social exploration in rats [33]. This suggests that central cytokines induced by peripheral inflammation can act within the brain to elicit at least part of the behavioral effects associated with sickness.

Using expression of the early gene c-fos as a marker of neuronal activation, it was shown that intraperitoneal injection of LPS activates the primary projection area of the vagus nerve in the brain, the nucleus tractus solitarius, and the secondary projections of this nerve, including the parabrachial nucleus, the hypothalamic paraventricular and supraoptic nuclei, the central nucleus of the amygdala, and the bed nucleus of the stria terminalis [47]. A subdiaphragmatic vagotomy abrogated the expression of Fos in the brain after this intraperitoneal stimulus. The key role of the vagus nerve in the transmission of peripheral immune signals to the brain was further confirmed by the demonstration that vagotomy attenuates the behavioral actions of peripheral cytokines [18, 48].

Nadjar *et al.* [49] have shown that cerebral NFκB activation is a crucial step in the transmission of immune signals from the periphery to the brain. Injection of the NEMO Binding Domain peptide into the lateral ventricle blocked the behavioral effects of intraperitoneal IL-1β injection in the form of social withdrawal and decreased food intake. This treatment also abolished NFκB activation and Cox-2 synthesis in the brain microvasculature, and reduced c-Fos expression in various regions of the brain. This report shows then that the intracellular NFκB signaling pathway is involved in IL-1β-induced sickness behavior.

The data presented so far suggests that peripheral inflammation elicits sickness behavior by activating the vagus nerve and its projections. This activation induces central expression of pro-inflammatory cytokines that, probably, lead to NFκB activation. Nevertheless, more research in trying to solve the mechanisms of peripheral inflammation inducing sickness behavior are needed.

As mentioned before, one feature of sickness behavior is depressed cognitive functioning. Using a behavioral task called autoshaping, Aubert *et al.* [50] demonstrated the existence of specific cognitive deficits in rats, independent of other effects of different pyrogens. Autoshaping consists of presenting hungry rats with a stimulus (introduction of a retractable lever) that predicted food delivery. Control rats quickly learned to press the lever, although this response does not influence the probability of food delivery. When LPS, IL-1 or yeast were injected i.p. to rats during acquisition of the task, treatment severely disrupted acquisition, as indexed by increased latencies of the conditioned response among treatment groups relative to controls. This deficit in acquisition persisted throughout 12 days of training, although the acute effects of immune stimulation persisted for fewer than 24 h. This suggests that treatment impaired learning in early trials, which affected performance throughout the remaining training period. In contrast to the effects of immune activation on autoshaping learning, stable autoshaped performance of a previously learned response was not affected by immune stimulation which, the authors reason, indicates a specific effect of immune activation on associative learning rather than on performance factors such as the anorectic or locomotor suppressive effects of inflammation. However, these results might also be explained in terms of treatment-induced deficits in attention.

Peripheral administration of LPS impairs contextual fear conditioning [51]. Intraperitoneal injection of LPS in rats after the standard conditioning procedure resulted in impairment in hippocampal-dependent contextual fear conditioning. This treatment had no effect on hippocampal-independent auditory-cue fear conditioning. Moreover, using a variation of the fear conditioning paradigm, Pugh *et al.* [52] showed that LPS administered after context pre-exposure eliminated the pre-exposure beneficial effect on subsequent contextual fear conditioning. Pre-exposure is thought to facilitate contextual fear conditioning by allowing the rat to construct a memory representation of the context before conditioning occurs, a process thought to depend on the hippocampus [53].

Intraperitoneal injections of IL-1β daily for 6 days also has been shown to significantly impair spatial working memory in mice tested in the Morris water maze [54]. Mice injected with a sub-lethal dose of the gram-negative bacteria, *Legionella pneumophila* (Lp), also showed attenuated learning in the water maze. However, administration of Lp concurrently with intraperitoneal IL-1β antibodies (IL-1β Ab) that block the bioactive effects of IL-1β released by virus-stimulated immune cells, resulted in learning rates equal to saline-treated control mice. These results suggest that learning impairments produced by Lp infection are mediated in part by IL-1β released by stimulated immune cells. Although IL-1β Ab restored normal learning in Lp infected mice, it did not block Lp-induced fever, again suggesting that the thermoregulatory and cognitive effects of inflammation are not linked. It is worth to mention, however, that IL-1β-injected animals showed nonspecific symptoms of sickness, such as reduced activity and anorexia. As it was later shown for peripheral LPS, these treatments can have performance effects that make it difficult to specifically evaluate learning in tests like the Morris water maze where swimming is required [55].

Banks *et al.* [56] showed that the CNS effect of IL-1α administered intravenously (i.v.) was dependent in large part on the ability of that cytokine to cross the BBB. They injected i.v. human IL-1α immediately after training and observed a significant impairment in retention on a T-maze footshock avoidance apparatus. It was previously shown that the transport of IL-1α across the blood-brain barrier is particularly high into the posterior division of the septum [57]. Injecting antibodies specific to human IL-1α directly into the posterior division of the septum, Banks *et al.* showed that memory impairment could be reversed. As these antibodies do not neutralize murine IL-1α, authors demonstrated that blood-borne IL-1α acts on the posterior division of the septum to block memory formation. Interestingly, i.v. human IL-1β also impaired retention of the task, but animals injected in the posterior division of the septum with neutralizing antibodies specific to human IL-1β showed the same level of impairment in retention than i.v. human IL-1β alone.

To examine the functional role of IL-6 in hippocampus-mediated cognitive impairments associated with peripheral inflammation, IL-6 KO mice were trained in a matching-to-place version of the water maze [58]. In wild-type mice, LPS administered after the training phase reduced the efficiency in mice locating the platform. IL-6 KO mice, on the contrary, appeared refractory to LPS-induced impairments in spatial working memory. Because authors observed a normal activation of the NTS after peripheral LPS, they concluded that humoral and neural immune-to-brain communication pathways appear to be independent of IL-6.

In summary, it has been shown that different peripheral inflammatory stimuli can impair acquisition and/or retention of hippocampal-dependent tasks. Although the precise mechanisms of this modulation have not been elucidated, these and similar studies have suggested that cytokines within the brain can modulate learning, independently of the other behavioral deficits observed during sickness behavior. Further studies injecting cytokines in the lateral ventricles or in specific regions of the brain have proven a specific role of certain cytokines in learning and memory formation. This evidence will be discussed below (Cytokines in health: Role in learning and memory).

Neurodegeneration

In addition to being induced after peripheral inflammation, cytokines have been detected in the brain during various neurodegenerative diseases, including AIDS Dementia Complex, brain trauma, Alzheimer's disease, Multiple Sclerosis, Human Prion Disease and Parkinson's Disease. In these pathologies activated microglia and/or astrocytes have also been detected.

It is important to note that presence of activated glial cells does not imply that the disease is an immune disorder. Different stimuli can result in glial activation, and this in turn can elicit an immune response that could further damage the diseased brain. Some authors have proposed immune-mediated neurotoxicity as a unifying hypothesis of neurodegenerative diseases, in the sense that neurodegenerative syndromes of diverse etiology may share the feature of inflammatory neuronal damage as the final pathway leading to clinical impairments [59, 60]. We will discuss here the immune-mediated pathogenesis in Alzheimer's disease, because one of the main consequences of brain inflammation in this disease is to affect cognition.

Alzheimer's disease is a primary degenerative disease of the central nervous system, which is characterized by widespread cortical atrophy, and enlargement of the ventricles [61]. The progression of Alzheimer's disease ultimately leads to dementia, and behavioral and cognitive impairments are often the basis for patients' initial medical referral leading to the diagnosis [62]. The histopathological hallmark of Alzheimer's disease is the presence of β-amyloid (Aβ) plaques forming insoluble aggregates in the cortex [61].

The Aβ plaques in the brains of Alzheimer's disease patients are consistently associated with activated microglia and microglial-derived molecules [63-67]. Aβ plaques consist of a central core of aggregated amyloid peptide surrounded by activated glial cells. Although Aβ plaques are the defining histopathological feature of Alzheimer's disease pathophysiology, the Aβ peptide has not consistently been demonstrated to be neurotoxic [64, 68] or to cause learning or memory deficits [69].

Moreover, the presence of activated microglia in the brains of Alzheimer's patients does not in itself imply that these cells contribute to the clinical neuropathology. Indeed, considering the phagocytic function of microglial cells, it is not surprising that these cells are present in the vicinity of amyloid plaques. Thus, the co-localization of activated microglia cells and senile plaques has been interpreted as a secondary consequence of Alzheimer's disease pathogenic processes.

In addition to the phagocytic response to extracellular Aβ, microglia may become activated to synthesize and secrete cytokines upon binding of Aβ to a second-messenger coupled membrane receptor [70]. In fact, the aggregating form of the Aβ peptide induces TNF-α production by a human microglia cell line, THP-1 [71]. Subfragments of the Aβ peptide have also been shown to induce or enhance microglial synthesis of other cytokines, including IL-1, as well as the complement protein C3 and nitric-oxide, and Aβ can induce increased intracellular Ca^{2+} concentrations in cultured rodent microglia [72].

Early onset Alzheimer's disease associated with genetic variants of the apolipoprotein gene may also involve Aβ and brain inflammation in the pathogenic cascade. The espilon3 variant of apolipoprotein E (ApoE3) has been shown to block Aβ-induced microglia activation *in vitro* whereas ApoE4, coded by an ApoE allele which is a known genetic risk factor for familiar early onset Alzheimer's disease [73], does not protect against microglial activation [74]. This finding suggests that the cognitive deficits and cortical neuropathology associated with the ApoE4 allele may be caused by inflammatory mechanisms.

Hsiao *et al.* [75] drew a more direct link among brain inflammation, amyloidosis and behavioral deficits using a transgenic mouse model of Alzheimer's-like amyloidosis based on overexpression of the amyloid precursor protein gene (APP mice). APP mice have multiple copies of the APP gene and over-express APP in the brain. By 10 months of age, APP mice develop consolidated Aβ plaques analogous to Aβ plaques present in the brains of Alzheimer's patients. APP mice showed age-dependent impairments in spatial learning in the Morris water maze and deficits in spontaneous alternation in a T-maze. Moreover, the emergence of these behavioral deficits correlated with Aβ plaque formation. Amyloid plaques in the brains of APP mice were co-localized with activated astrocytes and glial cells, indicating the presence of brain inflammation. Although the effects of brain inflammation on amyloidosis and behavior were not explicitly examined in this study, the findings are consistent with the possibility that inflammatory processes contribute both to the development of Aβ plaques and to the cognitive/behavioral impairments observed in these mice.

Among inflammatory molecules, cytokines are the best candidates to contribute to the development of cognitive dysfunction because they can modulate neurotransmitter and second-messenger signal transduction systems, which are known to subserve certain cognitive processes. Along this line, cytokines have been shown to affect noradrenalin, serotonin, acetylcholine (Ach), glutamate, nitric oxide (NO), and dopamine neurotransmission, and the cAMP, IP-3, and Ca2+-dependent intracellular transduction pathways [3, 76, 77].

There is some evidence that NO dysregulation is a factor in Alzheimer's disease and that NO dysregulation is related to CNS inflammation. Cerebrospinal fluid from Alzheimer's disease patients has significantly lower levels of nitrate, a metabolic product of NO, than cerebrospinal fluid from aged-matched controls [78]. Furthermore, there is decreased staining of NAPDH-diaphorase, an index of NO synthase (NOS) levels, in the hippocampus of Alzheimer's disease patients, and the degree of NOS deficit has been found to be correlated with severity of cognitive deficits measured prior to death [79]. However, not all investigators have found significant alterations in NO activity in the brains of Alzheimer's disease patients [80, 81].

Disruption of brain NO concentrations has also been reported to produce Alzheimer's disease-like behavioral deficits in experimental animals, particularly on measures of learning and memory functions [82]. For example, intracranial administration of NOS blockers causes impairments in spatial working memory in the Morris water maze in mice and rats [83, 84] and impairments in learning in the radial arm maze in rats [85]. These behavioral effects of NO blockade are transient and can occur without permanent damage to neurons [82].

However, when abnormalities in brain NO activity have been demonstrated in brain or cerebrospinal fluid of Alzheimer's patients, these were decreased NO levels, whereas stimulation of glial cells with cytokines *in vitro* increases NO release. Similarly, while disruptions in learning, memory and other behaviors have been shown in experimental animals after blockade of NO synthesis, there are no reports directly linking NO hyperfunction to behavioral impairment.

A partial explanation to these discrepancies would be the different NO effects in young healthy cells versus those already at risk. For example, Ohno *et al.* [86] showed deficits in working memory in rats after intrahippocampal injection of the NOS inhibitor, L-NAME, and, in a later paper [84] this same group showed that intrahippocampal injection of L-NAME prevented deficits in working memory when administered 24 h after induction of cerebral ischemia. Significantly, cerebral ischemia is known to activate glial cells and glial iNOS [87]. These opposite effects of NOS blockade on memory performance when administered after ischemic challenge or in healthy animals may reflect activation of different cellular sources of NO.

In summary, while the relationship among cytokine-mediated NO hyperfunction, the evidence of NO dysregulation in Alzheimer's disease brains, and the behavioral effects of NOS inhibition in experimental animals cannot be definitively resolved based on the data currently available, the findings reviewed above suggest that NO may be one pathogenic agent in immune-mediated cognitive dysfuncion in Alzheimer's disease.

Numerous studies in experimental animals and humans have supported the theory that age-related deficits in acetylcholine (ACh) neurotransmission produce cognitive impairments consistent with Alzheimer's pathology [88]. This theory became known as the 'cholinergic hypothesis' of Alzheimer's disease in the 1980's. This hypothesis is based on an observed decrease in Ach release from cholinergic neurons projecting to the basal forebrain, hippocampus, and, to a lesser extent, in other CNS cholinergic circuits [89]. Ach dysregulation has been associated with behavioral dysfunction in animal experiments using a variety of behavioral measures [90-92]. Intracerebroventricular injection of the carboxyl-terminal fragment of APP significantly impaired cued, spatial, and working memory performance of mice in Y-maze and water maze tasks and showed decreases in Ach levels in the cerebral cortex and hippocampus compared with the saline controls [93].

The decrease in cholinergic activity in the brain has been attributed to hyperactivity of a post-synaptic enzyme that terminates cholinergic synaptic transmission through hydrolysis of acetylcholine, acetylcholinesterase (AChE; [94]). AChE is overexpressed by neuritis associated with β-amyloid plaques in Alzheimer brain [95-97]. AChE, in turn, has been shown to regulate processing of the β-amyloid precursor protein [98] and to accelerate assembly of amyloid peptide into β-amyloid fibrils [99, 100], suggesting a link between AChE overexpression and β-amyloid formation. Overexpression of human AChE in neurons of transgenic mice produces progressive cognitive deterioration, as assessed by the Morris water maze [101]. Therapeutic interventions based on increasing CNS Ach neurotransmission has been reported to ameliorate mental dysfunction in animal models of Alzheimer's pathology [89] and in human patients [102].

Several studies have linked the cytokine IL-2 to cholinergic neurotransmission in the rat brain [7, 103-106]. Under normal physiological conditions, brain concentration of IL-2 is low, and IL-2 is unlikely to play an important role in normal ongoing brain processes. However, during conditions of CNS inflammation, IL-2 and IL-2 receptors are strongly up-regulated and may reach concentrations sufficient to modify Ach neurotransmission with consequent effects on cognitive functioning and behavior [103]. In brain slices, IL-2 had no effect on spontaneous Ach release from neurons in hippocampus, cortex or striatum [103], however IL-2 did significantly suppress K^+-evoked Ach release in hippocampal and striatal slices. This effect of IL-2 was dose dependent and was detectable at relatively low concentrations in hippocampal slices. Hanisch *et al.* [104] also tested the ability of other cytokines to modulate Ach release from hippocampal, striatal, or cortical slices, and found IL-1α, IL-1β, IL-3, IL-5, IL-6 and TNF-α all to be ineffective.

A more recent report, however, has shown a central role of IL-1 as the cytokine inducing self-propagating neuronal injury and consequent microglia activation, along with further IL-1 overexpression [107]. In particular, authors showed that IL-1 increases AChE levels in the brain. Moreover, *in vitro* secreted APP fragments can activate microglia, which then secretes

IL-1. This IL-1 in turn promotes AChE expression, proving a pathway of inflammation-mediated alteration of neuronal function.

In summary, there are three types of evidence supporting the role of inflammatory processes in Alzheimer's disease pathology: (1) the co-regulatory interactions among Aβ, proteases and protease inhibitors, and glia-derived inflammatory mediators, that contribute to neurotoxicity, (2) the modulation of neurotransmitters by inflammatory mediators, that can be induced by amyloid proteins, and (3) the induction of Alzheimer's-like cognitive/behavioral effects by immune factors. The theory of immunopathogenesis of Alzheimer's disease has clear therapeutic implications: anti-inflammatory drugs taken at critical times in the disease process may protect against the development or progression of the disease [108, 109]. Indeed, several studies have already sought to assess the therapeutic potential of anti-inflammatory drugs for Alzheimer's disease.

For example, Rich *et al.* [110] found that Alzheimer's patients who had been taking non-steroidal anti-inflammatory drugs (NSAID) daily for 12 months has a shorter duration of illness relative to age and performed better on tests of cognitive functioning (including memory) than Alzheimer's disease patients without a history of consistent NSAID use. Further, patients taking NSAID showed a slower rate of cognitive decline over 1 year of periodic testing than did non-NSAID patients in this study.

Moreover, Rogers *et al.* [111] reported similar findings in a 6-month, double-blind prospective study comparing Alzheimer's patients treated with the potent anti-inflammatory drug, indomethacin, with matched, placebo-treated control subjects. By the end of 6 months, indomethacin treated patients showed slight overall improvements in measures of cognitive functioning, whereas control subjects showed significant cognitive decline.

Cytokines in Health: Role in Learning and Memory

Interleukin-1 (IL-1)

The interleukin-1 (IL-1) is a cytokine produced by a number of peripheral cell types and plays a variety of roles in immune and inflammatory responses [112-114]. IL-1 action is regulated by a complex network of molecules that includes multiple ligands (IL-1α, IL-1β, and the endogenous IL-1 receptor antagonist [IL-1ra]), several binding sites (IL-1 receptor [IL-1R] type I, IL-1R type II, IL-1 accessory protein, soluble receptors), and a key regulatory enzyme (IL-1-converting enzyme). As mentioned before, most of these molecules have been localized in the brain under varying conditions, both in neurons and in glial cells [115, 116].

The first unequivocal evidence showing that IL-1 was active in the brain was published in 1986 [1]. It was shown that administration of subpyrogenic doses of both purified and recombinant IL-1 to mice and rats increased blood levels of adrenocorticotropic hormone (ACTH) and glucocorticoids. Because the same effect was found in athymic nude mice, authors concluded that the effect observed supported the existence of an immunoregulatory feedback circuit on the hypothalamic-pituitary-adrenal (HPA) axis. In fact, they later showed that IL-1 activates the corticotrophin-releasing factor containing neurons in the paraventricular nucleus of the hypothalamus [117].

It was subsequently shown that exogenously applied IL-1 can modulate neuronal activity inhibiting calcium influx [118, 119], protein kinase C [118], or the release of acetylcholine [120] and glutamate [118] in the normal hippocampus. In addition, IL-1 modulates a process related to learning, such as long-term potentiation (LTP) *in vivo* [121-126]. In this model, as in other models in the periphery, physiological low levels of IL-1 could have opposite effects to those observed when larger amounts are induced or applied exogenously [51].

Oitz *et al.* [127] reported for the first time impaired memory performance in rats in the Morris water maze after treatment with proinflammatory cytokines. IL-1β or IL-6 were injected into the cerebral ventricles of rats 60 minutes prior to water maze training, using a procedure designed to test spatial learning. While treatment with IL-6 had no effect, water maze performance of IL-1β treated rats was significantly impaired relative to saline treated controls. Both IL-6 and IL-1β significantly increased body temperature, suggesting that cognitive effects of IL-1β are not a consequence of the immune thermoregulatory response.

In the same line, Pugh *et al.* [128] showed that administration of the HIV protein gp120 into the lateral ventricle immediately following fear conditioning, impaired contextual fear conditioning, while having no effect on auditory-cue fear conditioning. As gp120 induces IL-1β mRNA in the brain [129], authors tested whether IL-1 antagonism could block this effect on memory. IL-1ra i.c.v. given after conditioning but before gp120 administration blocked the effect of gp120 on conditioning.

Matsumoto *et al.* [130] studied the effect of exogenous IL-1β on working memory performance of rats. Using a three-panel runaway task, the authors showed that IL-1β injected laterally into the dorsal hippocampus significantly increased the working memory errors in this test, while the number of errors in the first trial or the latencies to obtain food pellets were not affected. Moreover, the combined injection of IL-1β and IL-1ra into the hippocampus significantly decreased the working memory deficit. Finally, authors proposed that IL-1β effect is mediated by acetylcholine and/or glutamate in the hippocampus, as both a cholinesterase inhibitor and a NMDA partial agonist revert IL-1β-induced working memory deficits.

Pre-exposure of rats to the context has a facilitatory effect on contextual fear conditioning 24 h later. Barrientos *et al.* [131] showed that IL-1β injected into the dorsal hippocampus after pre-exposure to a conditioning context, interferes with the context pre-exposure facilitation effect. Interestingly, IL-1β blocks context conditioning independently of corticosteroid induction in the periphery. These results suggest that intra-hippocampal IL-1β interferes with memory consolidation of contextual representation. Moreover, they showed that IL-1β can affect memory consolidation both immediately after context exposure and 3 or 24 h later.

Using a different approach, Palin *et al.* [132] studied the role of IL-1 in the in the memory impairment associated with a second exposure to bacillus Calmette-Guerin (BCG). Animals were primed with an injection of BCG into the dorsal hippocampus and challenged 4 weeks later with BCG administered subcutaneously. This challenge was associated with impaired spatial memory in a Y-maze and with increases of IL-1β levels in the hippocampus. The chronic subcutaneous administration of IL-1ra abrogated these effects. These results show that increases of IL-1β during inflammation can result in cognitive impairments.

Trying to identify the molecular mechanisms of IL-1 modulation of learning, Hein *et al.* [133] showed that prostaglandins are necessary and sufficient to impair contextual fear conditioning after IL-1β treatment. Cox-2 was induced after IL-1β injection into the dorsal hippocampus and prostaglandin E_2 (PGE_2) reduced freezing during testing. Finally, PGE_2 injected during the 2 h post-conditioning reduced the conditioning-induced increase in brain-derived neurotrophic factor (BDNF), a molecule previously shown to be necessary after training to form a long-term memory. Therefore, IL-1 can regulate memory formation through the induction of neurotrophins.

Although these reports demonstrated that IL-1 could play a role in learning and memory processes during inflammation in the brain, they did not address the question of whether endogenous hippocampal IL-1 modulates memory acquisition and consolidation during nonpathological situations.

To examine the hypothesis that IL-1 signaling is involved in learning and memory, Yirmiya *et al.* [134] injected rats i.c.v. with IL-1ra and tested their performance in the Morris water maze (MWM) and passive avoidance test. They found that IL-1ra caused memory impairment in the passive avoidance test and the standard version of the MWM, which assesses spatial memory. It is interesting to note that even though these authors analyze hippocampus-dependent behavior, they inject the IL-1ra into the ventricles. I.c.v. injection distributes proteins to different regions of the brain, and has strong effects on the ventricles walls [135]. In fact, among generalized effects on behavior, authors report an increase in anorexia. However, the influence of these unspecific effects on learning has not been analyzed.

Avital *et al.* [136] showed that previously generated type I IL-1 receptor knockout mice (IL-1rKO; [137]) show learning deficiencies. IL-1rKO mice displayed a slower rate of learning in the spatial memory version of the MWM and impaired contextual fear conditioning. In contrast, IL-1rKO mice showed normal hippocampal-independent memory in the visually guided task of the water maze and in the auditory-cued fear conditioning. However, IL-1rKO mice show slower speed of swimming, suggesting that they have motor impairments, and reduced pain sensibility [138]. This suggests that IL-1rKO mice not only have compromised hippocampal plasticity but that also other systems are affected.

To study the role of IL-1 system in learning, we chose a fear-motivated learning task that is hippocampal-dependent and is acquired in a single and brief training session [139]. We first analyzed the expression of IL-1α, IL-1β, and IL-1ra during the posttraining time window previously shown to be involved in the memory consolidation process [140-142]. We observed a transient increment in IL-1α mRNA levels 4 h after training. The IL-1α increment observed was specific for the training and was not related to the stress of the procedure, because control animals submitted to the same shock and handling, but incapable of making the stepping down-shock association, showed no alterations of their IL-1α mRNA levels. In our experiments, IL-1β mRNA levels were not altered.

As described before, IL-1 expression is induced by stress in some brain areas but detected only in adrenalectomized animals, since glucocorticoids downregulates IL-1α levels in shocked animals [143]. It is interesting to highlight that, in our experiments, IL-1α expression was refractory to the inhibitory action of stress through glucocorticoids, strengthening a possible specific role of the *de novo* production of this cytokine in learning. Thus, these results showed a learning-specific regulation of IL-1α, suggesting that IL-1α could be involved in memory formation. This prompted us to further investigate the role of endogenous IL-1α in hippocampal memory processing.

Using an adenoviral vector that expresses the natural antagonist of the IL-1 receptor (IL-1ra), we were able to block IL-1 function specifically in the dorsal hippocampus and to show that this blockade has a facilitatory effect on short-term memory (STM) and long-term memory (LTM) in an inhibitory avoidance learning task. These results cannot be explained by the IL-1α capability of modulating nociceptive information [144, 145], because all experimental groups had similar current thresholds for jumping and vocalization [146, 147]. Moreover, we showed that IL-1ra expression in the dorsal hippocampus had no effect on the number of crossings and rearings in an open field, so that the adenoviral vector does not affect locomotor activity. Given that the increase in stepping-down latency could not be due to increased shock sensitivity or to the reduction of locomotor activity, our results strongly suggest that blockade of hippocampal IL-1 receptor has a learning-specific effect on the inhibitory avoidance learning task.

However, given that animals were trained and tested under the influence of AdIL-1ra, we were unable to elucidate whether endogenous IL-1 is involved in acquisition, consolidation, and/or retrieval during hippocampal memory processing. Some reports have emphasized the physiological importance of learning and memory suppressors [148]. Thus, we postulated that endogenous IL-1α in the hippocampus could act as a modulator to physiologically constrain memory formation or retrieval, or both. However, this does not rule out that different forms of memory can be modulated differently by IL-1 or by different IL-1 levels, so that endogenous IL-1 could actually be facilitatory in other learning tasks.

To evaluate whether IL-1 receptor blockade had similar effects on a nonassociative learning task [149-151], we evaluated AdIL-1ra animals during one of the most elementary nonassociative learning tasks, i.e., the behavioral habituation to a novel environment. In this paradigm, the blockade of IL-1 receptor had no effect on LTM. So we demonstrated that two hippocampal-dependent memories, one requiring association to an aversive stimulus and other nonassociative, have different sensitivity to IL-1. Namely, IL-1ra facilitates the inhibitory avoidance task but has no effect in the habituation to a novel environment.

Taken together, our results suggest a specific role of the endogenous proinflammatory cytokine IL-1α in the formation and/or retrieval of an associative memory. This shows a modulatory function of a cytokine similar to those previously shown for neurotrophins (e.g., [140]), neurotransmitters and hormones [152, 153].

Goshen *et al.* [154] also studied the physiological role of IL-1 in learning and memory. As we showed before, authors found that learning of a hippocampal-dependent task induces IL-1 gene expression in the hippocampus. Mice that express the IL-1ra under the GFAP promoter (Tg IL-1ra mice) show disrupted hippocampal-dependent memory in both contextual-fear conditioning paradigm and MWM. It was later shown that Tg IL-1ra mice present changes in BDNF-ERK1/2 and Src signalling pathways, suggesting an underlying mechanisms of IL-1 modulation of memory formation [155]. Considering their results, Goshen *et al.* suggested an inverted U-shaped pattern of IL-1 modulation of memory processes, i.e., physiological levels of IL-1 are needed for memory formation, and a slight increase in brain IL-1 levels can even improve memory, whereas any deviation from physiological range, either by excess elevation in IL-1 or by blockade of IL-1 signaling, results in impaired memory.

Genetic studies in humans showed that individuals carrying interleukin-converting enzyme polymorphisms that are accompanied by lower IL-1β levels (e.g. 10643C and 5352A) performed better on all cognitive tests [156]. A biallelic functional polymorphism in the promoter region (position -511) of the IL-1β gene is associated with cognitive performance in elderly males [157]. C/C genotype showed better cognitive function test results than T/T carriers. This latter group secretes significantly more IL-1β than -511C carriers [158], suggesting again that high IL-1 levels are detrimental to cognitive performance.

In summary, there is consensus that that high IL-1 expression in the brain (and particularly in the hippocampus) blocks learning and memory consolidation of hippocampus-dependent tasks. The research has focused mainly on IL-1β, while the specific role of pathological levels of IL-1α has not been evaluated.

The role of endogenous, physiological levels of IL-1 is, however, less clear. The analysis of IL-1R KO mice and GFAP TgIL-1ra mice suggest that IL-1 may be necessary for learning and/or memory formation. However, these mice lack IL-1 signalling from conception or early development, and other unspecific effects cannot be ruled out. In fact motor and nociceptive deficits have been reported. To our knowledge, our paper is the only one reporting a facilitatory effect of endogenous IL-1 blockade. Two particular facts are worth to mention. First, the treatment with adenoviral vectors expressing IL-1ra is limited to the adult animal and the dorsal hippocampus. This is a clear difference with knockout and transgenic mice. Second, in our paradigm IL-1α, and not IL-1β, appeared involved in memory consolidation. These differences could account for the otherwise controversial results. Moreover, species-specific differences could also be cited.

Interleukin-6 (IL-6)

IL-6 regulates immune responses, acute phase reactions and hematopoiesis, and plays a central role in host defence mechanisms. IL-6 is a pleiotropic cytokine that is produced in a variety of cells and acts on a wide range of tissues, exerting growth-inducing, growth-inhibitory and differentiation-inducing effects, depending on the nature of the target cells [159]

IL-6 is expressed in the embryonic cortex and adult hippocampus of the rat brain [160]. Also IL-6 receptor (IL-6R) mRNA has been detected in the adult hippocampus and striatum [161, 162], specifically in the granular layer of the dentate gyrus, in the fimbria, and in large pyramidal neurons of the CA1 to CA4 hippocampal fields. Moreover, both IL-6 and IL-6R mRNAs are expressed in the granular cell layer of the cerebellum. Membrane depolarization induces IL-6 mRNA accumulation in primary cortical cells and is increased *in vivo* after epileptic seizures [163]. However, IL-6 can also enhance the survival of several classes of neurons in culture [164, 165].

IL-6 exerts pronounced effects on the CNS: stimulates neuronal growth [166, 167], reduces food intake [168], induces fever [169] and activates the hypothalamic-pituitary-adrenal (HPA) system [170]. Transgenic mice with high levels of IL-6 expression develop severe neurologic disease characterized by tremor, ataxia, and seizure [171]. These mice also exhibit neurodegeneration, astrocytosis, and angiogenesis.

Heyser *et al.* [172] used a transgenic mouse model of chronic CNS inflammation to study the effects of brain inflammation on spatial learning in a Y-maze. Transgenic mice (GFAP-IL-6 mice) express IL-6 chronically in astrocytes, due to fusing the gene coding for IL-6 to the promoter of the normally expressed astrocytic protein, glial fibrillary acidic protein GFAP. The brains of GFAP-IL-6 mice are characterized by localized inflammation and localized, age-dependent neurodegeneration in the hippocampus and cerebellum, as well as increased BBB permeability. GFAP-IL-6 mice also show microglia activation and increased cytokine production by microglia and astrocytes in the hippocampus. While GFAP-IL-6 mice aged less than 6 months showed normal avoidance learning, GFAP-IL-6 mice aged 6 months or older were found to be significantly impaired in a Y-maze active avoidance learning task compared to wild-type control mice. The age dependence on learning deficits in GFAP-IL-6 mice suggests a temporal accumulation of inflammatory neurotoxicity, and, according to the authors, represents a plausible model for the progressive degenerative behavioral disorders in Alzheimer's and other human dementias involving chronic CNS inflammation.

In line with these results, Braida *et al.* [173] found facilitation in learning over 30 days in IL-6 KO mice. IL-6 KO mice showed reduced number of working memory errors in a radial maze. Moreover, these mice showed normal spontaneous motor activity, suggesting that the effect is not due to unspecific differences in motor function. This revealed a facilitatory effect of IL-6 gene deletion on spatial learning, as opposed to the detrimental effect of IL-6 over-expression demonstrated before.

However, other authors have found impaired memory in IL-6 KO mice, both in the MWM and in the novel object recognition test [174]. In the MWM, IL-6 KO mice displayed both reduced acquisition and impaired reversal learning. Moreover, IL-6 KO mice showed reduced exploratory behavior.

The disturbance of IL-6 signaling in IL-6 KO mice is very likely to affect brain development and the development of the immune system and its connections with the brain. As a consequence, neuronal functions correlated with memory processes would be compromised. Furthermore, disturbed IL-6 signaling leads to behavioral changes (reduced exploratory behavior, increased stress susceptibility) that have negative impact on memory formation. In conclusion, new tools should be generated that block IL-6 signaling specifically in the brain and in a restricted period of time.

Human studies have shown that high IL-6 plasma levels are associated with risk in decline on cognitive function in elderly people [175]. Moreover, a study among newborns reported a relationship between specific IL-6 genotypes and cognitive function showing that the 572C-allele of IL-6 (CC/GC genotypes) is associated with impaired cognitive development among children [176].

In summary, although there is less work studying the role of IL-6 in learning and memory in comparison with IL-1, all evidence suggests that increased IL-6 into the brain is detrimental to learning. Again, the role of endogenous IL-6 is less clear, some evidence showing that blockade of basal IL-6 signaling facilitates learning and other suggesting that basal IL-6 activity is required to learn.

Tumor Necrosis Factor-Alpha (TNF-α)

TNF-α is a cytokine produced by activated cells of the immune system, mainly by macrophages [177]. It is produced mostly as a 17 kD secreted protein, although a membrane-bound variant of the protein has citotoxic activity and an important role in cellular communication. There are two types of TNF receptors, TNF-RI (55-60 kDa) and TNF-RII (75-80 kDa), which can be shed, therefore existing in soluble form [178]. TNF-α binds both receptors with approximately equal affinity. These two distinct receptors have been shown to elicit different molecular and cellular responses [179-181]. For example, binding to the TNF-RI initiates the activation of caspases and can ultimately lead to apoptosis [181]. Conversely, TNF-RII appears to inhibit the activation of caspases and protect against apoptosis. TNF-α production in the periphery is induced by different stimuli, including mitogens, IL-1, IL-2 and interferons.

TNF-α is expressed at very low levels in basal conditions in the CNS. In contrast, astrocytes, microglia and neurons have been described to produce TNF-α upon exposure to multiple physiological and pathological stimuli (e.g. CNS infection and brain injury) [178]. In the brain, as opposed to what has been described in the periphery, IL-1 fails to induce TNF-α expression, and TNF-α does not induce either itself or IL-1 [182, 183].

Transgenic mice, specifically overexpressing murine TNF-α in the CNS either in neurons or in astrocytes, and at different stages of development, spontaneously develop chronic CNS inflammation. This is characterized by widespread reactive astrocytosis and microgliosis, meningeal and parenchymal infiltration by activated T-cells and macrophages, loss of white matter and neurodegeneration [184]. On the contrary, mice lacking TNF-α or both receptors show exacerbated neuronal damage elicited by different neurotoxic stimuli [185, 186]. Therefore, TNF-α can be neurotoxic or have neuroprotective effects depending on the level of expression, the type of neurons affected and other factors.

TNF-α blocks LTP in slices [121], at least partly through p38 MAPK and metabotropic glutamate receptors [187, 188]. It has been suggested that the continual presence of TNF-α is required for preservation of synaptic strengths at the excitatory synapse [189] and that neurotransmitter metabolism and neurodevelopmental processes were altered by TNF-α [190].

As mentioned before, TNF-α transgenic mice that express the cytokine in the brain develop neurologic symptoms, including CNS inflammation and demyelination [184]. These mice show a retardation of passive avoidance acquisition, with no effects during the retention phase [191]. However, as these mice show reduced body weight, reduced exploratory activity and analgesia, the specificity of the learning deficits is not clear.

Comparing that same mouse line with a different transgenic line that presents no neurological or phenotypical alterations, Aloe *et al.* [192] showed that both lines exhibit impairments in learning in the MWM. More specifically, both transgenic lines showed increased escape latency during the test. It is worth to mention that both lines exhibited reduced swimming speed, while the distance travelled was the same. This suggests that transgenic mice were less effective than wild type animals in using the acquired positional information either because of forgetting or of motivational changes caused by the new stressing environmental situation. Alternatively, transgenic mice could be more distractible in learning a task, which requires more complex informational processing as retrieving the platform position. These mice also present reduced neurotrophic factors levels in the hippocampus (namely, NGF and BDNF), suggesting a possible mechanism of this effect. Finally, learning deficits in TNF-α Tg mice appear only at 30-35 days of age [193], suggesting that this phenotype might be influenced by the TNF-α produced in specific brain regions during the adult life.

Again, the role of the endogenous cytokine levels is less clear. One report showed that TNF-α KO mice have no phenotype in the Y-maze or the MWM [194], suggesting that this cytokine is not necessary for memory formation in these tests. In contrast, other work demonstrated that TNF-α KO mice show a deficiency in spatial memory when young, but with age TNF deficiency leads to facilitation in spatial memory [195].

A significant association between the TNF-α 308G to A polymorphism and processing speed was observed, indicating better performance for heterozygous or homozygous carriers of the A allele in elderly people [196]. This polymorphism, however, was not associated with altered cytokine plasma levels.

CONCLUSION

Pro-inflammatory cytokines are expressed within the brain in health and in disease. All evidence suggests that IL-1, IL-6 and TNF-α can be induced in the brain under various pathological conditions and that this up-regulation results in detrimental effects on learning and memory. This is normally observed during sickness, when cognitive impairment is associated with a need to save energy to fight infection. However, neuropathological conditions that lead to increased cytokine production in the brain can also result in cognitive impairment. For example, in Alzheimer's disease amyloid plaques are accompanied by gliosis, cytokine increments and cognitive impairment.

The role of low, endogenous levels of brain cytokines in learning and memory is less clear. Only few reports have studied the role of pro-inflammatory cytokines under these conditions, and results are controversial. It is essential to develop new genetic tools to elucidate the role of cytokines in the normal brain, without the confounding effects of inflammation.

ABBREVIATIONS

ACTH, adrenocorticotropic hormone
APP, amyloid precursor protein
BBB, blood-brain barrier
CNS, central nervous system
GFAP, glial fibrillary acidic protein
HPA, hypothalamus-pituitary-adrenal
i.c.v., intracerebroventricular
i.p., intraperitoneal
i.v., intravenous
IL-1, interleukin 1
IL-1R, IL-1 receptor
IL-6, interleukin 6
IL-6R, IL-6 receptor
KO, knockout
LPS, lipopolysaccharide

LTM, long-term memory
LTP, long-term potentiation
MWM, Morris water maze
NO, nitric oxide
STM, short-term memory
TNF-alpha, tumor necrosis factor alpha
TNF-R, TNF-alpha receptor

REFERENCES

Besedovsky, H; del Rey, A; Sorkin, E; Dinarello, CA. Immunoregulatory feedback between interleukin-1 and glucocorticoid hormones. *Science*, 1986, 233(4764), 652-654.

Hopkins, SJ; Rothwell, NJ. Cytokines and the nervous system. I: Expression and recognition. *Trends in Neurosciences*, 1995, 18(2), 83-88.

Rothwell, NJ; Hopkins, SJ. Cytokines and the nervous system II: Actions and mechanisms of action. *Trends in Neurosciences*, 1995, 18(3), 130-136.

Cunningham, C; Campion, S; Teeling, J; Felton, L; Perry, VH. The sickness behaviour and CNS inflammatory mediator profile induced by systemic challenge of mice with synthetic double-stranded RNA (poly I:C). *Brain, Behavior, and Immunity*, 2007, 21(4), 490-502.

Gilmore, JH; Jarskog, LF. Exposure to infection and brain development: cytokines in the pathogenesis of schizophrenia. *Schizophr Res*, 1997, 24(3), 365-367.

Akashi, S; Shimazu, R; Ogata, H; Nagai, Y; Takeda, K; Kimoto, M; Miyake, K. Cutting edge: cell surface expression and lipopolysaccharide signaling via the toll-like receptor 4-MD-2 complex on mouse peritoneal macrophages. *The Journal of Immunology*, 2000, 164(7), 3471-3475.

Carlson, SL; Beiting, DJ; Kiani, CA; Abell, KM; McGillis, JP. Catecholamines decrease lymphocyte adhesion to cytokine-activated endothelial cells. *Brain, Behavior, and Immunity*, 1996, 10(1), 55-67.

Merrill, JE; Murphy, SP. Inflammatory events at the blood brain barrier: regulation of adhesion molecules, cytokines, and chemokines by reactive nitrogen and oxygen species. *Brain, Behavior, and Immunity*, 1997, 11(4), 245-263.

Banks, WA; Plotkin, SR; Kastin, AJ. Permeability of the blood-brain barrier to soluble cytokine receptors. *Neuroimmunomodulation*, 1995, 2(3), 161-165.

Ellison, MD; Povlishock, JT; Merchant, RE. Blood-brain barrier dysfunction in cats following recombinant interleukin-2 infusion. *Cancer Res*, 1987, 47(21), 5765-5770.

Saija, A; Princi, P; Lanza, M; Scalese, M; Aramnejad, E; De Sarro, A. Systemic cytokine administration can affect blood-brain barrier permeability in the rat. *Life Sci*, 1995, 56(10), 775-784.

Luheshi, GN; Hammond, E; Van Dam, AM. Cytokines as messengers of neuroimmune interactions. *Trends in Neurosciences*, 1996, 19(2), 46-47.

Banks, WA; Farr, SA; Morley, JE. Entry of blood-borne cytokines into the central nervous system: effects on cognitive processes. *Neuroimmunomodulation*, 2002, 10(6), 319-327.

Ek, M; Kurosawa, M; Lundeberg, T; Ericsson, A. Activation of vagal afferents after intravenous injection of interleukin-1beta: role of endogenous prostaglandins. *The Journal of Neuroscience*, 1998, 18(22), 9471-9479.

Dantzer, R; Bluthe, RM; Laye, S; Bret-Dibat, JL; Parnet, P; Kelley, KW. Cytokines and sickness behavior. *Ann N Y Acad Sci*, 1998, 840, 586-590.

Maier, SF; Goehler, LE; Fleshner, M; Watkins, LR. The role of the vagus nerve in cytokine-to-brain communication. *Ann N Y Acad Sci*, 1998, 840, 289-300.

Toulmond, S; Parnet, P; Linthorst, ACE. When cytokines get on your nerves: cytokine networks and CNS pathologies. *Trends in Neurosciences*, 1996, 19(10), 409-410.

Bluthe, RM; Michaud, B; Kelley, KW; Dantzer, R. Vagotomy attenuates behavioural effects of interleukin-1 injected peripherally but not centrally. *NeuroReport*, 1996, 7(9), 1485-1488.

Fleshner, M; Goehler, LE; Schwartz, BA; McGorry, M; Martin, D; Maier, SF; Watkins, LR. Thermogenic and corticosterone responses to intravenous cytokines (IL-1beta and TNF-alpha) are attenuated by subdiaphragmatic vagotomy. *Journal of Neuroimmunology*, 1998, 86(2), 134-141.

Bluthe, RM; Michaud, B; Kelley, KW; Dantzer, R. Vagotomy blocks behavioural effects of interleukin-1 injected via the intraperitoneal route but not via other systemic routes. *NeuroReport*, 1996, 7(15-17), 2823-2827.

Bret-Dibat, JL; Bluthe, RM; Kent, S; Kelley, KW; Dantzer, R. Lipopolysaccharide and interleukin-1 depress food-motivated behavior in mice by a vagal-mediated mechanism. *Brain, Behavior, and Immunity*, 1995, 9(3), 242-246.

Hansen, MK; Taishi, P; Chen, Z; Krueger, JM. Vagotomy blocks the induction of interleukin-1beta (IL-1beta) mRNA in the brain of rats in response to systemic IL-1beta. *The Journal of Neuroscience*, 1998, 18(6), 2247-2253.

Laye, S; Bluthe, RM; Kent, S; Combe, C; Medina, C; Parnet, P; Kelley, K; Dantzer, R. Subdiaphragmatic vagotomy blocks induction of IL-1 beta mRNA in mice brain in response to peripheral LPS. *American Journal of Physiology*, 1995, 268(5 Pt 2), R1327-1331.

Luheshi, GN; Bluthe, RM; Rushforth, D; Mulcahy, N; Konsman, JP; Goldbach, M; Dantzer, R. Vagotomy attenuates the behavioural but not the pyrogenic effects of interleukin-1 in rats. *Auton Neurosci*, 2000, 85(1-3), 127-132.

Ban, E; Haour, F; Lenstra, R. Brain interleukin 1 gene expression induced by peripheral lipopolysaccharide administration. *Cytokine*, 1992, 4(1), 48-54.

Perry, V; Andersson, P-B; Gordon, S. Macrophages and inflammation in the central nervous system. *Trends in Neuroscience*, 1993, 16(7), 268-273.

Rothwell, NJ; Luheshi, G; Toulmond, S. Cytokines and their receptors in the central nervous system: physiology, pharmacology, and pathology. *Pharmacol Ther*, 1996, 69(2), 85-95.

Dantzer, R. Cytokine-induced sickness behavior: mechanisms and implications. *Ann N Y Acad Sci*, 2001, 933, 222-234.

Konsman, JP; Parnet, P; Dantzer, R. Cytokine-induced sickness behaviour: mechanisms and implications. *Trends in Neurosciences*, 2002, 25(3), 154-159.

Dantzer, R; Kelley, KW. Twenty years of research on cytokine-induced sickness behavior. *Brain, Behavior, and Immunity*, 2007, 21(2), 153-160.

Dantzer, R; Kelley, KW. Stress and immunity: an integrated view of relationships between the brain and the immune system. *Life Sci*, 1989, 44(26), 1995-2008.

Hart, BL. Biological basis of the behavior of sick animals. *Neurosci Biobehav Rev*, 1988, 12(2), 123-137.

Kent, S; Bluthe, RM; Dantzer, R; Hardwick, AJ; Kelley, KW; Rothwell, NJ; Vannice, JL. Different receptor mechanisms mediate the pyrogenic and behavioral effects of interleukin 1. *Proc Natl Acad Sci,* U S A, 1992, 89(19), 9117-9120.

Maier, SF; Wiertelak, EP; Martin, D; Watkins, LR. Interleukin-1 mediates the behavioral hyperalgesia produced by lithium chloride and endotoxin. *Brain Research*, 1993, 623(2), 321-324.

Watkins, LR; Maier, SF. The pain of being sick: implications of immune-to-brain communication for understanding pain. *Annu Rev Psychol*, 2000, 51, 29-57.

Bluthe, RM; Crestani, F; Kelley, KW; Dantzer, R. Mechanisms of the behavioral effects of interleukin 1. Role of prostaglandins and CRF. *Ann N Y Acad Sci*, 1992, 650, 268-275.

Bluthe, RM; Dantzer, R; Kelley, KW. Effects of interleukin-1 receptor antagonist on the behavioral effects of lipopolysaccharide in rat. *Brain Research*, 1992, 573(2), 318-320.

Bluthe, RM; Pawlowski, M; Suarez, S; Parnet, P; Pittman, Q; Kelley, KW; Dantzer, R. Synergy between tumor necrosis factor alpha and interleukin-1 in the induction of sickness behavior in mice. *Psychoneuroendocrinology*, 1994, 19(2), 197-207.

Kent, S; Bret-Dibat, JL; Kelley, KW; Dantzer, R. Mechanisms of sickness-induced decreases in food-motivated behavior. *Neurosci Biobehav Rev*, 1996, 20(1), 171-175.

Plata-Salaman, CR. Cytokines and feeding suppression: an integrative view from neurologic to molecular levels. *Nutrition*, 1995, 11(5 Suppl), 674-677.

Plata-Salaman, CR. Cytokines and feeding. *Int J Obes Relat Metab Disord*, 2001, 25 Suppl 5, S48-52.

Deacon, RM. Burrowing: a sensitive behavioural assay, tested in five species of laboratory rodents. *Behavioural Brain Research*, 2009, 200(1), 128-133.

Gatti, S; Bartfai, T. Induction of tumor necrosis factor-alpha mRNA in the brain after peripheral endotoxin treatment: comparison with interleukin-1 family and interleukin-6. *Brain Research*, 1993, 624(1-2), 291-294.

Laye, S; Parnet, P; Goujon, E; Dantzer, R. Peripheral administration of lipopolysaccharide induces the expression of cytokine transcripts in the brain and pituitary of mice. *Brain Res Mol Brain Res*, 1994, 27(1), 157-162.

Pitossi, F; del Rey, A; Kabiersch, A; Besedovsky, H. Induction of cytokine transcripts in the central nervous system and pituitary following peripheral administration of endotoxin to mice. *Journal of Neuroscience Research*, 1997, 48(4), 287-298.

van Dam, AM; Brouns, M; Louisse, S; Berkenbosch, F. Appearance of interleukin-1 in macrophages and in ramified microglia in the brain of endotoxin-treated rats: a pathway for the induction of non-specific symptoms of sickness? *Brain Research*, 1992, 588(2), 291-296.

Wan, W; Wetmore, L; Sorensen, CM; Greenberg, AH; Nance, DM. Neural and biochemical mediators of endotoxin and stress-induced c-fos expression in the rat brain. *Brain Research Bulletin*, 1994, 34(1), 7-14.

Bluthe, RM; Walter, V; Parnet, P; Laye, S; Lestage, J; Verrier, D; Poole, S; Stenning, BE; Kelley, KW; Dantzer, R. Lipopolysaccharide induces sickness behaviour in rats by a vagal mediated mechanism. *C R Acad Sci III*, 1994, 317(6), 499-503.

Nadjar, A; Bluthe, RM; May, MJ; Dantzer, R; Parnet, P. Inactivation of the cerebral NFkappaB pathway inhibits interleukin-1beta-induced sickness behavior and c-Fos expression in various brain nuclei. *Neuropsychopharmacology*, 2005, 30(8), 1492-1499.

Aubert, A; Vega, C; Dantzer, R; Goodall, G. Pyrogens specifically disrupt the acquisition of a task involving cognitive processing in the rat. *Brain, Behavior, and Immunity*, 1995, 9, 129-148.

Pugh, RC; Fleshner, M; Watkins, LR; Maier, SF; Rudy, JW. The immune system and memory consolidation: a role for the cytokine IL-1beta. *Neurosci Biobehav Rev*, 2001, 25(1), 29-41.

Pugh, CR; Kumagawa, K; Fleshner, M; Watkins, LR; Maier, SF; Rudy, JW. Selective effects of peripheral lipopolysaccharide administration on contextual and auditory-cue fear conditioning. *Brain, Behavior, and Immunity*, 1998, 12(3), 212-229.

Rudy, JW; O'Reilly, RC. Contextual fear conditioning, conjunctive representations, pattern completion, and the hippocampus. *Behav Neurosci*, 1999, 113(5), 867-880.

Gibertini, M; Newton, C; Friedman, H; Klein, TW. Spatial learning impairment in mice infected with Legionella pneumophila or administered exogenous interleukin-1-beta. *Brain, Behavior, and Immunity*, 1995, 9(2), 113-128.

Sparkman, NL; Kohman, RA; Scott, VJ; Boehm, GW. Bacterial endotoxin-induced behavioral alterations in two variations of the Morris water maze. *Physiology & Behavoir*, 2005, 86(1-2), 244-251.

Banks, W; Farr, S; La Scola, M; Morley, J. Intravenous human interleukin-1a impairs memory processing in mice: Dependence on blood-brain barrier transport into posterior division of the septum. *The Journal of Pharmacology and Experimental Therapeutics*, 2001, 299(2), 536-541.

Maness, LM; Banks, WA; Zadina, JE; Kastin, AJ. Selective transport of blood-borne interleukin-1 alpha into the posterior division of the septum of the mouse brain. *Brain Research*, 1995, 700(1-2), 83-88.

Sparkman, NL; Buchanan, JB; Heyen, JR; Chen, J; Beverly, JL; Johnson, RW. Interleukin-6 facilitates lipopolysaccharide-induced disruption in working memory and expression of other proinflammatory cytokines in hippocampal neuronal cell layers. *The Journal of Neuroscience*, 2006, 26(42), 10709-10716.

Oken, RJ. Towards a unifying hypothesis of neurodegenerative diseases and a concomitant rational strategy for their prophylaxis and therapy. *Med Hypotheses*, 1995, 45(4), 341-342.

Toulmond, S; Parnet, P; Linthorst, AC. When cytokines get on your nerves: cytokine networks and CNS pathologies. *Trends in Neurosciences*, 1996, 19(10), 409-410.

Hart, S; Semple, JM. Neuropsychology and the Dementias. 1990, London, UK: Taylor and Francis.

Mirra, SS; Hart, MN; Terry, RD. Making the diagnosis of Alzheimer's disease. A primer for practicing pathologists. *Arch Pathol Lab Med*, 1993, 117(2), 132-144.

Eikelenboom, P; Rozemuller, JM; Kraal, G; Stam, FC; McBride, PA; Bruce, ME; Fraser, H. Cerebral amyloid plaques in Alzheimer's disease but not in scrapie-affected mice are closely associated with a local inflammatory process. *Virchows Arch B Cell Pathol Incl Mol Pathol*, 1991, 60(5), 329-336.

Ishii, T; Haga, S. Complements, microglial cells and amyloid fibril formation. *Res Immunol*, 1992, 143(6), 614-616.

Rozemuller, JM; Eikelenboom, P; Pals, ST; Stam, FC. Microglial cells around amyloid plaques in Alzheimer's disease express leucocyte adhesion molecules of the LFA-1 family. *Neurosci Lett*, 1989, 101(3), 288-292.

Rozemuller, JM; van der Valk, P; Eikelenboom, P. Activated microglia and cerebral amyloid deposits in Alzheimer's disease. *Res Immunol*, 1992, 143(6), 646-649.

Weldon, DT; Rogers, SD; Ghilardi, JR; Finke, MP; Cleary, JP; O'Hare, E; Esler, WP; Maggio, JE; Mantyh, PW. Fibrillar beta-amyloid induces microglial phagocytosis, expression of inducible nitric oxide synthase, and loss of a select population of neurons in the rat CNS in vivo. *The Journal of Neuroscience*, 1998. 18(6), 2161-2173.

Vandenabeele, P; Fiers, W. Is amyloidogenesis during Alzheimer´s disease due to an IL-1/IL-6-mediated ´acute phase response´ in the brain? *Immunology Today*, 1991, 12(7), 217-219.

McDonald, MP; Overmier, JB; Bandyopadhyay, S; Babcock, D; Cleary, J. Reversal of beta-amyloid-induced retention deficit after exposure to training and state cues. *Neurobiology of Learning and Memory*, 1996, 65(1), 35-47.

Yan, SD; Chen, X; Fu, J; Chen, M; Zhu, H; Roher, A; Slattery, T; Zhao, L; Nagashima, M; Morser, J; Migheli, A; Nawroth, P; Stern, D; Schmidt, AM. RAGE and amyloid-beta peptide neurotoxicity in Alzheimer's disease. *Nature*, 1996, 382(6593), 685-691.

Klegeris, A; Walker, DG; McGeer, PL. Interaction of Alzheimer beta-amyloid peptide with the human monocytic cell line THP-1 results in a protein kinase C-dependent secretion of tumor necrosis factor-alpha. *Brain Research*, 1997, 747(1), 114-121.

Klegeris, A; McGeer, PL. beta-amyloid protein enhances macrophage production of oxygen free radicals and glutamate. *Journal of Neuroscience Research*, 1997, 49(2), 229-235.

Houlden, H; Crook, R; Backhovens, H; Prihar, G; Baker, M; Hutton, M; Rossor, M; Martin, JJ; Van Broeckhoven, C; Hardy, J. ApoE genotype is a risk factor in nonpresenilin early-onset Alzheimer's disease families. *Am J Med Genet*, 1998, 81(1), 117-121.

Barger, SW; Harmon, AD. Microglial activation by Alzheimer amyloid precursor protein and modulation by apolipoprotein E. *Nature*, 1997, 388(6645), 878-881.

Hsiao, K; Chapman, P; Nilsen, S; Eckman, C; Harigaya, Y; Younkin, S; Yang, F; Cole, G. Correlative memory deficits, Abeta elevation, and amyloid plaques in transgenic mice. *Science*, 1996, 274(5284), 99-102.

Miller, B; Sarantis, M; Traynelis, SF; Attwell, D. Potentiation of NMDA receptor currents by arachidonic acid. *Nature*, 1992, 355(6362), 722-725.

Molina-Holgado, F; Guaza, C. Endotoxin administration induced differential neurochemical activation of the rat brain stem nuclei. *Brain Research Bulletin*, 1996, 40(3), 151-156.

Kuiper, MA; Visser, JJ; Bergmans, PL; Scheltens, P; Wolters, EC. Decreased cerebrospinal fluid nitrate levels in Parkinson's disease, Alzheimer's disease and multiple system atrophy patients. *J Neurol Sci*, 1994, 121(1), 46-49.

Rebeck, GW; Marzloff, K; Hyman, BT. The pattern of NADPH-diaphorase staining, a marker of nitric oxide synthase activity, is altered in the perforant pathway terminal zone in Alzheimer's disease. *Neurosci Lett*, 1993, 152(1-2), 165-168.

Milstien, S; Sakai, N; Brew, BJ; Krieger, C; Vickers, JH; Saito, K; Heyes, MP. Cerebrospinal fluid nitrite/nitrate levels in neurologic diseases. *Journal of Neurochemistry*, 1994, 63(3), 1178-1180.

Navarro, JA; Molina, JA; Jimenez-Jimenez, FJ; Benito-Leon, J; Orti-Pareja, M; Gasalla, T; Cabrera-Valdivia, F; Vargas, C; de Bustos, F; Arenas, J. Cerebrospinal fluid nitrate levels in patients with Alzheimer's disease. *Acta Neurologica Scandinavica*, 1996, 94(6), 411-414.

Medina, JH; Izquierdo, I. Retrograde messengers, long-term potentiation and memory. *Brain Res Brain Res Rev*, 1995, 21(2), 185-194.

Myslivecek, J; Hassmannova, J; Barcal, J; Safanda, J; Zalud, V. Inhibitory learning and memory in newborn rats influenced by nitric oxide. *Neuroscience*, 1996, 71(2), 299-312.

Ohno, M; Yamamoto, T; Watanabe, S. Intrahippocampal administration of the NO synthase inhibitor L-NAME prevents working memory deficits in rats exposed to transient cerebral ischemia. *Brain Research*, 1994, 634(1), 173-177.

Noda, Y; Yamada, K; Nabeshima, T. Role of nitric oxide in the effect of aging on spatial memory in rats. *Behavioural Brain Research*, 1997, 83(1-2), 153-158.

Ohno, M; Yamamoto, T; Watanabe, S. Deficits in working memory following inhibition of hippocampal nitric oxide synthesis in the rat. *Brain Research*, 1993, 632(1-2), 36-40.

Paakkari, I; Lindsberg, P. Nitric oxide in the central nervous system. *Ann Med*, 1995, 27(3), 369-377.

Fudenberg, HH; Whitten, HD; Arnaud, P; Khansari, N. Is Alzheimer's disease an immunological disorder? Observations and speculations. *Clin Immunol Immunopathol*, 1984, 32(2), 127-131.

Ingram, DK; Spangler, EL; Iijima, S; Ikari, H; Kuo, H; Greig, NH; London, ED. Rodent models of memory dysfunction in Alzheimer's disease and normal aging: moving beyond the cholinergic hypothesis. *Life Sci*, 1994, 55(25-26), 2037-2049.

Dubovik, V; Faigon, M; Feldon, J; Michaelson, DM. Decreased density of forebrain cholinergic neurons in experimental autoimmune dementia. *Neuroscience*, 1993, 56(1), 75-82.

Miyagawa, K; Narita, M; Akama, H; Suzuki, T. Memory impairment associated with a dysfunction of the hippocampal cholinergic system induced by prenatal and neonatal exposures to bisphenol-A. *Neurosci Lett*, 2007, 418(3), 236-241.

Walsh, TJ; Herzog, CD; Gandhi, C; Stackman, RW; Wiley, RG. Injection of IgG 192-saporin into the medial septum produces cholinergic hypofunction and dose-dependent working memory deficits. *Brain Research*, 1996, 726(1-2), 69-79.

Choi, SH; Park, CH; Koo, JW; Seo, JH; Kim, HS; Jeong, SJ; Lee, JH; Kim, SS; Suh, YH. Memory impairment and cholinergic dysfunction by centrally administered Abeta and carboxyl-terminal fragment of Alzheimer's APP in mice. *FASEB Journal*, 2001, 15(10), 1816-1818.

Hall, ZW; Kelly, RB. Enzymatic detachment of endplate acetylcholinesterase from muscle. *Nat New Biol*, 1971, 232(28), 62-63.

Alvarez, A; Opazo, C; Alarcon, R; Garrido, J; Inestrosa, NC. Acetylcholinesterase promotes the aggregation of amyloid-beta-peptide fragments by forming a complex with the growing fibrils. *Journal of Molecular Biology*, 1997, 272(3), 348-361.

Mesulam, MM. Alzheimer plaques and cortical cholinergic innervation. *Neuroscience*, 1986, 17(1), 275-276.

Moran, MA; Mufson, EJ; Gomez-Ramos, P. Colocalization of cholinesterases with beta amyloid protein in aged and Alzheimer's brains. *Acta Neuropathol*, 1993, 85(4), 362-369.

Mori, F; Lai, CC; Fusi, F; Giacobini, E. Cholinesterase inhibitors increase secretion of APPs in rat brain cortex. *NeuroReport*, 1995, 6(4), 633-636.

Inestrosa, NC; Alvarez, A; Calderon, F. Acetylcholinesterase is a senile plaque component that promotes assembly of amyloid beta-peptide into Alzheimer's filaments. *Mol Psychiatry*, 1996, 1(5), 359-361.

Inestrosa, NC; Alvarez, A; Perez, CA; Moreno, RD; Vicente, M; Linker, C; Casanueva, OI; Soto, C; Garrido, J. Acetylcholinesterase accelerates assembly of amyloid-beta-peptides into Alzheimer's fibrils: possible role of the peripheral site of the enzyme. *Neuron*, 1996, 16(4), 881-891.

Beeri, R; Andres, C; Lev-Lehman, E; Timberg, R; Huberman, T; Shani, M; Soreq, H. Transgenic expression of human acetylcholinesterase induces progressive cognitive deterioration in mice. *Current Biology*, 1995, 5(9), 1063-1071.

Sihver, W; Gunther, P; Schliebs, R; Bigl, V. Repeated administration of tacrine to normal rats: effects on cholinergic, glutamatergic, and GABAergic receptor subtypes in rat brain using receptor autoradiography. *Neurochemistry International*, 1997, 31(5), 693-703.

Araujo, DM; Lapchak, PA; Collier, B; Quirion, R. Localization of interleukin-2 immunoreactivity and interleukin-2 receptors in the rat brain: interaction with the cholinergic system. *Brain Research*, 1989, 498(2), 257-266.

Hanisch, UK; Seto, D; Quirion, R. Modulation of hippocampal acetylcholine release: a potent central action of interleukin-2. *The Journal of Neuroscience*, 1993, 13(8), 3368-3374.

Lapchak, PA; Araujo, DM; Quirion, R; Beaudet, A. Immunoautoradiographic localization of interleukin 2-like immunoreactivity and interleukin 2 receptors (Tac antigen-like immunoreactivity) in the rat brain. *Neuroscience*, 1991, 44(1), 173-184.

Nistico, G; De Sarro, G. Is interleukin 2 a neuromodulator in the brain? *Trends in Neurosciences*, 1991, 14(4), 146-150.

Li, Y; Liu, L; Kang, J; Sheng, JG; Barger, SW; Mrak, RE; Griffin, WS. Neuronal-glial interactions mediated by interleukin-1 enhance neuronal acetylcholinesterase activity and mRNA expression. *The Journal of Neuroscience*, 2000, 20(1), 149-155.

Aisen, PS; Davis, KL. Inflammatory mechanisms in Alzheimer's disease: implications for therapy. *America Journal of Psychiatry*, 1994, 151(8), 1105-1113.

McGeer, PL; Rogers, J. Anti-inflammatory agents as a therapeutic approach to Alzheimer's disease. *Neurology*, 1992, 42(2), 447-449.

Rich, JB; Rasmusson, DX; Folstein, MF; Carson, KA; Kawas, C; Brandt, J. Nonsteroidal anti-inflammatory drugs in Alzheimer's disease. *Neurology*, 1995, 45(1), 51-55.

Rogers, J; Kirby, LC; Hempelman, SR; Berry, DL; McGeer, PL; Kaszniak, AW; Zalinski, J; Cofield, M; Mansukhani, L; Willson, P; et al. Clinical trial of indomethacin in Alzheimer's disease. *Neurology*, 1993, 43(8), 1609-1611.

Burger, D; Dayer, JM. IL-1Ra, in *Cytokine Reference*, O.J.a.F. M, Editor., 2000, Academic Press: Orlando, FL. 319-336.

Dinarello, C. IL-1a, in *Cytokine Reference*, O.J.a.F. M, Editor. 2000, Academic Press: Orlando, FL. 307-318.

Dinarello, C. IL-1b, in *Cytokine Reference*, O.J.a.F. M, Editor. 2000, Academic Press: Orlando, FL. 351-374.

Loddick, SA; Liu, C; Takao, T; Hashimoto, K; De Souza, EB. Interleukin-1 receptors: cloning studies and role in central nervous system disorders. *Brain Res Brain Res Rev*, 1998, 26(2-3), 306-319.

Vitkovic, L; Bockaert, J; Jacque, C. "Inflammatory" cytokines: neuromodulators in normal brain? *Journal of Neurochemistry*, 2000, 74(2), 457-471.

Berkenbosch, F; van Oers, J; del Rey, A; Tilders, F; Besedovsky, H. Corticotropin-releasing factor-producing neurons in the rat activated by interleukin-1. *Science*, 1987, 238(4826), 524-526.

Murray, C; McGahon, B; McBennet, S; Lynch, M. Interleukin-1b inhibits glutamate release in hippocampus of young, but not aged, rats. *Neurobiology of Aging*, 1997, 18, 343-348.

Plata-Salaman, CR; ffrench-Mullen, JM. Interleukin-1 beta inhibits Ca2+ channel currents in hippocampal neurons through protein kinase C. *European Journal of Pharmacology*, 1994, 266(1), 1-10.

Rada, P; Mark, GP; Vitek, MP; Mangano, RM; Blume, AJ; Beer, B; Hoebel, BG. Interleukin-1 beta decreases acetylcholine measured by microdialysis in the hippocampus of freely moving rats. *Brain Research*, 1991, 550(2), 287-290.

Cunningham, AJ; Murray, CA; O'Neill, LA; Lynch, MA; O'Connor, JJ. Interleukin-1 beta (IL-1 beta) and tumour necrosis factor (TNF) inhibit long-term potentiation in the rat dentate gyrus in vitro. *Neurosci Lett*, 1996, 203(1), 17-20.

Bellinger, F; Madamba, S; Siggins, G. Interleukin-1b inhibits synaptic strength and long-term potentiation in the rat CA1 hippocampus. *Brain Research*, 1993, 628, 227-234.

Katsuki, H; Nakai, S; Hirai, Y; Akaji, K; Kiso, Y; Satoh, M. Interleukin-1b inhibits long-term potentiation in the CA3 region of mouse hippocampal slices. *European Journal of Neuroscience*, 1990, 181, 323-326.

Murray, C; Lynch, M. Evidence that increased hippocampal expression of the cytokine interleukin-1b is a common trigger for age- and stress-induced impairments in long-term potentiation. *The Journal of Neuroscience*, 1998, 18(8), 2974-2981.

Schneider, H; Pitossi, F; Balschun, D; Wagner, A; del Rey, A; Besedovsky, HO. A neuromodulatory role of interleukin-1beta in the hippocampus. *Proc Natl Acad Sci,* U S A, 1998, 95(13), 7778-7783.

Vereker, E; O´Donnell, E; Lynch, A; Kelly, A; Nolan, Y; Lynch, M. Evidence that interleukin-1b and reactive oxygen species production play a pivotal role in stress-induced impairment of LTP in the rat dentate gyrus. *European Journal of Neuroscience*, 2001, 14, 1809-1819.

Oitzl, MS; van Oers, H; Schobitz, B; de Kloet, ER. Interleukin-1 beta, but not interleukin-6, impairs spatial navigation learning. *Brain Research*, 1993, 613(1), 160-163.

Pugh, CR; Johnson, JD; Martin, D; Rudy, JW; Maier, SF; Watkins, LR. Human immunodeficiency virus-1 coat protein gp120 impairs contextual fear conditioning: a potential role in AIDS related learning and memory impairments. *Brain Research*, 2000, 861(1), 8-15.

Opp, MR; Rady, PL; Hughes, TK, Jr. Cadet, P; Tyring, SK; Smith, EM. Human immunodeficiency virus envelope glycoprotein 120 alters sleep and induces cytokine mRNA expression in rats [published errata appear in Am J Physiol 1996, Aug; 271(2 Pt 2), section R following table of contents and 1996 Dec;271(6 Pt 3), section R following table of contents]. *American Journal of Physiology*, 1996, 270(5 Pt 2), R963-970.

Matsumoto, Y; Yoshida, M; Watanabe, S; Yamamoto, T. Involvement of cholinergic and glutamatergic functions in working memory impairment induced by interleukin-1b in rats. *European Journal of Pharmacology*, 2001, 430, 283-288.

Barrientos, R; Higgins, E; Sprunger, D; Watkins, L; Rudy, J; Maier, S. Memory for context is impaired by a post context exposure injection of interleukin-1 beta into dorsal hippocampus. *Behavioural Brain Research*, 2002, 134, 291-298.

Palin, K; Bluthe, RM; Verrier, D; Tridon, V; Dantzer, R; Lestage, J. Interleukin-1beta mediates the memory impairment associated with a delayed type hypersensitivity response to bacillus Calmette-Guerin in the rat hippocampus. *Brain, Behavior, and Immunity*, 2004, 18(3), 223-230.

Hein, AM; Stutzman, DL; Bland, ST; Barrientos, RM; Watkins, LR; Rudy, JW; Maier, SF. Prostaglandins are necessary and sufficient to induce contextual fear learning impairments after interleukin-1 beta injections into the dorsal hippocampus. *Neuroscience*, 2007, 150(4), 754-763.

Yirmiya, R; Winocur, G; Goshen, I. Brain interleukin-1 is involved in spatial memory and passive avoidance conditioning. *Neurobiology of Learning and Memory*, 2002, 78(2), 379-389.

Konsman, J; Tridon, V; Dantzer, R. Difussion and action or intracerebroventricularly injected interleukin-1 in the CNS. *Neuroscience*, 2000, 101(4), 957-967.

Avital, A; Goshen, I; Kamsler, A; Segal, M; Iverfeldt, K; Richter-Levin, G; Yirmiya, R. Impaired interleukin-1 signaling is associated with deficits in hippocampal memory processes and neural plasticity. *Hippocampus*, 2003, 13(7), 826-834.

Labow, M; Shuster, D; Zetterstorm, M; Nunes, P; Terry, R; Cullinan, E; Bartfei, T; Solorzano, C; Moldawer, L; Chizzonite, R; McIntyre, K. Absence of IL-1 signaling and reduced inflammatory response in IL-1 type I receptor-deficient mice. *The Journal of Immunology*, 1997, 159, 2452-2461.

Wolf, G; Yirmiya, R; Goshen, I; Iverfeldt, K; Holmlund, L; Takeda, K; Shavit, Y. Impairment of interleukin-1 (IL-1) signaling reduces basal pain sensitivity in mice: genetic, pharmacological and developmental aspects. *Pain*, 2003, 104, 471-480.

Depino, AM; Alonso, M; Ferrari, C; del Rey, A; Anthony, D; Besedovsky, H; Medina, JH; Pitossi, F. Learning modulation by endogenous hippocampal IL-1: blockade of endogenous IL-1 facilitates memory formation. *Hippocampus*, 2004, 14(4), 526-535.

Alonso, M; Vianna, MR; Depino, AM; Mello e Souza, T; Pereira, P; Szapiro, G; Viola, H; Pitossi, F; Izquierdo, I; Medina, JH. BDNF-triggered events in the rat hippocampus are required for both short- and long-term memory formation. *Hippocampus*, 2002, 12(4), 551-560.

Izquierdo, I; Medina, J. Memory formation: The sequence of biochemical events in the hippocampus and its connection to activity in other brain structures. *Neurobiology of Learning and Memory*, 1997, 68, 285-316.

Igaz, L; Vianna, M; Medina, J; Izquierdo, I. Two time periods of hippocampal mRNA synthesis are required for memory consolidation of fear-motivated learning. *The Journal of Neuroscience*, 2002, 22(15), 6781-6789.

Nguyen, K; Deak, T; Owens, S; Kohno, T; Fleshner, M; Watkins, L; Maier, S. Exposure to acute stress induces brain interleukin-1b protein in rat. *The Journal of Neuroscience*, 1998, 18(6), 2239-2246.

Bianchi, M; Dib, B; Panerai, A. Interleukin-1 and nociception in the rat. *Journal of Neuroscience Research*, 1998, 53, 645-650.

Zou, CJ; Liu, JD; Zhou, YC. Roles of central interleukin-1 on stress-induced-hypertension and footshock-induced-analgesia in rats. *Neurosci Lett*, 2001, 311(1), 41-44.

Pittenger, C; Huang, YY; Paletzki, RF; Bourtchouladze, R; Scanlin, H; Vronskaya, S; Kandel, ER. Reversible inhibition of CREB/ATF transcription factors in region CA1 of the dorsal hippocampus disrupts hippocampus-dependent spatial memory. *Neuron*, 2002, 34, 447-462.

Shimizu, E; Tang, YP; Rampon, C; Tsien, J. NMDA receptor-dependent synaptic reinforcement as a crucial process for memory consolidation. *Science*, 2000, 290, 1170-1174.

Genoux, D; Haditsch, U; Knobloch, M; Michalon, A; Storm, D; Mansuy, I. Protein phosphatase 1 is a molecular constraint on learning and memory. *Nature*, 2002, 418, 970-975.

Acquas, E; Wilson, C; Fibiger, H. Conditioned and unconditioned stimuli increase frontal cortical and hippocampal acetylcholine release: Effects of novelty, habituation, and fear. *The Journal of Neuroscience*, 1996, 16(9), 3089-3096.

Thiel, C; Huston, J; Schwarting, R. Hippocampal acetylcholine and habituation learning. *Neuroscience*, 1998, 85(4), 1253-1262.

Vianna, M; Alonso, M; Viola, H; Quevedo, J; de Paris, F; Furman, M; Levi de Stein, M; Medina, J; Izquierdo, I. Role of hippocampal signaling pathways in long-term memory formation of a nonassociative learning task in the rat. *Learning & Memory*, 2000, 7, 333-340.

Izquierdo, I; Medina, J. The biochemistry of memory formation and its regulation by hormones and neurotransmitters. *Psychobiology*, 1997, 25, 1-9.

McGaugh, J; Roozendaal, B. Role of adrenal stress hormones in forming lasting memories in the brain. *Current Opinion in Neurobiology*, 2002, 12, 205-210.

Goshen, I; Kreisel, T; Ounallah-Saad, H; Renbaum, P; Zalzstein, Y; Ben-Hur, T; Levy-Lahad, E; Yirmiya, R. A dual role for interleukin-1 in hippocampal-dependent memory processes. *Psychoneuroendocrinology*, 2007, 32(8-10), 1106-1115.

Spulber, S; Mateos, L; Oprica, M; Cedazo-Minguez, A; Bartfai, T; Winblad, B; Schultzberg, M. Impaired long term memory consolidation in transgenic mice overexpressing the human soluble form of IL-1ra in the brain. *Journal of Neuroimmunology*, 2009, 208(1-2), 46-53.

Trompet, S; de Craen, AJ; Slagboom, P; Shepherd, J; Blauw, GJ; Murphy, MB; Bollen, EL; Buckley, BM; Ford, I; Gaw, A; Macfarlane, PW; Packard, CJ; Stott, DJ; Jukema, JW; Westendorp, RG. Genetic variation in the interleukin-1 beta-converting enzyme associates with cognitive function. The PROSPER study. *Brain*, 2008, 131(Pt 4), 1069-1077.

Tsai, SJ; Hong, CJ; Liu, ME; Hou, SJ; Yen, FC; Hsieh, CH; Liou, YJ. Interleukin-1 beta (C-511T) genetic polymorphism is associated with cognitive performance in elderly males without dementia. *Neurobiology of Aging*, 2008.

Pociot, F; Molvig, J; Wogensen, L; Worsaae, H; Nerup, J. A TaqI polymorphism in the human interleukin-1 beta (IL-1 beta) gene correlates with IL-1 beta secretion in vitro. *Eur J Clin Invest*, 1992, 22(6), 396-402.

Hirano, T; Akira, S; Taga, T; Kishimoto, T. Biological and clinical aspects of interleukin 6. *Immunology Today*, 1990, 11(12), 443-449.

Pousset, F. Developmental expression of cytokine genesin the cortex and hippocampus of the rat central nervous system. *Developmental Brain Research*, 1994, 81, 143-146.

Gadient, RA; Otten, U. Expression of interleukin-6 (IL-6) and interleukin-6 receptor (IL-6R) mRNAs in rat brain during postnatal development. *Brain Research*, 1994, 637, 10-14.

Schöbitz, B; de Kloet, ER; Sutanto, W; Holsboer, F. Cellular localization of interleukin 6 mRNA and interleukin 6 receptor mRNA in rat brain. *European Journal of Neuroscience*, 1993, 5, 1426-1435.

Sallmann, S; Juttler, E; Prinz, S; Petersen, N; Knopf, U; Weiser, T; Schwaninger, M. Induction of interleukin-6 by depolarization of neurons. *The Journal of Neuroscience*, 2000, 20(23), 8637-8642.

Kushima, Y; Hama, T; Hatanaka, H. Interleukin-6 as a neurotrophic factor for promoting the survival of cultured catecholaminergic neurons in a chemically defined medium from fetal and postnatal rat midbrains. *Neurosci Res*, 1992, 13(4), 267-280.

Kushima, Y; Hatanaka, H. Interleukin-6 and leukemia inhibitory factor promote the survival of acetylcholinesterase-positive neurons in culture from embryonic rat spinal cord. *Neurosci Lett*, 1992, 143(1-2), 110-114.

Hama, T; Kushima, Y; Miyamoto, M; Kubota, M; Takei, N; Hatanaka, H. Interleukin-6 improves the survival of mesencephalic catecholaminergic and septal cholinergic neurons from postnatal, two-week-old rats in cultures. *Neuroscience*, 1991, 40(2), 445-452.

Satoh, T; Nakamura, S; Taga, T; Matsuda, T; Hirano, T; Kishimoto, T; Kaziro, Y. Induction of neuronal differentiation in PC12 cells by B-cell stimulatory factor 2/interleukin 6. *Mol Cell Biol*, 1988, 8(8), 3546-3549.

Plata-Salaman, CR. Food intake suppression by growth factors and platelet peptides by direct action in the central nervous system. *Neurosci Lett*, 1988, 94(1-2), 161-166.

LeMay, LG; Vander, AJ; Kluger, MJ. Role of interleukin 6 in fever in rats. *American Journal of Physiology*, 1990, 258(3 Pt 2), R798-803.

Naitoh, Y; Fukata, J; Tominaga, T; Nakai, Y; Tamai, S; Mori, K; Imura, H. Interleukin-6 stimulates the secretion of adrenocorticotropic hormone in conscious, freely-moving rats. *Biochem Biophys Res Commun*, 1988, 155(3), 1459-1463.

Campbell, IL; Abraham, CR; Masliah, E; Kemper, P; Inglis, JD; Oldstone, MBA; Mucke, L. Neurologic disease induced in transgenic mice by cerebral overexpression of interleukin 6. *Proceedings of National Academy of Sciences*, 1993, 90, 10061-10065.

Heyser, CJ; Masliah, E; Samimi, A; Campbell, IL; Gold, LH. Progressive decline in avoidance learning paralleled by inflammatory neurodegeneration in transgenic mice expressing interleukin 6 in the brain. *Proc Natl Acad Sci,* U S A, 1997, 94(4), 1500-1505.

Braida, D; Sacerdote, P; Panerai, AE; Bianchi, M; Aloisi, AM; Iosue, S; Sala, M. Cognitive function in young and adult IL (interleukin)-6 deficient mice. *Behavioural Brain Research*, 2004, 153(2), 423-429.

Baier, PC; May, U; Scheller, J; Rose-John, S; Schiffelholz, T. Impaired hippocampus-dependent and -independent learning in IL-6 deficient mice. *Behavioural Brain Research*, 2009, 200(1), 192-196.

Weaver, JD; Huang, MH; Albert, M; Harris, T; Rowe, JW; Seeman, TE. Interleukin-6 and risk of cognitive decline: MacArthur studies of successful aging. *Neurology*, 2002, 59(3), 371-378.

Harding, DR; Humphries, SE; Whitelaw, A; Marlow, N; Montgomery, HE. Cognitive outcome and cyclo-oxygenase-2 gene (-765 G/C) variation in the preterm infant. *Arch Dis Child Fetal Neonatal Ed*, 2007, 92(2), F108-112.

Mattson, MP; Bruce, AJ; Blane, EM, Cellular actions of tumor necrosis factor in ischemic brain injury., in *Pharmacology of Cerebral Ischemia.*, J; Krieglstein, Editor. 1996, 93-105.

Munoz-Fernandez, MA; Fresno, M. The role of tumour necrosis factor, interleukin 6, interferon-gamma and inducible nitric oxide synthase in the development and pathology of the nervous system. *Progress in Neurobiology*, 1998, 56(3), 307-340.

Chen, G; Goeddel, DV. TNF-R1 signaling: a beautiful pathway. *Science*, 2002, 296(5573), 1634-1635.

Baud, V; Karin, M. Signal transduction by tumor necrosis factor and its relatives. *Trends Cell Biol*, 2001, 11(9), 372-377.

MacEwan, DJ. TNF receptor subtype signalling: differences and cellular consequences. *Cell Signal*, 2002, 14(6), 477-492.

Blond, D; Campbell, SJ; Butchart, AG; Perry, VH; Anthony, DC. Differential induction of interleukin-1beta and tumour necrosis factor-alpha may account for specific patterns of leukocyte recruitment in the brain. *Brain Research*, 2002, 958(1), 89-99.

Depino, A; Ferrari, C; Pott Godoy, MC; Tarelli, R; Pitossi, FJ. Differential effects of interleukin-1beta on neurotoxicity, cytokine induction and glial reaction in specific brain regions. *Journal of Neuroimmunology*, 2005, 168(1-2), 96-110.

Probert, L; Akassoglou, K; Pasparakis, M; Kontogeorgos, G; Kollias, G. Spontaneous inflammatory demyelinating disease in transgenic mice showing central nervous system-specific expression of tumor necrosis factor alpha. *Proc Natl Acad Sci* U S A, 1995, 92(24), 11294-11298.

Bruce, AJ; Boling, W; Kindy, MS; Peschon, J; Kraemer, PJ; Carpenter, MK; Holtsberg, FW; Mattson, MP. Altered neuronal and microglial responses to excitotoxic and ischemic brain injury in mice lacking TNF receptors. *Nat Med*, 1996, 2(7), 788-794.

Liu, J; Marino, MW; Wong, G; Grail, D; Dunn, A; Bettadapura, J; Slavin, AJ; Old, L; Bernard, CC. TNF is a potent anti-inflammatory cytokine in autoimmune-mediated demyelination. *Nat Med*, 1998, 4(1), 78-83.

Butler, MP; O'Connor, JJ; Moynagh, PN. Dissection of tumor-necrosis factor-alpha inhibition of long-term potentiation (LTP) reveals a p38 mitogen-activated protein kinase-dependent mechanism which maps to early-but not late-phase LTP. *Neuroscience*, 2004, 124(2), 319-326.

Cumiskey, D; Butler, MP; Moynagh, PN; O'Connor J, J. Evidence for a role for the group I metabotropic glutamate receptor in the inhibitory effect of tumor necrosis factor-alpha on long-term potentiation. *Brain Research*, 2007, 1136(1), 13-19.

Beattie, EC; Stellwagen, D; Morishita, W; Bresnahan, JC; Ha, BK; Von Zastrow, M; Beattie, MS; Malenka, RC. Control of synaptic strength by glial TNFalpha. *Science*, 2002, 295(5563), 2282-2285.

Stellwagen, D; Malenka, RC. Synaptic scaling mediated by glial TNF-alpha. *Nature*, 2006, 440(7087), 1054-1059.

Fiore, M; Probert, L; Kollias, G; Akassoglou, K; Alleva, E; Aloe, L. Neurobehavioral alterations in developing transgenic mice expressing TNF-alpha in the brain. *Brain, Behavior, and Immunity*, 1996, 10(2), 126-138.

Aloe, L; Properzi, F; Probert, L; Akassoglou, K; Kassiotis, G; Micera, A; Fiore, M. Learning abilities, NGF and BDNF brain levels in two lines of TNF-alpha transgenic mice, one characterized by neurological disorders, the other phenotypically normal. *Brain Research*, 1999, 840(1-2), 125-137.

Fiore, M; Angelucci, F; Alleva, E; Branchi, I; Probert, L; Aloe, L. Learning performances, brain NGF distribution and NPY levels in transgenic mice expressing TNF-alpha. *Behavioural Brain Research*, 2000, 112(1-2), 165-175.

Iida, R; Saito, K; Yamada, K; Basile, AS; Sekikawa, K; Takemura, M; Fujii, H; Wada, H; Seishima, M; Nabeshima, T. Suppression of neurocognitive damage in LP-BM5-infected mice with a targeted deletion of the TNF-alpha gene. *FASEB Journal*, 2000, 14(7), 1023-1031.

McAfoose, J; Koerner, H; Baune, BT. The effects of TNF deficiency on age-related cognitive performance. *Psychoneuroendocrinology*, 2009, 34(4), 615-619.

Baune, BT; Ponath, G; Rothermundt, M; Riess, O; Funke, H; Berger, K. Association between genetic variants of IL-1beta, IL-6 and TNF-alpha cytokines and cognitive performance in the elderly general population of the MEMO-study. *Psychoneuroendocrinology*, 2008, 33(1), 68-76.

In: Learning and Memory Developments...
Editors: L. C. Eklund, A. S. Nyman, pp. 103-126
ISBN: 978-1-60876-397-9

Chapter 4

PERCEPTIONS OF FORGETFULNESS IN ADULTHOOD: DOES MEMORY KNOWLEDGE MATTER?

Susan Brigman and Katie E. Cherry*
Louisiana State University.

ABSTRACT

We examined the effects of age and knowledge of memory aging on subjective appraisals of memory in forgetful others using a person perception paradigm. Younger and older adults were tested in one of three information conditions: no information control group, grandparent seminar group, and memory aging seminar group. All completed the Knowledge Memory of Aging Questionnaire (KMAQ; Cherry, Brigman, Hawley, & Reese, 2003) at pretest and posttest to evaluate changes in memory aging knowledge. All read vignettes that described forgetful younger (in their 20's to 30's) or older characters (in their 60's to 70's). Attribution ratings on the potential causes of the forgetful behavior and memory opinion ratings were solicited. All completed the Memory Functioning Questionnaire (MFQ; Gilewski, Zelinski, & Schaie, 1990) at posttest to measure self-perceived memory ability. Both age groups showed an age-based double standard in memory appraisal. Attribution and memory opinion ratings did not vary across the information groups. Only the memory aging seminar participants showed significant pre- to posttest gains on the KMAQ. Self-perceived memory functioning was significantly correlated with perceptions of forgetful characters. These data indicate that although memory knowledge improved following instruction, perceptions of forgetfulness in older adults were not influenced by increased knowledge of normative age-associated memory changes.

* Corresponding author: Department of Psychology, Louisiana State University, Baton Rouge, LA, 70803-5501, (225) 578-8745, fax: (225) 578-4125, email: pskatie@lsu.edu.

INTRODUCTION

People of all ages experience forgetfulness in daily life, although lapses of memory occur more frequently in late adulthood. To be precise, adult age differences in self-perceived memory functioning have been documented in survey and questionnaire studies (e.g., Reese & Cherry, 2006) and in the types of everyday information that younger and older people find difficult to recall (Reese & Cherry, 2004). Other evidence has shown that declining memory ability and forgetfulness is expected in older persons (Ryan, 1992; Ryan & Kwong See, 1993). Hummert (1999) has suggested that age is one category upon which schemas are based, activating positive as well as negative aging stereotypes. Consequently, an older person who is forgetful may activate a negative aging stereotype in others that can subsequently influence the social judgments we make about that person. Understanding the variables that influence people's perceptions of the causes of forgetful behavior, as well as their opinions of the forgetful person, is an important challenge for applied researchers.

Erber and her colleagues have examined people's views of everyday memory failures in forgetful, fictitious characters using a person perception paradigm where participants rate the perceived causes of forgetful behavior along six dimensions. In many studies, Erber and her colleagues found an age-based double standard where forgetful behavior is evaluated differently depending upon the age of the forgetful person (see Erber & Prager, 1999, for review). For instance, Erber, Szuchman, and Rothberg (1990a, 1990b) found that forgetfulness in younger fictitious characters was more often attributed to lack of effort and attention compared to the same memory failures in older characters, which were likely to be attributed to lack of ability, an internal stable factor (see also Erber & Rothberg, 1991; Parr & Siegert, 1993). Age of the participant has also been shown to be important with younger adults, compared to older adults, rating memory failures in older fictitious characters as more serious (Erber, 1989), as a greater sign of mental difficulty, and in need of professional evaluation (Erber et al., 1990a).

The present research was designed to examine the influence of younger and older adults' knowledge of memory aging on their appraisals of fictitious forgetful persons using an adapted version of Erber et al.'s (1990a) person perception paradigm. Cherry and her associates have made the point that understanding the difference between normal and pathological memory aging is necessary for people to have appropriate expectations for elderly persons and avoid ageist stereotypes that depict a negative image of cognitive capability in late life. In particular, normal memory aging is the result of natural maturational processes, while pathological memory aging is due to non-normative factors such as disease or trauma to the brain (see Cherry & Smith, 1998, for discussion). Ample experimental evidence has shown that people are less knowledgeable about normative age-related memory changes compared to pathological memory deficits using the Knowledge of Memory Aging Questionnaire (KMAQ; Cherry, Brigman, Hawley, & Reese, 2003; see also Hawley, Cherry, Su, Chiu, & Jazwinski, 2006; Reese, Cherry, & Copeland, 2000). Whether individuals' knowledge of normative age-related memory changes affects their perceptions of forgetful behavior in others is not clear, as this issue has not been systematically examined in previous research to date.

In this study, we examine the contribution of age and memory knowledge to memory appraisal of forgetful others using both an experimental and individual difference approach to the research problem. The experimental approach involved testing participants in one of three information conditions: a no information control group, a grandparent seminar group who received information concerning social functioning in later adulthood, or a memory seminar group who were given specific information about normative cognitive functioning in later adulthood. All participants read short vignettes depicting either younger (25-35 years old) or older (65-75 years old) target characters experiencing identical instances of everyday forgetting (e.g., forgetting the name of a new acquaintance). They made attribution judgments regarding the perceived causes of the forgetting along six dimensions: lack of ability, effort, task difficulty, bad luck, and two measures of attention (external and internal distractions). They also evaluated the target characters' memory in terms of whether the forgetting was (a) a sign of mental difficulty, (b) in need of memory training, and (c) in need of professional evaluation (either medical or psychological).

We also included an individual difference approach to the study of memory appraisal in late adulthood. Appraisals of forgetful others may be influenced by participants' veridical knowledge of memory aging and by subjective beliefs about their own memory functioning. To test this notion, participants in this study completed the KMAQ (Cherry et al., 2003) and the Memory Functioning Questionnaire (MFQ; Gilewski, Zelinski, & Schaie, 1990). Together, these measures should provide new insight into the role of memory knowledge and self-perceived memory functioning as individual difference variables in younger and older adults' appraisals of fictitious forgetful characters.

To summarize, we hypothesized that knowledge of normative, age-related memory changes in later adulthood would be associated with more positive memory appraisals of forgetful older targets. Specifically, those attending the memory aging seminar were expected to show more positive perceptions of forgetful older adults than those in the two comparison groups who were expected to demonstrate the age-based double standard in perceptions of forgetfulness (Erber & Prager, 1999). Additionally, greater knowledge of normative memory aging issues and higher self-perceived memory functioning were expected to be associated with more positive perceptions of forgetful older adults. Such a pattern of outcomes would provide important new evidence on the hypothesized relationship between memory knowledge and memory appraisal in adulthood.

METHOD

Participants

In all, 192 individuals participated in this study. There were 96 undergraduate students (M = 20.04 years, SD = 1.60) who received extra credit in a psychology course. There were 96 community-dwelling older adults (M = 72.36 years, SD = 5.54) who were paid \$10.00 each for their participation. The majority of younger adults were female (87.5%), white (82.3%), and single (100%), and the majority of older adults were female (72.9%), white (97.9%), and married (65.6%). Participants' responses to a demographic questionnaire that contained a subset of self-perceived health questions from the Older American Resources and Services Multidimensional Functional Assessment Questionnaire (Duke University Center for the Study of Aging and Human Development, 1975) indicated that most were generally in good health. Older adults' mean self-perceived health score was somewhat lower compared to the younger adults with means of 2.07 and 1.80, respectively, $t(190) = -2.27$, $p = 0.02$. Older adults ($M = 1.90$) were more likely than younger adults ($M = 1.53$) to report that their health interfered with activities, $t(190) = -2.75$, $p = 0.007$. When evaluating their health in comparison to others their age, older adults ($M = 1.83$) gave lower ratings than younger adults ($M = 2.69$), $t(190) = 6.45$, $p < 0.001$, suggesting that the older adults in this study maintained an optimistic view of their current health status in comparison to age matched peers. Older adults ($M = 5.70$) reported higher educational attainment relative the younger adults' same-sex parent ($M = 5.40$), $t(186) = -2.07$, $p = 0.04$; with non-significant age group differences for occupational level ($p = 0.06$).

On a measure of verbal ability (Gardner & Monge, 1977), older adults ($M = 19.73$) scored higher than younger adults ($M = 12.61$), $t(190) = -10.80$, $p < 0.001$. Older adults ($M = 1.09$) scored significantly lower on the Geriatric Depression Scale-Short Form (GDS; Yesavage et al., 1983) than younger adults ($M = 2.26$), $t(189) = 3.60$, $p < 0.001$, although both age groups were well below the cutoff score of 6 representing mild depression. All demonstrated at least 20/30 corrected visual acuity assessed by a standard Snellen eye chart.

MATERIALS

Knowledge of Memory Aging Questionnaire. The KMAQ (Cherry et al., 2003) is a 28-item true/false/don't know measure of laypersons' knowledge of memory changes in adulthood for educational or research purposes. Half of the questions address knowledge of normal memory changes that occur in later life as a result of maturational processes (i.e., normal memory aging). The other half address knowledge of pathological memory changes that may be due to non-normative factors that affect memory functioning in older adults (i.e., physiological or psychopathological conditions, pharmacological agents, and/or adult dementia) yielding normal and pathological subscales. Initial work on the psychometric properties of the KMAQ yields evidence of convergent and discriminant validity (Cherry, West, Reese, Santa Maria, & Yassuda, 2000). Subsequent work has demonstrated content validity (Jackson, Cherry, Smitherman, & Hawley, 2008) and satisfactory internal consistency reliability (.76), though somewhat lower than standard conventions (.80) probably due to the diversity of topics that represent normal and pathological aging (Cherry, Allen, Olinde, Robichaux, & Hawley, 2008).

Self-Perceived Memory Functioning. The MFQ (Gilewski et al., 1990) was used as a self-report measure of perceived memory ability in this study. The MFQ assesses four areas of memory functioning: (a) frequency of specific types of forgetting (e.g., names, appointments, frequently used phone numbers, etc.), (b) seriousness of these same instances of forgetting, (c) current memory functioning in comparison to memory functioning in the past (e.g., 1 year ago, 5 years ago, 10 years ago, 20 years ago), and (d) usage of various mnemonic strategies (e.g., keeping an appointment book, making lists, etc). Higher scores on the MFQ reflect higher levels of perceived memory functioning (i.e., less forgetfulness, less serious perceptions of the forgetting, improvement in [or maintenance of] memory ability compared to earlier in life, and less use of mnemonics). Past research confirms that the MFQ possesses high internal consistency reliability (Gilewski et al., 1990) and adequate concurrent validity with other measures of memory (Zelinski, Gilewski, & Anthony-Bergstone, 1990; but see Zelinski, Gilewski, & Schaie, 1993).

Overview of Seminars. Participants in the grandparent seminar group watched a film entitled, "The Bond between the Generations" (33:32 running time), and participants in the memory aging seminar group watched a film entitled, "Memory and Aging" (36:47 running time). The first author developed, wrote, and performed both lectures presented in the films, which were edited to Digital Video Display (DVD). Films were presented on a 27" television set located approximately 2 feet in front of the table where participants were seated. The content of the films was made as comparable as possible and were similar to lectures one might receive in an introductory developmental psychology course.

To ensure participants were attentive during the showing of the films, they completed guided notes, which required them to answer basic questions as topics were introduced in the films. For example, the guided notes for the memory aging seminar asked, "*What are the 3 stages of memory?*", a topic explicitly covered in the film both verbally and visually with slides, and participants were to write in the blanks provided, "*sensory memory, short-term memory, and long-term memory*". A post-experimental review revealed that all but one older adult research participant correctly completed the majority of questions on the guided notes.

Grandparent Seminar. The content of the grandparent lecture focused on the unique relationship between grandparents and grandchildren, describing factors that influence emotional closeness between the generations. The grandparent seminar was designed to provide a lecture on an "aging" issue stylistically similar to the memory aging lecture, but focusing on a different content area in adulthood (i.e., social functioning versus cognitive functioning). The style and format of the two seminars were made as comparable as possible in that every effort was made to include the same number of topics as presented in the memory aging lecture described next.

Memory Aging Seminar. The content of the memory aging seminar was developed using the KMAQ as a guide (Cherry et al., 2003). The KMAQ is comprised of items that pertain to both normal memory changes that occur in later adulthood and pathological memory deficits due to non-normative factors affecting memory in older adults, such as adult dementia. Based on an item analyses from a sample of older adults ($N = 80$) who took the KMAQ as part of another experiment, seven normal memory aging items that were less well-known by participants were selected for inclusion in the lecture. Consequently, participants were expected to benefit from instruction on these items and decrease the likelihood that performance on these items would be at ceiling. Only older adults' scores on the KMAQ were included in this analysis because prior research documents age effects favoring older adults on the KMAQ (e.g., Cherry et al., 2003; Reese et al., 2000). Selecting items based on older adults' knowledge of memory aging increases the likelihood that these items are not well-known by this specific age group.

In the introduction of the lecture the distinction between normative memory changes associated with growing older and pathological memory deficits that are a result of disease was discussed. The lecture concluded with the "take home" message that memory is a skill that can be improved with effort and maintained throughout the life course (e.g., Lachman, Weaver, Bandura, Elliott, & Lewkowicz's, 1992, adaptive view of memory aging). Pilot studies confirmed the effectiveness of the lectures as instructional aids.

Vignettes. In all, eight vignettes modeled after Erber et al. (1990) were developed for this study (see Appendix). Each vignette described a target person experiencing a single instance of forgetting that matched one of Herrmann and Neisser's (1978) eight factors of everyday forgetting (e.g., rote, absentminded, names, people, conversation, errands, retrieval, and place). To control for possible gender-based attribution bias, half described a male target and the other half described a female target. Pilot testing confirmed that the forgetting described in each vignette was highly typical and perceived as equally likely to happen to both younger and older adults, to both males and females, and that there were no or only minor consequences as a result of the forgetting. To ensure that age of the target character was salient, a projector displayed a slide containing a photograph of the fictitious target person on a screen while participants read the vignettes. The photographs were taken from a pictorial church directory from a different city and state to ensure anonymity of the person in the photograph. Pilot work confirmed the approximate age of the individuals depicted in the photographs. All photographs were rated similarly in terms of perceived attractiveness, amount of social activity, degree of forgetfulness, level of independence/self-sufficiency, and degree of physical/mental disability.

Design and Procedure

The design was a 2 x 2 x 3 factorial with participant age (young, old), target characters' age (young, old), and information group (control, grandparent, memory aging) as between-group factors. Sixteen participants were tested in each condition. Participants were randomly assigned to one of the three information groups. They were tested in small groups of up to 4 persons across two testing sessions. In the first session, the individual difference measures were given. Afterward, those in the control group were dismissed for the day. Those assigned to the seminar information groups watched an educational video on their respective topic.

One week later, participants returned for the second session to complete the vignette rating task. Two practice vignettes were given to familiarize persons with the rating scales. Following practice, participants responded to six vignettes where fictitious, forgetful target characters were described. For each vignette, participants completed six causal attribution scales and three memory opinion scales. Half of the participants read vignettes about a target character in his/her 20-30's and the other half read about a person in his/her 60-70's.

All vignettes were read aloud by the experimenter. As each vignette was read, a slide containing a photograph of the fictitious target was displayed on a screen. The target's name and age introduced each new vignette (e.g., *This is a picture of Bill. Bill is a 76-year-old man who...*). To control for potential order effects, two presentation orders were used. Presentation order was counterbalanced so that each sequence appeared an equal number of times across participants and groups. Participants were instructed to complete the rating scales at their own pace, and it was stressed to participants that their opinions were the primary concern of the study. This task was followed by the second administration of the KMAQ. Debriefing followed.

Causal Attribution Ratings. Following Erber et al. (1990), participants rated the likelihood of six possible reasons of forgetting described in the vignettes: (a) poor memory ability, (b) lack of effort, (c) difficulty remembering that type of thing (i.e., task difficulty), (d) bad luck, and two attention attributions: (e) other things that might have been going on around the central character (external distraction), and (f) all the other things on the central character's mind (internal distraction). Attribution ratings were made using separate 7-point Likert scales, where 1 = *not at all a cause* and 7 = *very much a cause*.

Memory Opinion Ratings. The three memory opinion scales were: (a) how much do you think the central character's forgetting is a sign of mental difficulty (1 = *no indication of mental difficulty*; 7 = *without a doubt a sign of mental difficulty*), (b) how much do you think the central character should seek memory training techniques to improve his/her memory (1 = *definite need for memory training*; 7 = *no need for memory training*), and (c) at what point do you think evaluation should be recommended to determine whether the central character's forgetting was caused by medical and/or psychological problems (1 = *I see no need for evaluation no matter how often it happens*; 2 = *If it happens several times a day*; 3 = *If it happens once a day*; 4 = *If it happens several times a week*; 5 = *It if happens once a week*; 6 = *If it happens once a month*; 7 = *I recommend evaluation the first time it happens*). Higher ratings on the memory opinion scales suggest a poorer opinion of the target persons' memory.

RESULTS

Overview of Scoring and Analyses

These data were analyzed according to the following plan. For each participant, separate proportion correct scores for the KMAQ normal and pathological question types were calculated and submitted to a 2 (Participant Age) x 3 (Information Group) x 2 (Question Type) x 2 (Time of Test) mixed analysis of variance (ANOVA). MFQ ratings were submitted to a 2 (Participant Age) x 3 (Information Group) x 4 (MFQ Scale) mixed ANOVA[1]. Next, causal attribution and memory opinion ratings were submitted to separate 2 (Participant Age) x 2 (Target Age) x 3 (Information Group) x 6 (Vignette) repeated multivariate analyses of variance (MANOVA), using the Wilk's Λ test of significance. For MANOVA effects that reached significance (alpha = .05), univariate ANOVAs for each dependent measure were conducted and follow-up *t*-tests using Bonferroni corrections were performed. Participants' ratings on each of the nine 7-point Likert scales (causal attribution and memory opinion) for each of the six forgetting vignettes served as the dependent measures[2]. Partial correlation analyses were conducted to examine relationships among memory knowledge, self-perceived memory functioning, and causal attribution and memory opinion ratings, statistically controlling for age.

---

1 Because younger adults in this study ranged in age from 18 to 26 years, their scores to the retrospective functioning subscale were calculated omitting responses to the question, "*How is your memory compared to the way it was 20 years ago?*"

2 Missing values were replaced with the average rating for that scale using ratings from the remaining vignettes that were answered. Twenty-seven data points (less than .01% of the total data points) for 17 older participants were estimated in this manner.

Memory Knowledge

KMAQ means appear in Table 1. Replicating previous work (e.g., Cherry et al, 2003; Reese et al., 2000) older adults (M = .77) scored better then younger adults (M = .71), F(1, 186) = 21.32, p < .001. Fewer normal memory aging items (M = .71) were answered correctly than pathological memory aging items (M = .77), F(1, 186) = 34.23, p < .001. Posttest performance on the KMAQ (M = .75) exceeded pretest performance (M = .72), F(1, 186) = 12.29, p = .001. The Participant Age x Question Type interaction was also significant, F(1, 186) = 27.79, MS_e = .48, p < .001. Follow-up ANOVAs revealed no significant differences between younger and older adults on the normal memory aging KMAQ items (p = .56), however older adults (M = .82) scored significantly higher than younger adults (M = .71) on pathological memory aging items, F(1, 191) = 51.25, MS_e = .58, p < .001. The Time of Testing x Question Type interaction was also significant, F(1, 186) = 5.23, MS_e = .04, p = .02. Paired t-tests revealed a significant pre- to posttest improvement for normal memory aging items (M_{pre} = .69 vs. M_{post} = .76), t(191) = -3.64, p < .001, but not for pathological memory aging items (M_{pre} = .73 vs. M_{post} = .77, p = .17). There was a significant Information Group x Question Type interaction, F(2, 186) = 3.47, MS_e = .06, p = .03. Paired t-tests showed significant differences between normal and pathological memory aging items for participants in the control group (M_{norm} = .71 vs. M_{path} = .76), t(63) = -3.22, p = .002, and grandparent seminar group (M_{norm} = .69 vs. M_{path} = .78), t(63) = -4.58, p < .001. There was no significant difference between normal and pathological items for participants in the memory aging seminar group (M_{norm} = .73 vs. M_{path} = .76, p = .12).

Table 1. Mean Proportion Correct on Knowledge of Memory Aging Questionnaire

	Younger Adults				Older Adults			
	Pretest		Posttest		Pretest		Posttest	
Question Type	*M*	*SD*	*M*	*SD*	*M*	*SD*	*M*	*SD*
Control Group								
Normal	.73	0.09	.70	0.13	.68	0.18	.73	0.11
Pathological	.71	0.16	.74	0.11	.77	0.16	.82	0.13
Grandparent Group								
Normal	.68	0.14	.66	0.16	.68	0.18	.73	0.11
Pathological	.72	0.11	.70	0.14	.84	0.14	.85	0.10
Memory Aging Group								
Normal	.67	0.15	.79	0.13	.70	0.15	.77	0.10
Pathological	.70	0.11	.71	0.09	.82	0.10	.82	0.09

Interpretation of these effects was qualified by the significant Information Group x Question Type x Time of Testing interaction effect, F(2, 186) = 6.02, MS_e = .05, p = .003. Using a Bonferroni corrected alpha = .008, separate paired sample t-tests were conducted on proportion correct normal and pathological scores from pretest to posttest for each group. Only one significant difference was revealed: those in the memory aging seminar group showed a significant pre- to posttest improvement on normal memory aging items (M_{pre} = .69 vs. M_{post} = .78), t(63) = -4.44, p < .001. Participants in the control and grandparent groups did not show significant improvement on normal KMAQ items at posttest and none of the groups significantly improved at posttest on pathological KMAQ items.

To assess pre- to posttest improvement on KMAQ normal memory aging items addressed specifically in the memory aging video, a 2 (Time of Test) x 2 (Item: covered vs. not covered) repeated measures ANOVA was conducted on proportion correct scores for participants in the memory aging group. Significant main effects of time of testing, $F(1, 63) = 23.35$, $MS_e = .70$, $p < .001$, and item, $F(1, 63) = 14.48$, $MS_e = .50$, $p < .001$, were found. The Time x Item interaction was not significant ($p = .07$). Posttest performance (.78) was significantly greater than pretest performance (.68) on both items covered in the seminar as well as items not covered. Proportion correct was higher for items not covered in the seminar (.76) than for items covered in the seminar (.69), most likely because only items that were not well-known to participants were selected for inclusion in the seminar.

Self-Perceived Memory Functioning

MFQ means appear in Table 2. Younger adults' mean rating (4.17) exceeded the older adults' mean rating (3.93), a significant difference, $F(1, 177) = 9.38$, $MS_e = 10.80$, $p = .003$. The information group main effect was non-significant ($p = .57$), suggesting that the memory seminar did not influence participants' perceptions of their own memory ability. The main effect of subscale was significant, $F(3, 531) = 272.36$, $MS_e = 211.84$, $p < .001$. Mean ratings were highest for the frequency of forgetting subscale (5.19), followed by seriousness of forgetting (4.43), retrospective functioning (3.95), and mnemonics usage (2.63), which were all significantly different from one another. The interpretation of these effects was qualified by a significant Participant Age x Subscale interaction, $F(3, 531) = 18.30$, $MS_e = 14.23$, $p < .001$. Using a Bonferroni corrected alpha = .013, separate ANOVAs were conducted on each subscale. The only significant difference was on the retrospective memory functioning subscale, $F(1, 182) = 62.56$, $MS_e = 49.40$, $p < .001$. Younger adults ($M = 4.46$) reported slightly better current memory functioning compared to past memory functioning, whereas older adults ($M = 3.43$) reported slightly worse current compared to past memory functioning. Taken together, these results suggest that younger and older adults differ in their perceptions of past compared to present memory performance; however, the two age groups had similar views regarding the frequency and seriousness of current forgetting and reported comparable mnemonics usage.

Memory Appraisals

Causal Attribution Ratings. Mean attribution ratings appear in Table 3. The participant age main effect was significant, $F(6, 175) = 5.33$, $p < .001$. Replicating Parr and Siegert (1993), older participants gave higher ratings ($M = 3.11$) than did younger participants ($M = 2.56$) to the effort scale, $p = .003$, suggesting that older adults were more likely to endorse lack of effort as a cause for memory failures. The target age main effect was also significant, $F(6, 175) = 6.31$, $p < .001$. Five of the univariates were significant: ability, task difficulty, luck, and the two attention scales (external and internal). Old targets' memory failures ($M =$

4.12) were rated higher on the ability scale than young targets (M = 3.48), $F(1, 180) = 15.45$, $MS_e = 19.90$, $p < .001$. Old targets (M = 3.99) also received higher ratings on task difficulty than young targets (M = 3.65), $F(1, 180) = 5.27$, $MS_e = 5.53$, $p = .02$. In contrast, young targets (M = 1.89) were rated higher than old targets (M = 1.46) on bad luck, $F(1, 180) = 6.74$, $MS_e = 8.96$, $p = .01$, and both of the attention scales. Young targets (M = 4.41) received higher ratings for "other things going on around the central character" than old targets (M = 4.07), $F(1, 180) = 4.16$, $MS_e = 5.39$, $p = .04$. Young targets (M = 4.66) also received higher ratings for "other things on the central character's mind" than old targets (M = 4.18), $F(1, 180) = 7.60$, $MS_e = 11.10$, $p = .006$. Together, these findings replicate the age-based double standard (Erber et al., 1990a; Erber & Rothberg, 1991). Contrary to expectations, the MANOVA main effect of information group was not significant ($p = .53$, $\eta^2 = .03$, $1 - \beta = .54$) and did not participate in any significant interaction effects.

Table 2. Mean Ratings on the Memory Functioning Questionnaire.

	Participant Age			
	Younger Adults		Older Adults	
Subscale	M	SD	M	SD
Control Group				
Frequency of Forgetting	5.28	0.66	5.14	0.67
Seriousness of Forgetting	4.29	0.78	4.58	1.10
Retrospective Functioning	4.40	0.82	3.48	0.90
Mnemonics Usage	2.93	1.14	2.76	1.04
Grandparent Group				
Frequency of Forgetting	5.38	0.70	5.05	0.69
Seriousness of Forgetting	4.31	0.92	4.54	1.18
Retrospective Functioning	4.48	0.73	3.36	1.02
Mnemonics Usage	2.56	1.06	2.55	0.98
Memory Aging Group				
Frequency of Forgetting	5.22	0.68	5.06	0.55
Seriousness of Forgetting	4.44	1.22	4.44	1.12
Retrospective Functioning	4.54	1.04	3.46	0.84
Mnemonics Usage	2.22	0.95	2.73	1.17

Note. Higher scores reflect higher levels of perceived memory functioning (i.e., less forgetfulness, less serious perceptions of the forgetting, improvement in memory ability compared to earlier in life, and less use of mnemonics).

The vignette main effect was significant, $F(30, 151) = 10.72$, $p < .001$. The univariates for all six causal attribution rating scales were significant ($ps < .01$). To determine the locus of differences across the six vignettes, pairwise comparisons were performed on each univariate. On the ability scale, the mean rating for the people vignette was significantly higher (4.59) than the other vignettes, suggesting that participants were more likely to perceive forgetting a name to a familiar face was caused by poor memory ability. The vignettes receiving the lowest ability mean ratings were the absentmindedness (3.71), names (3.64), conversation (3.40), and rote (3.34) vignettes, which did not significantly differ from each other, suggesting that these types of memory failures (e.g., forgetting what one intended to do in another room, the name of a new acquaintance, what one was about to say in a conversation, and a phone number before dialing) were least likely to be perceived as due to lack of ability.

Table 3. Means for Attribution and Memory Opinion Scales.

	Younger Adults				Older Adults			
	Yng Targets		Old Targets		Yng Targets		Old Targets	
Rating Scale	*M*	*SD*	*M*	*SD*	*M*	*SD*	*M*	SD
Control Group								
Causal-Attribution								
Ability	3.80	0.86	4.06	1.22	3.55	0.71	4.32	1.29
Effort	2.72	0.97	2.42	1.16	3.10	1.41	3.21	1.86
Task Difficulty	3.82	0.95	3.81	0.89	3.93	0.77	4.53	1.12
Luck	1.95	1.23	1.53	0.66	1.92	1.49	1.74	1.40
Attention (External)	4.74	1.12	4.20	1.15	4.32	1.33	4.19	1.30
Attention (Internal)	4.70	1.43	4.40	0.99	4.82	1.18	4.08	1.54
Memory Opinion								
Mental Difficulty	2.77	0.70	3.22	1.26	2.38	0.83	3.71	1.31
Need for Training	2.55	0.51	2.94	1.11	2.93	0.91	3.85	1.41
Need for Evaluation	3.00	1.06	3.00	0.87	2.82	1.09	2.79	0.99
Grandparent Group								
Causal-Attribution								
Ability	3.83	1.31	4.21	1.02	3.15	1.18	4.23	1.56
Effort	2.63	1.00	2.45	1.13	3.04	0.92	2.96	1.30
Task Difficulty	3.81	0.79	3.78	1.04	3.16	0.85	4.23	1.28
Luck	1.84	1.24	1.67	0.92	1.48	0.63	1.34	1.03
Younger Adults	Older Adults							
Yng Targets	Old Targets	Yng Targets	Old Targets					
Rating Scale	*M*	*SD*	*M*	*SD*	*M*	*SD*	*M*	SD
Attention (External)	4.38	0.98	4.08	1.29	3.85	1.03	3.77	1.22
Attention (Internal)	4.67	1.03	4.07	1.39	4.08	1.20	4.09	1.25
Memory Opinion								
Mental Difficulty	2.92	1.10	3.57	1.16	2.42	1.09	3.15	1.08
Need for Training	2.66	1.33	3.18	1.08	2.69	1.19	3.14	1.35
Need for Evaluation	2.63	0.91	3.35	0.96	2.53	1.10	3.15	0.93
Memory Aging Group								
Causal-Attribution								
Ability	3.42	1.21	4.05	0.49	3.13	1.14	3.86	1.21
Effort	2.86	0.96	2.44	1.06	3.10	1.24	3.24	1.12
Task Difficulty	3.63	1.10	3.76	1.02	3.56	0.96	3.83	1.34
Luck	2.31	1.46	1.44	1.07	1.84	1.63	1.03	0.13
Attention (External)	4.77	0.92	4.21	1.04	4.39	1.22	3.99	0.95
Attention (Internal)	4.88	0.89	4.17	1.06	4.80	1.39	4.25	0.97
Memory Opinion								
Mental Difficulty	2.70	1.06	3.27	0.64	2.72	1.28	3.06	1.07
Need for Training	3.02	1.42	3.14	1.25	3.61	1.37	3.45	1.28
Need for Evaluation	2.90	0.92	2.97	0.99	3.33	0.85	2.69	1.13

On the effort scale, the retrieval (3.19) and names (3.25) vignettes received the highest mean ratings, suggesting that forgetting the name of a new acquaintance and forgetting a person one met only once before were more likely to be perceived as due to lack of effort. The remaining vignettes received significantly lower ratings on the effort scale. On the task difficulty scale, the rote (4.25), retrieval (4.19), and names (4.14) vignettes received the highest mean ratings, suggesting that these types of memory failures (e.g., forgetting a person one met only once before, the name of a new acquaintance, and a phone number before dialing) were more likely to be perceived as due to difficulty of the memory task. The absentmindedness (3.34) and conversation (3.17) vignettes received the lowest mean ratings for task difficulty (and did not significantly differ from each other).

On the bad luck scale, the names (1.81), conversation (1.77), and rote (1.72) vignettes received the highest mean ratings, suggesting that these types of memory failures (e.g., forgetting the name of a new acquaintance, what one was about to say in a conversation, and a phone number before dialing) were more likely perceived as due to bad luck compared to the other types of forgetting. However, it should also be noted that bad luck received the lowest ratings across all the vignettes. In contrast, the two attention (internal and external) attribution scales received the highest overall ratings. Specifically, the rote (4.67), conversation (4.67) and names (4.28) vignettes received the highest mean ratings on the scale of external attention, suggesting that these types of memory failures (e.g., forgetting a phone number, what one was about to say in a conversation, and the name of a new acquaintance) were perceived as due to external distractions (e.g., "other things going on around the central character"). For the internal attention scale, the rote (4.89), absentmindedness (4.72), and conversation (4.67) vignettes received the highest mean ratings, suggesting that these types of memory failures (e.g., forgetting a phone number, what one intended to do in another room, and what one was about to say in a conversation) were likely to be perceived as due to internal distractions (e.g., "other things going on in the central character's mind). Our findings for the vignettes do not replicate Erber et al. (1990a) who found very few differences among the various forms of everyday forgetting. Methodological differences across the two studies may account for these differences (e.g., differences in participants, vignette properties, minor procedural variations).

The Vignette x Participant Age interaction was significant, $F(30, 151) = 2.36$, $p < .001$. Four Vignette x Participant Age interaction univariates were significant: ability ($p < .001$), task difficulty ($p = .004$), luck ($p = .02$), and the two measures of attention (external, $p = .04$, and internal, $p = .01$). Follow-up t-tests were conducted on the significant univariates to determine the locus of the interaction. Despite four significant univariates, only two vignettes stood out as different from the others. Younger and older participants differed in perceptions regarding the causes of forgetfulness on the people vignette and the rote vignette. That is, younger participants ($M = 5.02$) gave significantly higher "lack of ability" ratings than older participants ($M = 4.17$) to the people vignette, $t(190) = 3.92$, $p < .001$, suggesting that younger participants were more likely than older participants to perceive ability as the primary cause of forgetting a name to a familiar face. Younger and older participants did not rate this vignette differently on any of the other causal attribution scales. On the rote vignette, younger participants (5.02) gave higher mean ratings than older participants (4.35) to the attribution scale of "other things on the central character's mind", $t(190) = 2.67$, $p = .008$, suggesting that younger adults were more likely than older adults to attribute rote types of forgetting to internal distractions. Younger and older participants did not rate this vignette any differently on the other attribution scales. These data provide new evidence of age-related differences in how younger and older adults view specific types of forgetting.

Memory Opinion Ratings. There was a significant main effect of participant age, $F(3, 178) = 6.67$, $p < .001$. Only one of the three univariates was significant. Older participants gave higher ratings ($M = 3.28$) than did younger participants ($M = 2.91$) on the "need for memory training" scale, $F(1, 180) = 4.36$, $MS_e = 38.33$, $p = .04$, suggesting that older adults perceived a higher need for memory training for the forgetful individuals compared to younger adults. This result conflicts with Erber et al. (1990a) who reported non-significant participant age group differences on the need for memory training scale, as discussed more fully in the General Discussion. The main effect of target age was significant, $F(3, 178) = 7.76$, $p < .001$. Two of the univariates were significant: mental difficulty and memory training. Replicating Erber et al. (1990a), memory failures of older targets ($M = 3.33$) were seen as indicating greater mental difficulty than younger targets ($M = 2.65$), $F(1, 180) = 19.46$, $MS_e = 133.49$, $p < .001$, and the recommendation for memory training was significantly higher for older targets ($M = 3.28$) than younger targets ($M = 2.91$), $F(1, 180) = 4.58$, $MS_e = 40.34$, $p = .03$. Contrary to expectations, but consistent with outcomes of the causal attribution evaluations, the information group main effect was non-significant and did not participate in any significant group interaction effects on the memory opinion rating scales.

There was a significant main effect of vignette, $F(15, 166) = 15.11$, $p < .001$. All of the univariates were significant ($ps < .01$). Pairwise comparisons were performed on each of the univariates to determine the locus of the significant difference across the six vignettes on each memory opinion rating scale. The people vignette was rated significantly higher on the memory opinion scale of mental difficulty ($M = 3.72$) than the other vignettes, suggesting that forgetting a name to a familiar face is more likely to be perceived as a sign of failing mental ability. The names ($M = 2.70$) and rote ($M = 2.52$) vignettes received the lowest mental difficulty ratings. Similarly, the people vignette also received the highest ratings ($M = 3.60$) on the memory opinion scale of "need for memory training". The conversation ($M = 2.74$) and rote ($M = 2.88$) vignettes received the lowest ratings on this scale. For the memory opinion scale of "need for evaluation", the people ($M = 3.55$) and retrieval ($M = 3.31$) vignettes received the highest ratings, whereas the absentminded ($M = 2.74$), names ($M = 2.74$), and rote ($M = 2.47$) received significantly lower ratings on this scale. Taken together, these data suggest that forgetting a name to a familiar face (i.e., people forgetting) was perceived as the most troubling to participants. These results are consistent with the causal attribution evaluations in which the people vignette received higher lack of ability ratings.

The Vignette x Participant Age interaction was also significant, $F(15, 166) = 3.30$, $p < .001$. All three Vignette x Participant Age interaction univariates reached significance ($ps = .002$). Follow-up *t*-tests were conducted on the significant univariates to determine the locus of the interaction. Only two vignettes stood out as different from the others. Younger and older participants differed in perceptions regarding memory opinions on the people vignette and the rote vignettes. Younger participants ($M = 4.03$) gave significantly higher mental difficulty ratings than older participants ($M = 3.40$) to the people vignette, $t(190) = 2.84$, $p = .005$, suggesting that younger participants were more likely than older participants to perceive forgetting a name to a familiar face as a sign of mental difficulty. Younger and older adults did not differ in their perceptions on the remaining two memory opinion scales on this vignette. Compared to younger participants ($M = 2.49$), older participants ($M = 3.26$) gave significantly higher need for memory training ratings to rote forgetting (e.g., forgetting a phone number before dialing), $t(190) = -3.47$, $p = .001$, and older participants ($M = 2.71$) gave higher ratings on the "need for evaluation" scale compared to younger participants ($M = 2.24$), $t(190) = -2.79$, $p = .006$. Younger and older adults did not differ in perceptions on the mental difficulty scale for this vignette.

Summary. The primary aim of this study was to determine whether knowledge of normal memory aging contributes to how forgetful older persons are perceived in social contexts. Analyses of KMAQ performance revealed that older adults were more knowledgeable than younger adults about memory aging overall. Participants correctly answered fewer normal memory aging items than pathological memory aging items, as in previous research (e.g., Hawley et al., 2006; Reese et al., 2000). A critical three-way interaction indicated that the memory seminar group showed an advantage in proportion correct for normal memory aging items at posttest relative to pretest whereas the other groups did not, confirming that KMAQ scores improved with instruction on normal memory aging issues. Contrary to expectation, the information groups did not differ in causal attributions or memory opinions of the forgetful target individual. This result was obtained for younger and older target characters across 6 different types of forgetting, thus the finding appears to be reliable. Overall, the results of the experimental approach imply that declarative memory knowledge appears to have very little effect on participants' causal attribution and memory opinion ratings.

In the next section, we employ an individual differences approach to the research problem. In particular, we conducted partial correlations to examine interrelationships among memory knowledge, self-reported memory ability, causal attribution and memory opinion data while statistically controlling for the variance associated with age. Partial correlations statistically controlling for age were desirable because significant age group effects occurred in the KMAQ, causal attribution, and memory opinion analyses. We also collapsed over information group, including only those in the no information control and grandparenting seminar groups in the analyses that follow. Our rationale for excluding the memory aging seminar participants in these analyses was to provide a clearer assessment of the interrelationships among the individual difference variables and memory appraisals unconfounded by changes in memory aging knowledge due to exposure to the information provided in the seminar.

Relationships Among Memory Knowledge, Self-Perceived Memory Functioning, and Memory Appraisals

Knowledge of Memory Aging and Self-Perceived Memory Functioning. Inspection of Table 4 indicates that KMAQ normal and pathological scores were significantly correlated ($r = .35$, $p < .001$). The MFQ frequency of forgetting subscale was significantly correlated with the seriousness of forgetting subscale ($r = .18$, $p = .05$) and the retrospective functioning subscale ($r = .41$, $p < .001$). The seriousness subscale was also correlated with the retrospective functioning subscale ($r = .20$, $p = .03$). These data show that knowledge of normal and pathological memory aging was not significantly correlated with self-perceived memory functioning, implying that these two aspects of metamemory (memory knowledge and memory beliefs) are conceptually distinct. This aspect of the data is consistent with prior research which has shown that memory knowledge and memory beliefs have a differential relationship with objective memory performance (e.g., Hertzog, Dixon, & Hultsch, 1990; Reese & Cherry, 2006).

Table 4. Partial correlations among KMAQ, MFQ, and Causal Attribution and Memory Opinion Ratings.

Variable	1	2	3	4	5	6
1. KMAQ Normal	--					
2. KMAQ Pathological	.35**	--				
3. MFQ Frequency	.08	.07	--			
4. MFQ Seriousness	-.02	.09	.18*	--		
5. MFQ Retrospective	-.03	-.08	.41**	.20*	--	
6. MFQ Mnemonics	.00	-.10	.07	.03	.00	--
7. Ability	-.11	-.20*	-.18*	-.18*	-.15	-.07
8. Effort	-.17	-.24**	-.12	-.12	.05	.05
9. Task Difficulty	-.10	-.08	-.10	-.07	-.04	.03
10. Luck	-.14	-.03	.06	.01	.03	.02
11. Attention (External)	-.03	-.07	-.09	-.09	.10	.00
12. Attention (Internal)	.00	-.10	-.13	-.15	.06	-.04
13. Mental Difficulty	-.14	-.12	-.24**	-.16	-.11	.03
14. Training	-.05	-.14	-.22*	-.09	-.06	-.01
15. Evaluation	.02	.03	-.05	-.13	.05	-.07

Variable	7	8	9	10	11	12	13	14	15
7. Ability	--								
8. Effort	.19*	--							
9. Task Difficulty	.46**	.35**	--						
10. Luck	-.18*	.17	.17	--					
11. Attention (External)	.05	.30**	.23**	.25**	--				
12. Attention (Internal)	.09	.27**	.26**	.18	.86**	--			
13. Mental Difficulty	.76**	.18*	.48**	-.07	.11	.04	--		
14. Training	.68**	.15	.44**	-.14	.14	.08	.85**	--	
15. Evaluation	.30**	.01	.22*	-.04	.11	.08	.37**	.36**	--

* $p \leq 0.05$. ** $p \leq 0.01$

Knowledge of Memory Aging, Self-Perceived Memory Functioning, Causal Attribution and Memory Opinion Ratings. The KMAQ normal memory aging scores were not significantly correlated with any of the causal attribution or memory opinion scales (see Table 4). In contrast, the pathological scores were negatively correlated with ratings on the ability scale (r = -.20, p = .03) and the effort scale (r = -.24, p = .009), suggesting that greater knowledge of pathological memory aging is associated with lower ratings on the ability and effort attribution scales. Several subscales of the MFQ were correlated with the causal attribution and memory opinion ratings scales (see Table 4, boxed portion). The frequency of forgetting and seriousness of forgetting subscales were negatively correlated with ability, although the size of the correlation coefficients was small (both r's = -.18, p's = .05). Of greater interest was that the frequency of forgetting subscale was negatively correlated with mental difficulty (r = -.24, p = .009) and memory training (r = -.22, p = .02), replicating the earlier Cherry and Brigman (2005) report. The finding that higher scores on the frequency of forgetting subscale were associated with lower lack of ability, sign of mental difficulty, and need for memory training evaluations implies that a more positive view of one's own memory is associated with less harsh evaluations of others' memory failures, regardless of age of perceiver. Interpretative caution is warranted, however; the MFQ was administered after the vignette rating task raising concerns about possible reactivity in the dependent measures[3]. With this caveat in mind, the present findings point to a potential avenue for future research: the relationship between implicit views of one's own forgetting and perceptions of forgetfulness in others.

General Discussion

This study examined the contribution of age and memory knowledge to memory appraisal of forgetful others using both an experimental and an individual difference approach to the research problem. Three main findings emerged from the analyses. First, we found that increased declarative knowledge of age-related memory changes did not lead to changes in causal attributions or memory opinions of forgetful characters. Second, there was strong evidence of an age-based double standard in participants' perceptions of memory failures in fictitious others. Specifically, older characters who experienced a single instance of forgetting were evaluated more negatively than their younger counterparts who experienced the very same forgetting, as in earlier research (Erber & Prager, 1999; Erber & Rothberg, 1991; Erber et al., 1990a). Third, individual differences in memory aging knowledge were not related to participants' perceptions of forgetful others. However, perceptions of one's own memory functioning were correlated with evaluations made of other people's memory failures. These findings are discussed more fully in the sections that follow.

Changing Knowledge, Not Perceptions

The present study addressed the question: does lack of memory aging knowledge account for how older persons are perceived in the context of forgetting? We addressed this question with an experimental approach that included two control groups and one experimental group who viewed an educational video addressing normative memory changes associated with later adulthood. Those persons in the memory seminar groups showed significant pre- to posttest gains on KMAQ normal memory aging items, indicating that declarative knowledge of memory aging is malleable. Despite exhibiting greater knowledge of normative age-associated memory changes as a result of instruction, changes in how older forgetful adults were perceived did not follow. In fact, those in the memory aging seminar group showed the same age-based double standard in perceptions of older adults' memory failures as did participants in the control and grandparent seminar comparison groups (see Erber et al., 1990; Erber & Prager, 1999).

---

3 The MFQ requires participants to rate the frequency of specific instances of forgetting (e.g., forgetting names, faces, phone numbers, etc.). Five of the forgetting episodes depicted in the vignettes were identical to the types of forgetting assessed using the MFQ. Completing the vignette rating task prior to the MFQ may have influenced how participants evaluated their memory functioning.

Our KMAQ findings are consistent with prior research where KMAQ performance improved as a result of specific instruction for college students (e.g., Cherry et al., 2003, Exp. 2) and mental health professionals (Jackson et al., 2008). This study is the first to demonstrate knowledge gains on the KMAQ for older adults as a result of instruction. Further, this improvement was noted one week following the informational seminar for both younger and older adults, suggesting that gains in memory aging knowledge were robust. For participants watching the memory aging video, performance gains were noted in both KMAQ items that were specifically addressed in the video and KMAQ items not addressed in the video. Improvements on items covered and not covered suggest that knowledge gained from the video may have transferred to other items on the questionnaire. Alternatively, it could also be that viewing the video encouraged participants to examine their assumptions about cognitive aging at posttest thereby improving the accuracy of their responses. As Hertzog and Hultsch (2000) note, there is little empirical data regarding declarative memory knowledge. Our findings suggest that although people know less about normal memory aging compared to pathological memory aging, this aspect of metamemory appears to be plastic and receptive to instruction.

Age-Based Double Standard in Perceptions of Forgetfulness

Causal Attributions and Memory Opinions. Participants' responses to the causal attribution and memory opinion scales revealed that young and old forgetful targets were perceived differently, despite being depicted in identical situations experiencing identical instances of forgetting. Old forgetful targets received higher ratings on the ability and task difficulty attribution scales compared to young forgetful targets, who received higher ratings on the luck and attention scales (external distractions as well as internal distractions). Thus, memory failures of older adults were more likely to be perceived as due to failing memory ability and task difficulty, whereas memory failures of younger adults were perceived as due to bad luck and inattention. These findings replicate the age-based double standard found by Erber et al. (1990a, see also Erber & Prager, 1999) and are consistent with Deaux's (1976) expectancy attribution bias in which expected behaviors of a stereotyped group are more likely to be attributed to stable causes, such as ability and task difficulty, and unexpected behaviors are more likely to be attributed to unstable causes, such as effort, luck, and attention. These data suggest that participants may have been using stereotypes, or at least implicit theories about the nature of cognitive aging, to evaluate older adults in stereotype-consistent contexts, although further research is necessary.

Our results also indicated that memory failures of old targets were more likely to be perceived as an indication of mental difficulty compared to memory failures of young targets, consistent with previous studies (Erber et al., 1990a). Old forgetful targets were also more likely to receive recommendations for memory training compared to young forgetful targets, but no differences were found on the rating scale assessing recommendations for medical or psychological evaluation for the forgetting (see also Erber et al. 1990a). These results are encouraging because they suggest that although older adults' forgetting is more likely to be perceived as a sign of failing mental ability, the memory failures were also perceived as malleable and not serious enough to deserve medical attention (i.e., not necessarily an indication of pathological memory deficits). Thus, participants appear to demonstrate views of memory consistent with Lachman et al.'s (1992) adaptive view of memory: memory is a skill that can be maintained and improved with effort.

Participant Age. Both younger and older adults had similar perceptions of forgetful target characters in that both age groups demonstrated the age-based double standard when making attribution evaluations. However, there were some differences in absolute ratings between younger and older participants on certain attribution and memory opinion scales. Specifically, older participants were more likely than younger participants to endorse lack of effort as a cause of memory failures, and older participants were more likely to recommend memory training for memory failures than younger participants. Although these data do not precisely replicate Erber et al.'s (1990s) findings in which older participants gave lower ratings than younger participants on the mental difficulty and medical evaluation scales and higher ratings on the task difficulty scale, our findings do provide a conceptual replication of the notion that older people may be more lenient in their evaluations of forgetful others than are younger people (see Erber & Prager, 1999, for discussion). Specifically, the finding that older adults were more likely to perceive lack of effort as a cause of everyday forgetting and that they were more likely to recommend memory training suggests that they endorse a more positive view of memory aging compared to younger adults. This suggestion is consistent with previous studies which have found that although older adults hold implicit views of cognitive decline, they also hold more elaborate conceptions about the course of cognitive development throughout the life span compared to younger adults (e.g., Lineweaver & Hertzog, 1998). Additionally, as Cuddy and Fiske (2002) note, people often make distinctions between "us" (i.e. in-group) and "them" (i.e., out-group) to promote positive evaluations of their own group, and consequently themselves. Thus, evaluating the forgetfulness of other older adults more leniently (i.e., more likely due to lack of effort and modifiable through training) would provide a means of framing one's own forgetting more positively.

Types of Forgetting. Examining ratings for each of the vignettes suggests that most of the everyday forgetting episodes were attributed to inattention (both internal and external). That is, most vignettes received the highest ratings on the two attribution scales measuring attention. In contrast, bad luck was least likely to be perceived as the cause for everyday kinds of forgetting. These finding are promising because they suggest that participants held realistic views of everyday memory failures – internal and external distractions often explain the majority of forgetting in day-to-day life.

Only one type of forgetting stood out as markedly different from the remaining forgetting episodes, forgetting a name to a familiar face (i.e., people forgetting), which was more likely to be perceived as due to lack of ability (see Table 3). Additionally, compared to the other kinds of forgetting, "people" memory failures received higher ratings on all three memory opinion scales: mental difficulty, need for memory training, and need for medical evaluation. This finding was qualified by a significant interaction with participant age on the ability and mental difficulty scale. Younger adults were more likely than older adults to evaluate forgetting a familiar face as due to lack of ability and as a sign of mental difficulty, suggesting that younger adults viewed this type of memory failure as more serious than did older adults. Erber et al. (1990a) reported very few differences among the everyday episodes of forgetting. In particular, the people vignette did not stand out on the attribution scale of ability. However, consistent with the present study, Erber et al. (1990) reported that the people forgetting did receive higher ratings on the memory opinion scale of "mental difficulty." It is not clear why this study found the people vignette to be more bothersome, but differences in how the specific instances of forgetting were perceived by participants could be due to differences in how the vignette scenarios were constructed as well as how judgments were made.

Role of Self-Perceived Memory Functioning in Memory Appraisal

Although normal memory aging knowledge was not related to causal attribution or memory opinion ratings, self-perceived memory functioning was significantly correlated with several of the attribution and memory opinion scales. Regardless of age of perceiver, a more positive perception of one's own memory functioning (i.e., less reported frequency of forgetting) was associated with less harsh evaluations of others' everyday memory failures (i.e., lower ratings on the ability, mental difficulty, and memory training scales). These results agree with Cherry and Brigman (2005) who found that the MFQ frequency of forgetting scale was negatively correlated with memory opinion ratings regarding mental difficulty and need for memory training when the consequences of the forgetful behavior were minor. Given that the same outcomes were obtained across two studies with different materials and procedural variations, the results appear to be reliable. Personal beliefs about one's own memory functioning, then, may have greater influence on his or her evaluation of forgetfulness of others, than does declarative knowledge of normative age-associated memory changes, although further research would be desirable before firm conclusions would bc warranted.

SUMMARY AND CONCLUSIONS

Two limitations of this study warrant brief mention. Although memory knowledge increased for participants viewing the memory aging video, the magnitude of the gain may not have been sufficient to influence causal attribution and memory opinion scale ratings. Additionally, we used convenience samples of younger and older adults, a typical practice in cognitive aging research. Older adults were well-educated, reported high occupational status, and had good cognitive functioning as measured by scores on the vocabulary assessment. Consequently, it is possible that participants in this study were not representative of the younger and older adult populations as a whole.

In closing, the present results imply that "knowledge" in the form of stereotypes about older adults and implicit theories of aging more strongly influence perceptions of older adults than declarative knowledge of age-related memory changes and that changes in one (increased declarative memory aging knowledge) do not necessarily lead to changes in the other (attributions of older adults reflected implicit views of cognitive aging). Future research to examine the relationship between declarative knowledge and implicit views of older adults would be desirable, possibly including a more comprehensive memory training program. For example, Caprio-Prevette and Fry (1993) found that cognitive restructuring techniques, in which participants identified maladaptive beliefs about memory, in addition to an educational component, which focused on educating participants about the various theories of forgetting, how memory works, and Alzheimer's disease and other causes of memory decline, resulted in the most robust changes in self-perceived memory functioning (changes in objective memory performance were also observed). A similar program may be effective in changing perceptions of forgetfulness as well. Future research to examine the relationship between knowledge of pathological memory aging and perceptions of older adults' forgetfulness may also be valuable.

REFERENCES

Caprio-Prevette, M. D. & Fry, P. S. (1996). Memory enhancement program for community-based older adults: Development and evaluation. *Experimental Aging Research, 22,* 281-303.

Cherry, K. E., Allen, P. D., Olinde, E. A., Robichaux, M. & Hawley, K. S. (2008). Knowledge of memory aging in students, caregivers and senior service providers. *Educational Gerontology.* Mannuscript in press.

Cherry, K. E. & Brigman, S. (2005). Memory failures appraisal in younger and older adults: Role of individual difference and event outcome variables. *Journal of Genetic Psychology, 166*, 435-450.

Cherry, K. E., Brigman, S., Hawley, K. S. & Reese, C. M. (2003). The knowledge of memory aging questionnaire: Effects of adding a "don't know" response option. *Educational Gerontology, 29*, 427-446.

Cherry, K. E. & Smith, A. D. (1998). Normal memory aging. In M. Hersen and V. B. Van Hasselt (Eds.), *Handbook of Clinical Geropsychology* (87-110). Plenum Press.

Cherry, K. E., West, R. L., Reese, C. M., Santa Maria, M. P. & Yassuda, M. (2000). The knowledge of memory aging questionnaire. *Educational Gerontology, 26.* 195-219.

Cuddy, A. J. C. & Fiske, S. T. (2002). Doddering but dear: Process, content, and function in stereotyping of older persons. In T. D., Nelson (Eds.), *Ageism: Stereotyping and prejudice against older persons* (3-26). Cambridge, MA: MIT Press.

Deaux, K. (1976). Sex: A perspective on the attribution process. In: J. F., Harvey, W. J., Ickes, & R. F., Kidd (Eds.), *New directions in attribution research: Vol. 1* (335-352). Hillsdale, NJ: Erlbaum.

Duke University Center for the Study of Aging and Human Development, (1975). *OARS: Multidimensional Functional Assessment Questionnaire.* Durham, NC: Author.

Erber, J. T. (1989). Young and older adults' appraisal of memory failures in young and older adult target persons. *Journal of Gerontology: Psychological Sciences, 6,* 170-175.

Erber, J. T. & Prager, I. G. (1999). Age and memory: Perceptions of forgetful young and older adults. In: T. M., Hess & F., Blanchard-Fields, (Eds.), *Social Cognition and Aging* (198-217). San Diego, CA: Academic Press.

Erber, J. T. & Rothberg, S. T. (1991). Here's looking at you: The relative effect of age and attractiveness on judgements about memory failure. *Journal of Gerontology: Psychological Sciences, 3,* 116-123.

Erber, J. T., Szuchman, L. T. & Rothberg, S. T. (1990a). Everyday memory failure: Age differences in appraisal and attribution. *Psychology and Aging, 5,* 236-241.

Erber, J. T., Szuchman, L. T. & Rothberg, S. T. (1990b). Age, gender, and individual differences in memory failure appraisal. *Psychology and Aging, 5,* 600-603.

Gardner, E. & Monge, R. (1977). Adult age differences in cognitive abilities and educational background. *Experimental Aging Research, 15,* 73-78.

Gilewski, M. J., Zelinski, E. M. & Schaie, K. W. (1990). The memory functioning questionnaire for assessment of memory complaints in adulthood and old age. *Psychology and Aging, 5,* 482-490.

Hawley, K. S., Cherry, K. E., Su, L. J., Chiu, Y. W. & Jazwinski, S. M. (2006). Knowledge of memory aging in adulthood. *International Journal of Aging and Human Development, 63,* 317-334

Herrmann, D. J. & Neisser, W. (1978). An inventory of everyday memory experiences. In M. M. Gruneberg, P. E. Morris, & R. N., Sykes, (Eds.), *Practical aspects of memory* (35-51). New York: Academic Press.

Hertzog, C., Dixon, R. A. & Hultsch, D. F. (1990). Metamemory in adulthood: Differentiating knowledge, belief, and behavior. In: T. M., Hess, (Ed.), *Aging and Cognition: Knowledge, organization, and utilization* (161-212). North-Holland: Elsevier Science Publisher.

Hertzog, C. & Hultsch, D. F. (2000). Metacognition in adulthood and old age. In: F. I. M., Craik, & T. A. Salthouse, (Eds.), *The Handbook of Aging and Cognition, 2nd Ed.* (417-466). Mahwah, NJ: Lawrence Erlbaum Associates.

Hummert, M. L. (1999). A social cognitive perspective on age stereotypes. In: T. M., Hess, & F., Blanchard-Fields, (Eds.), *Social cognition and aging* (pp. 175-196). San Diego, CA: Academic Press.

Jackson, E. M., Cherry, K. E., Smitherman, E. A. & Hawley, K. S. (2008). Knowledge of memory aging and Alzheimer's disease in college students and mental health professionals. *Aging and Mental Health,12,* 258-266.

Lachman, M. E., Weaver, S. L., Bandura, M., Elliott, E. & Lewkowicz, C. J. (1992). Improving memory and control beliefs through cognitive restructuring and self-generated strategies. *Journal of Gerontology: Psychological Sciences, 47,* P293-P299.

Lineweaver, T. T. & Hertzog, C. (1998). Adults' efficacy and control beliefs regarding memory and aging: Separating general from personal beliefs. *Aging, Neuropsychology, and Cognition, 5,* 264-269.

Parr, W. V. & Siegert, R. (1993). Adults' conceptions of everyday memory failures in others: Factors that mediate the effects of target age. *Psychology and Aging, 8,* 599-605.

Reese, C. M. & Cherry, K. E. (2004). Practical memory concerns across the lifespan. *International Journal of Aging and Human Development, 59,* 237-255.

Reese, C. M. & Cherry, K. E. (2006). Effects of age and ability on self-reported memory functioning and knowledge of memory aging. *Journal of Genetic Psychology, 167,* 221-240.

Reese, C. M., Cherry, K. E. & Copeland, A. L. (2000). Knowledge of normal versus pathological memory aging in younger and older adults. *Aging, Neuropsychology, and Cognition, 7,* 1-8.

Ryan, E. B. (1992). Beliefs about memory changes across the adult lifespan. *Journal of Gerontology: Psychological Sciences, 47,* P41-P46.

Ryan, E. B. & Kwong See, S. (1993). Age-based beliefs about memory changes for self and others across adulthood. *Journal of Gerontology: Psychological Sciences, 48,* P199-P201.

Yesavage, J. A., Brink, T. L., Rose, T. L., Lum, O., Huang, V., Adey, M. & Leirer, V. P. (1983). Development and validation of a geriatric screening scale: A preliminary report. *Journal of Psychiatric Research, 17,* 37-49.

Zelinski, E. M., Gilewski, M. J. & Anthony-Bergstone, C. R. (1990). Memory functioning questionnaire: Concurrent validity with memory performance and self-reported memory failures. *Psychology and Aging, 5*, 388-399.

Zelinski, E. M., Gilewski, M. J. & Schaie, K.W. (1993). Individual differences in cross-sectional and 3-year longitudinal memory performance across the adult life span. *Psychology and Aging, 8*, 176-186.

APPENDIX

Vignettes

Errands (Practice 1): George is a 25/65-year old man who is very active in his community and he enjoys doing volunteer work. He is involved in his neighborhood association. They are planning to build a new park in his neighborhood. George offered to serve on the planning committee, which meets the last Thursday of each month. George decided it would be nice to bring a snack to the next meeting. Before the meeting, he made his typical grocery store run. In addition to his regular shopping, he was going to buy paper plates, napkins, and cookies for the meeting. George forgot to buy the paper plates.

Place (Practice 2): Elizabeth is a 27/67-year old woman who is very conscientious. She enjoys doing helpful things for other people. Recently, Elizabeth took care of her neighbors' cat while they were away on vacation. She fed the cat and changed the litter box. As a way of saying thank you, the neighbor gave Elizabeth a gift certificate to one of her favorite stores. Elizabeth decided to put the gift certificate away for safekeeping until she was ready to go shopping. Later that month, she went to look for the gift certificate. She could not remember where she had put it.

Absentmindedness: Marjorie is a 30/70-year old woman who likes to spend the weekends working in her garden and taking care of household tasks before the new week begins. She spent last Saturday morning catching up on some personal correspondence. She wrote several letters to out-of-town friends and some notes to relatives thanking them for the gifts and cards they sent for her birthday. As soon as she had finished and sealed the last letter, she went upstairs to the study to get some postage stamps. She wanted to put the letters out for the mail carrier to pick up that day. When she got to the top of the steps, she forgot what she went upstairs to get.

Retrieval: Dean is a 36/76-year old man who enjoys spending time with his wife and family and he likes to read. He usually accompanies his wife to a continuing education course she is taking that meets every Saturday in a town that is 45-minutes away from the town in which they live. While his wife is in class, Dean often reads a book in the lobby. One Saturday Dean noticed another woman in the lobby. The two exchanged hellos and she told him that she was waiting for her husband who was taking the same course. They enjoyed a pleasant conversation while they waited. Recently Dean ran into the woman while at the local mall. The woman said hello to Dean and he returned the greeting, but Dean did not remember the woman.

Names: Bill is a 34/74-year old man who is very outgoing. He's an art and music enthusiast, but he also enjoys cooking and socializing at parties. Recently, Bill attended a party in the home of a friend in honor of the friend's birthday. During dinner, he sat beside a woman, Kathy, who recently moved to town. Bill and Kathy enjoyed a pleasant conversation during dinner and found that they had many interests in common. They talked at length about a museum exhibit they had both seen and really enjoyed. After dinner, Bill began to introduce Kathy to another person at the party, Jim. Bill could not remember Kathy's name.

Conversation: Mary Ann is a 32/72-year old woman who is a member of a local book club. Her favorite pastime is reading, and she enjoys talking about the books she has read. Once a month, the book club meets at the community library near her house to discuss a book that all the members have agreed to read. Last week at the meeting, they were taking turns discussing the most recent book they read, a murder mystery. One of the members made a comment about the main character in the book, which reminded Mary Ann of something that she wanted to say about the same character. However, when it was her turn to speak, she forgot what she had planned to say.

People: Ann is a 36/76-year old woman who is very active in her community. She is interested in current events and state and local politics. She often attends a monthly lecture series that meets at her neighborhood community center. The lecture topics include local politics, neighborhood improvement issues, and timely topics, such as tax law changes. At break, Ann usually visits with Nancy, another person that regularly attends the lecture series. Ann and Nancy do not know one another outside of the lecture series, but they enjoy discussing issues brought up at the lecture. Yesterday, Ann ran into Nancy while waiting in line at the deli counter at the grocery store. Nancy said, "Hello." Ann recognized Nancy's face, but she could not remember where she had seen her before.

Rote: Richard is a 23/63-year old man who has a lovely voice and often sings in the church choir. Last Saturday, he promised to drop off some materials at the choir director's home, but he was behind schedule in running errands. Richard decided to call the director to tell her that he would be a few minutes late, but he did not have her telephone number with him. Using his mobile phone, Richard called his wife at home and asked her for the phone number. He did not have a pen handy, so he quickly hung up and began dialing the number his wife had given him. After dialing the first three numbers, he forgot the rest of the phone number.

In: Learning and Memory Developments... ISBN: 978-1-60876-397-9
Editors: L. C. Eklund, A. S. Nyman, pp. 127-154

Chapter 5

MEMORY RECONSOLIDATION: HISTORY, RESEARCH, AND IMPLICATIONS FOR TREATMENT OF PSYCHIATRIC DISORDERS

Robert W. Flint, Jr., Karina H. Bengsz and Aeron E. Zamecnik
The College of Saint Rose, Albany, NY, USA

ABSTRACT

Since the 1960s, research has indicated that the acquisition of new information is followed by a time-limited period of memory consolidation. During this consolidation period, the new memory exists in a labile state, where enhancing or impairing treatments are capable of modulating the subsequent strength of the memory. Considerable evidence supports the existence of a period of memory consolidation; however, following the completion of the consolidation period many scientists believed that the new long-term memory became immune to memory enhancing or impairing treatments. Over the decades, isolated studies challenged this view and suggested that old memories may sometimes become malleable again under the right circumstances. During the last 10 years a substantial body of research has developed indicating that old, previously consolidated memories may enter a state of reconsolidation when retrieved from long-term memory. In other words, the retrieval of old memories may return them to a state where they are once again susceptible to memory modulation. This chapter will review the historical development of memory reconsolidation, summarize some of the tasks, species, and treatments used in research on reconsolidation, discuss some of the important behavioral characteristics and potential mechanisms of memory reconsolidation, and consider the possible implications of this research for treatment of psychiatric conditions such as post-traumatic stress disorder, phobias, and drug addiction.

INTRODUCTION

Difficulties in forming new memories or recalling old memories devastate the lives of many individuals who have suffered a traumatic brain injury or stroke, and are landmark characteristics of psychiatric disorders such as Alzheimer's disease and Korsakoff syndrome. Imagine, then, the paradoxical supposition that inducing selective memory impairment may be useful as a treatment for other psychiatric disorders. In this chapter we will follow the historical development of research on memory reconsolidation, briefly review the variety of species and paradigms that are being utilized to examine this phenomenon, consider some of the important issues challenging research on memory reconsolidation, and ponder the implications of these research endeavors for the treatment of disorders such as post-traumatic stress, phobias, and drug abuse.

Before launching into these topics, it is important to review some of the basic characteristics of how new memories are established. When learning occurs, sensory information is received, often in the form of auditory or visual input. While a number of theories argue for different stages or levels of processing of these inputs, it is generally believed that the information first undergoes a process of encoding, where sensory information is processed in preparation for further analysis (Flint & Zak, 2002). This information then undergoes consolidation, where it presumably becomes more stabilized. Neuroscientists have now identified two different consolidation processes: synaptic and systems. Synaptic consolidation occurs for only a few minutes or hours following learning and is believed to be associated with all forms of long-term memory (Dudai, 2004; Medina, Bekinschtein, Cammarota, & Izquierdo, 2008). During this period of synaptic consolidation the memory exists in a labile state where it is susceptible to a wide variety of treatments that may enhance (e.g., Dornelles et al., 2007; Ferry, Roozendaal, & McGaugh, 1999; Flint & Riccio, 1999; Mohanty & Flint, 2001; van der Staay et al., 2008) or impair (e.g., Desgranges, Levy, & Ferreira, 2008; Levesque et al., 2007; Lima et al., 2009) the target memory. Systems consolidation is a much longer process (years in humans) whereby hippocampus-dependent memories may be processed and moved from the hippocampus to the neocortex, thus becoming more independent of the hippocampus with time (Rasch & Born, 2007; Roediger, Dudai, & Fitzpatrick, 2007; Trifilieff, Calandreau, Herry, Mons, & Micheau, 2007). The ultimate goal of these neuronal activities is to establish and maintain a process of memory storage, whereby long-term memories are maintained in the brain in an accessible state so that they may be easily retrieved at a later time. It is at the point of subsequent memory retrieval that the process of reconsolidation becomes important. Research has demonstrated that upon retrieval, a long-term memory returns to a labile state where it is once again susceptible to memory modulating treatments and must undergo a process of reconsolidation, the focus of this chapter (see Figure 1).

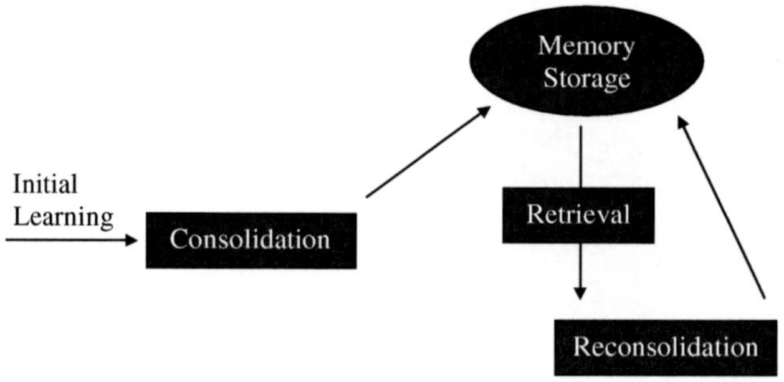

Figure 1. Schematic representation of the learning, consolidation, and reconsolidation processes.

HISTORY OF MEMORY RECONSOLIDATION

The concept of reconsolidation has not always been well accepted. For many decades evidence of reconsolidation conflicted with the mainstream consolidation hypothesis, which argued that consolidation occurs for a finite period of time following memory acquisition and occurs only a single time for any given memory (Dudai & Morris, 2001; McGaugh, 1966). While there is no doubt that immediate post-training or synaptic consolidation exists, the seemingly rigid adherence to the classic consolidation hypothesis precluded the consideration that such consolidation-like processes may exist following the retrieval of old stored memories. In addition to studies supporting the existence of reconsolidation processes, there have been a number of observations over the years that have challenged the consolidation hypothesis (Lewis, 1979; Riccio, Millin, & Gisquet-Verrier, 2003). For example, sometimes spontaneous or cue-induced recovery from amnesia may occur (Harrod, Metzger, & Riccio, 1996; Morgan, Flint, & Riccio, 1998; Quartermain, McEwen, & Azmitia, 1972; Riccio & Richardson, 1984), and clinical accounts as early as the mid 1960's have indicated that patients with retrograde amnesia often displayed evidence of islands of memory, or the sparing of some memories while other memories from the same time period or earlier are lost [(Landis, 1964; Whitty & Zangwill, 1966; Yacorzynski, 1965) as cited in Robbins & Meyer, 1970]. Such reports have been problematic for the classic consolidation hypothesis which argues, from a temporal perspective, that any not-yet-consolidated memories would likely be equally susceptible to amnesic agents.

During the reign of the consolidation hypothesis, hundreds of studies demonstrated the labile nature of memory during the immediate post-acquisition period as well as the temporal limitations of the consolidation period (e.g., Gold, 1986; Gold & van Buskirk, 1975). One major approach was to demonstrate that treatments such as electroconvulsive shock (Madsen & McGaugh, 1961; McGaugh, 1966; McGaugh & Alpern, 1966), hypothermia (Riccio, Gaebelein, & Cohen, 1968; Riccio, Hodges, & Randall, 1968) and a variety of pharmacological agents (McGaugh, 1989) are capable of disrupting memory consolidation processes. A second tactic has been to demonstrate that a variety of endogenous and exogenous compounds are capable of enhancing consolidation, and thus strengthening subsequent memory performance when administered immediately following learning (Castellano, Cabib, & Puglisi-Allegra, 1996; Gold, 1995; McGaugh, 1989).

The first demonstration of reconsolidation was made in 1968 by Misanin, Miller, and Lewis who showed that the reactivation of a previously consolidated memory rendered it susceptible to the memory impairing effects of electroconvulsive shock. This finding challenged the consolidation hypothesis because consolidation of the original memory from training had already ended (i.e., electroconvulsive shock alone had no effect) and that reactivation of the training memory was crucial for the electroconvulsive shock to induce amnesia. Despite this rather profound discovery, the consolidation hypothesis continued to dominate neuroscience for over thirty years.

Table 1. Research in Support of Memory Reconsolidation Between 1968 and 1999 (chronological order).

Year	Authors	Species	Task	Reconsolidation Modulator	Memory Status
1968	Misanin, Miller, & Lewis	Rat	Fear Conditioning	Electroconvulsive Shock	Impaired
1968	Schneider & Sherman	Rat	Passive Avoidance	Electroconvulsive Shock	Impaired
1969	Davis & Klinger	Goldfish	Shock Avoidance Training	KCl; Puromycin; Actoxycycloheximide	Impaired
1970	Robbins & Meyer	Rat	Two-Choice Discrimination	Electroconvulsive Shock	Impaired
1971	Howard & Meyer	Rat	Two-Choice Discrimination	Electroconvulsive Shock	Impaired
1972	DeVietti & Holliday	Rat	Fear Conditioning	Electroconvulsive Shock	Impaired
1972	Lewis, Bregman, & Mahan	Rat	Appetitive Maze	Electroconvulsive Shock	Impaired
1973	DeVietti, Holliday, & Larson	Rat	Fear Conditioning	Electroconvulsive Shock	Impaired
1973a	Gordon & Spear	Rat	Passive- to Active-Avoidance Negative Transfer Paradigm	Interference	Impaired
1973b	Gordon & Spear	Rat	Passive- to Active-Avoidance Negative Transfer Paradigm	Strychnine	Enhanced
1973	Lewis & Bregman	Rat	Appetitive Maze	Electroconvulsive Shock	Impaired
1976	Bregman, Nicholas, & Lewis	Rat	Appetitive Maze	Electroconvulsive Shock	Impaired
1976	DeVietti & Kirkpatrick	Rat	Fear Conditioning	Amygdaloid Complex Stimulation	Impaired
1977	DeVietti, Conger, & Kirkpatrick	Rat	Fear Conditioning	Mesencephalic Reticular Formation Stimulation	Enhanced
1977	DeVietti & Kirkpatrick	Rat	Fear Conditioning	Amygdaloid Complex Stimulation; Mesencephalic Reticular Formation Stimulation	Impaired; Enhanced
1977a	Gordon	Rat	Passive- to Active-Avoidance Negative Transfer Paradigm	Interference	Impaired
1977b	Gordon	Rat	Passive- to Active-Avoidance Negative Transfer Paradigm	Strychnine	Enhanced
1978	DeVietti & Kirkpatrick	Rat	Fear Conditioning	Mesencephalic Reticular Formation Stimulation	Enhanced
1979	Mactutus, Riccio, & Ferek	Rat	Passive Avoidance	Hypothermia	Impaired
1982	Judge & Quartermain	Mouse	Approach-Avoidance Learning	Anisomycin	Impaired
1993	Rodriguez, Van Ausdle, Dhanens, & Mondragon	Rat	Passive- to Active-Avoidance Negative Transfer Paradigm	Glucose	Enhanced
1997	Przybyslawski & Sara	Rat	Radial Arm Maze	MK-801	Impaired
1997	Summers, Crowe, & Ng	Chick	Passive Avoidance	AP5	Impaired
1999	Przybyslawski, Roullet, & Sara	Rat	Radial Arm Maze; CER Conditioning	Propranolol	Impaired
1999	Rodriguez, Horne, & Padilla	Rat	Passive Avoidance	Glucose	Enhanced
1999	Houpt & Berlin	Rat	Conditioned Taste Aversion	Cycloheximide	Impaired

The study by Misanin et al. (1968) was followed by more than 20 demonstrations of reconsolidation between 1968 and 1999 (see Table 1), but these results remained largely unappreciated by the broader scientific community. For example, in 1979, Mactutus, Riccio, and Ferek demonstrated that an old reactivated memory of passive avoidance conditioning in rats was susceptible to disruption with both mild and deep hypothermia, and in 1993, Rodriguez, Van Ausdle, Dhanens and Mondragon reported that post-reactivation administration of glucose enhanced memory of original training in rats, results that were subsequently expanded upon in later studies (Rodriguez, Horne, Haas, & Padilla, 2000; Rodriguez, Horne, & Padilla, 1999).

RESURGENCE OF MEMORY RECONSOLIDATION RESEARCH

Three separate studies appeared in the literature in 2000, marking what most neuroscientists recognize as the catalyst for the resurgence of interest in memory reconsolidation research. Litvin and Anokhin (2000) examined the effects of the protein synthesis inhibitor cycloheximide on passive-avoidance memory in chicks. They reported that intracerebral administration of cycloheximide five minutes prior to a reminder of training significantly disrupted retention, and they argued that the reactivation of a previously consolidated memory requires the synthesis of new proteins as it undergoes reconsolidation. Land, Bunsey, and Riccio (2000) used neurotoxic lesions of the hippocampal formation to examine retrograde amnesia for a Y-maze discrimination task. As would be expected, they found that animals given lesions immediately after training displayed amnesia in comparison to both sham control animals and animals that were given lesions 30-days following training (after consolidation was complete). However, Land et al. found that when hippocampal lesions were given immediately following a brief reminder administered 30-days after training, animals were severely impaired in comparison to those given sham lesions or those lesioned without a reminder treatment. It was argued that retrograde amnesia may not always be explained as a storage failure, and that the state of activity or recency of activation may be a relevant factor.

Probably the most widely referenced recent evidence of memory reconsolidation was reported by Nader, Schafe, and LeDoux (2000). In their study, rats were given auditory fear conditioning (tone-shock pairing) and then either one or 14 days later, some animals received a single presentation of the conditioned stimulus to reactivate the memory. Following reactivation, animals were given bilateral infusions of either artificial cerebrospinal fluid or the protein synthesis inhibitor anisomycin into the lateral and basal nuclei of the amygdala. Infusions of anisomycin immediately after memory reactivation impaired subsequent memory performance. The authors showed that this did not occur if the anisomycin infusion was delayed for six hours following memory reactivation and did not occur in the absence of memory reactivation.

Together, these three studies have resulted in numerous neuroscientists focusing their energy on elucidating the characteristics and mechanisms of memory reconsolidation over the last nine years. For some, this involves returning to an area of study with which they were already intimately familiar, while for others, this represents a pursuit into a novel area of neuroscience. The remainder of this chapter will review many of these characteristics and mechanisms of memory reconsolidation, with an emphasis on research with rodents, as the dominant animal model with which this phenomenon has been examined.

Table 2. Selected Citations Demonstrating the Range of Species within which Memory Reconsolidation has been Demonstrated (alphabetized by species).

Species	Task	Reconsolidation Modulator	Memory Status	Authors	Year
C. elegans	Habituation	Heat Shock	Impaired	Rose & Rankin	2006
Chick	Passive-Avoidance	Cycloheximide	Impaired	Litvin & Anokhin	2000
Crab	Context-Signal Memory	Cycloheximide	Impaired	Pedreira & Maldonado	2003
Drosophila	Olfactory Conditioning	Cycloheximide	Impaired	Lagasse, Devaud, & Mery	2009
Ewe	Social Recognition Memory	Cycloheximide	Impaired	Perrin, Ferreira, Meurisse, Verdin, Mouly, & Levy	2007
Goldfish	Shock Avoidance	KCl; Puromycin; Actoxycycloheximide	Impaired	Davis & Klinger	1969
Hermissenda	Pavlovian Conditioning	Anisomycin, Sensory Block, Actinomycin-D, RGD	Impaired	Child, Epstein, Kuzirian, & Alkon	2003
Honeybee	Appetitive Learning	Anisomycin	Impaired	Stollhoff, Menzel, & Eisenhardt	2005
Human	Motor Memory	Interference	Impaired	Walker, Brakefield, Hobson, & Stickgold	2003
Medaka Fish	Conditioned Fear	MS222	Impaired	Eisenberg & Dudai	2004
Mouse	Contextual Fear Conditioning	Rapamycin	Impaired	Blundell, Kouser, & Powell	2008
Rat	Conditioned Taste Aversion	Cycloheximide	Impaired	Flint & Marino	2007
Snail	Contextual Fear Conditioning	Anisomycin	Impaired	Gainutdinova et al.	2005

DIVERSITY OF SPECIES AND PARADIGMS

Animal Models

Two of the most important issues associated with scientific research are the extent to which it represents a phenomenon that is generalizable and reliable. In other words, are the characteristics and mechanisms of memory reconsolidation unique to a particular species or animal model used by one laboratory, or are these characteristics and mechanisms representative of reconsolidation across species and tasks in many different laboratories? To this end, recent research has demonstrated the existence of memory reconsolidation processes in no fewer than thirteen different species including snails, bees, fish, crabs, rats, sheep, and importantly, humans (see Table 2 for representative references from each species). More diverse than the species with which memory reconsolidation has been demonstrated are the types of memory paradigms that have been used to examine this phenomenon. The use of different paradigms increases the level of complexity because not all memories are the same. There are numerous different types of memory which depend upon many different and sometimes overlapping neural structures (Eichenbaum, 2003; Izquierdo et al., 2006; Squire, Stark, & Clark, 2004; Squire & Zola, 1998). The use of different tasks, within and across species, increases the generalizability of the phenomenon. Table 3 provides representative examples of more than fifteen paradigms that have been successfully used to demonstrate the existence of memory reconsolidation. To highlight a few and to demonstrate the breadth of these tasks we see that the paradigms include simple non-associative forms of learning such as habituation, associative tasks such as instrumental appetitive learning and Pavlovian fear conditioning tasks, declarative tasks such as paired-associate learning, and implicit tasks such as motor memory in humans.

Human Studies

Relatively little research has been conducted on human memory reconsolidation. Given that traditional research has focused on the use of drugs as inhibitors or stressors, non-human animals have been the obvious subject of choice. Studies carried out with human participants can be divided into two categories; those employing implicit memory tasks such as motor memory, and those employing explicit or declarative memory tasks such as paired-associate learning or word-recall tasks.

Walker, Brakefield, Hobson, and Stickgold (2003) were the first to provide evidence of memory reconsolidation for an implicit motor skill finger-tapping task in humans. The task required participants to press four numeric keys in a predetermined order (e.g., 4-1-3-2-4) using their non-dominant hand. Participants were instructed to repeat the sequence as many times as possible during multiple 30-second trials. Following acquisition, Walker et al. demonstrated that a single reactivation trial prior to learning a novel numeric sequence (e.g., 2-3-1-4-2) disrupted performance on a subsequent (24-hr delay) retention test for the original sequence. Importantly, the authors showed that the impairment did not occur unless learning the new sequence was preceded by a reactivation trial for the original sequence. In other words, the memory for the original sequence had to be reactivated so that the new sequence could sufficiently disrupt reconsolidation. These results appear to be the earliest support of memory reconsolidation in humans.

Evidence of reconsolidation involving explicit memory tasks using verbal material have been reported by Forcato et al. (2007) who used a paired-associate task. Participants learned an association between a cue syllable and respective response syllable within a particular context containing specific lighting, images, and sounds. Following training within specific contexts, participants were required to match the cue syllable (e.g., ITE, ASP) with the originally associated response syllable (e.g., OBN, UOD) within the appropriate context. The original memory was impaired when reminders were given prior to the second training, and also when the second training was given five minutes instead of 24 hours after the initial training. In a replication and extension, Forcato, Argibay, Pedreira, and Maldonado (2009) discovered that the omission of at least one component of the reminder context (i.e. light, image or sound) prevented the target memory from returning to a labile state, and as a result, new learning failed to impair the original memory.

Table 3. Selected Citations Demonstrating the Range of Procedures with which Memory Reconsolidation has been Demonstrated (alphabetized by task).

Task	Species	Reconsolidation Modulator	Memory Status	Authors	Year
Active-Avoidance (Two-Way)	Rat	Intracranial Self-Stimulation	Enhanced	Soriano-Mas, Redolar-Ripoll, Guillazo-Blanch, Morgado-Bernal, & Segura-Torres	2007
Appetitive Memory	Rat	MK-801	Impaired	Lee & Everitt	2008
Conditioned Place Preference	Rat	Scopolamine; Ketamine	Impaired	Zhai, Wu, Chen, Li, Liu, & Lu	2008
Conditioned Taste Aversion	Rat	Cycloheximide	Impaired	Flint & Marino	2007
Conditioned Withdrawal from Opiates	Rat	Zif268 Antisense Oligodeoxynucleotide	Impaired	Hellemans, Everitt, & Lee	2006
Context-Signal Memory	Crab	Cycloheximide	Impaired	Pedreira & Maldonado	2003
Contextual Memory for Cocaine-Induced Locomotor Activity	Rat	Anisomycin	Impaired	Bernardi, Lattal, & Berger	2007
Cue-Induced Cocaine-Seeking	Rat	Zif268 Antisense Oligodoxynucleotide	Impaired	Hellemans, Everitt, & Lee	2006
Delayed Matching-to-Place Task in the Water Maze	Rat	Anisomycin	Impaired	Morris et al.	2006
Eyeblink Conditioning	Mouse	Anisomycin	Impaired	Inda, Delgado-Garcia, & Carrion	2005
Fear Conditioning	Rat	Anisomycin	Impaired	Nader, Schafe, & LeDoux	2000
Habituation	*C. elegans*	Heat Shock	Impaired	Rose & Rankin	2006
Inhibitory (Passive) Avoidance	Mouse	Hemicholinium-3	Impaired	Boccia, Acosta, Blake, & Baratti	2004
Instrumental Incentive Learning	Rat	Anisomycin	Impaired	Wang, Ostlund, Nader, & Balleine	2005
Negative Transfer: Passive- to Active-Avoidance	Rat	Glucose	Enhanced	Rodriguez, Horne, Haas, & Padilla	2000
Object Recognition Memory	Rat	Anisomycin	Impaired	Rossato, Bevilaqua, Myskiw, Medina, Izquierdo, & Cammarota	2007
Paired-Associate Learning	Human	Interference	Impaired	Forcato, Burgos, Argibay, Molina, Pedreira, & Maldonado	2007
Reward-Related Memory	Rat	Propranolol	Impaired	Diergaarde, Schoffelmeer, & De Vries	2006
Social Recognition Memory	Ewe	Cycloheximide	Impaired	Perrin, Ferreira, Meurisse, Verdin, Mouly, & Levy	2007
Spatial Memory (Radial Maze)	Rat	MK-801	Impaired	Przybyslawski & Sara	1997
Spatial Memory (Water Maze)	Rat	Cycloheximide	Impaired	Flint, Valentine, & Papandrea	2007

Hupbach, Gomez, Hardt, and Nadel (2007) presented an explicit visual memory task involving word list recall. Similar to other paradigms, recall of items presented on day one was tested on day three following either (a) a reminder followed by new learning on day two or (b) no reminder with new learning trained on day two. Results of their study demonstrated that when given a reminder on day two, participants incorrectly recalled items from the second list during testing of the first list on day three. The impairment was found to be time dependent, in that memory for list two was not impaired on day three.

The existence of memory reconsolidation processes across species and paradigms implies that reconsolidation may occur for most species under many different mnemonic conditions (and likely, for many different forms of memory). The studies with humans, in particular, emphasize the susceptibility of old previously consolidated memories to disruption and may help explain some of the challenges faced by the traditional consolidation hypothesis. Despite the apparent breadth of research supporting the generalization of this phenomenon, there continues to be considerable debate regarding many of the characteristics and potential mechanisms of memory reconsolidation.

Characteristics of Memory Reconsolidation

Reactivating Old Memories

Can the environmental context alone sufficiently reactivate an old memory and elicit reconsolidation processes? Does new learning have to occur during memory reactivation in order to elicit memory reconsolidation? The literature addressing these issues is quite mixed. Several studies, including some from our lab, have suggested that a simple re-exposure to the original training context is sufficient to elicit protein synthesis-dependent memory reconsolidation (Artinian, De Jaeger, Fellini, de Saint Blanquat, & Roullet, 2007; Flint & Marino, 2007; Flint, Valentine, & Papandrea, 2007; Judge & Quartermain, 1982). Using rats and a conditioned taste aversion paradigm, Flint and Marino established a taste aversion to sucrose in a unique and salient context. Cycloheximide administered approximately 25-minutes prior to a brief re-exposure to the training context resulted in significant amnesia for the original taste aversion conditioning. In this study, animals were not re-administered the CS-US pairing (no opportunity for new learning) and they were not administered the CS (no opportunity for extinction). These results suggest that the simple re-exposure to the training context, in the absence of any explicit new learning, is sufficient to elicit a protein synthesis-dependent reconsolidation process.

In contrast to these findings, other evidence suggests that new learning may be necessary in order to elicit reconsolidation processes (Morris et al., 2006; Rossato et al., 2007). Using an object recognition task, Rossato et al. demonstrated that a reactivation condition consisting of one salient and behaviorally relevant novel object and one familiar object elicited reconsolidation for the familiar object which was impaired with infusion of anisomycin into CA1 of the hippocampus. Memory for the familiar object was not impaired by anisomycin when the reactivation condition included only familiar objects, only novel objects, only the training context, or in the absence of specific salient stimuli. According to these results, reconsolidation-dependent processes are activated only when new and relevant information is added at the time of retrieval.

Training Strength and Memory Age

Both the strength of initial training and the temporal delay between training and memory reactivation appear to be important factors in determining an organism's **susceptibility** to reconsolidation impairment. Schneider and Sherman (1968) provided the first evidence that the strength of original training might be important. They reported that electroconvulsive shock following a non-contingent reminder footshock produced permanent amnesia for weak conditioning, but only temporary amnesia for strong conditioning. Suzuki et al. (2004) showed that both the strength of the memory and its age are important for fear conditioning in mice. They demonstrated that older and stronger memories were more resistant to anisomycin-induced reconsolidation impairment in comparison to younger and weaker memories. Similar findings that remote memories are more resistant to reconsolidation-associated impairments than more recently formed memories have been reported in the medaka fish (Eisenberg & Dudai, 2004). Resistance to reconsolidation impairment may be partially due to the way the memory is distributed in the brain, as there have been differences reported with systemic and central administration of anisomycin (Frankland et al., 2006).

An important difference between weak and strong initial learning is the supposition that a reminder or reactivation treatment, often in the form of a training trial, will allow for new learning when original training was weak, but not if the original training was strong. As previously indicated, a number of studies have suggested that new learning is necessary in order to initiate the reconsolidation process (Morris et al., 2006). Rodriguez-Ortiz, Garcia-DeLaTorre, Benavidez, Ballesteros, and Bermudez-Rattoni (2008) have argued that memory updating (i.e., new learning) must take place in order for intrahippocampal anisomycin infusions to impair reconsolidation, a process that is presumed to be more closely linked with weaker memories. In their study of spatial memory they found that overtrained animals were not susceptible to the impairing effects of anisomycin.

A recent human study from our lab using an implicit skill finger-tapping task employed by Walker, Brakefield, Morgan, and Hobson, (2002) suggests a potential relationship between the age of the memory and its susceptibility to disruption when reactivated (Zamecnik, Bengsz, & Flint, 2009). In this study, participants in two of the groups were given either 16 training trials on day 1 followed by rest on days 2 through 5, or 12 training trials on day 1 and one trial each on days 2 through 5. On day 6, participants in these two groups were given a single trial to reactivate the memory and were then given 17 trials of a new finger-tapping sequence. We found evidence indicating that the first group with massed training on day 1 was not impaired on the retention test given on day 7 in comparison to other no-reminder groups; however, the second group which received trials every day was significantly impaired. These findings support the contention that the age or recency of activity of the target memory may play a role in determining its susceptibility to retrieval-induced reconsolidation.

Although there may be a tendency to view the evidence above as a clear relationship between the extent of training or its age and the susceptibility of that memory to subsequent disruption at the time of retrieval, other evidence suggests that such an interpretation may be overly simplistic. Abrari, Rashidy-Pour, Semnanian, and Fathollahi (2008) demonstrated that post-reactivation corticosterone disrupted memory reconsolidation for animals given fear conditioning with a high intensity shock, but not a low intensity shock. This finding suggests that more intense training may, under certain circumstances, be more susceptible to disruption following reactivation. In the Abrari et al. study the endogenous stress hormone corticosterone was used to impair memory reconsolidation. The relationships between the footshock used in fear conditioning paradigms and endogenous stress hormones may suggest a possible interaction between arousal and reconsolidation. Maroun and Akirav (2009) have suggested such a relationship based on their results of an object recognition experiment. In their study, infusions of a dopamine D1 receptor antagonist into the ventromedial prefrontal cortex impaired reconsolidation in rats that were not habituated to the apparatus, but had no effect on those that were habituated to the apparatus. They also found that a dopamine D1 receptor agonist and an MEK inhibitor impaired reconsolidation regardless of the arousal level.

Reconsolidation or Extinction

A number of studies have now demonstrated that the duration of the memory reactivation treatment (or number of trials) may be an important factor when attempting to elicit retrieval-induced reconsolidation processes. It appears as though one or a few brief reactivation trials are more likely to activate memory reconsolidation processes, whereas long or many reactivation trials are more apt to activate extinction processes (Berman & Dudai, 2001; De Oliveira Alvares, Pasqualini Genro, Diehl, Molina, & Quillfeldt, 2008; Eisenhardt & Menzel, 2007; Lattal, Honarvar, & Abel, 2004; Lee, Milton, & Everitt, 2006b; Mamiya et al., 2009; Pedreira & Maldonado, 2003; Power, Berlau, McGaugh, & Steward, 2006). Suzuki et al. (2004) reported that retrieval could induce either extinction or reconsolidation, each with their own distinct biochemical signatures. Antagonism of the cannabinoid receptor 1 or L-type-voltage-gated calcium channels had no effect on reconsolidation, but effectively blocked extinction processes. Bahar, Dorfman, and Dudai (2004) demonstrated that the neuroanatomical substrates of taste aversion consolidation, extinction, and reconsolidation are different. Using infusions of the protein synthesis inhibitor anisomycin they found that consolidation was dependent upon the central nucleus of the amygdala and extinction was dependent upon the basolateral nuclei of the amygdala, but that protein synthesis inhibition in either of these nuclei had no effect on reconsolidation. These studies demonstrate that extinction and reconsolidation processes may be elicited by different behavioral procedures and may involve different biochemical and neuroanatomical substrates. This does not mean, however, that such processes may not be simultaneously activated. Duvarci, Mamou, and Nader (2006) have shown that reconsolidation processes may be initiated even in the presence of extinction.

Neurobiological Factors

The use of many treatments such as electroconvulsive shock, broad spectrum pharmacological agents like protein synthesis inhibitors, or the systemic administration of drugs, make it difficult to discern the underlying neurobiological mechanisms associated with reconsolidation. It is on this front that there is currently the greatest activity and will likely be the source of the greatest amount of variability, given that different types of memory involve different neural substrates and biochemical systems. For example, there may be great differences between the mechanisms of reconsolidation for conditioned taste aversion per se and the mechanisms of reconsolidation for spatial memory. As a result of this variability, finding common ground for the mechanisms of reconsolidation at the molecular or cellular level across paradigms is likely an unrealistic endeavor.

Table 4. Some Pharmacological Agents and their Routes of Administration for Modulating Memory Reconsolidation in Rodents (alphabetized by drug then route of administration).

Drug	Route of Administration	Species	Memory Status	Authors	Year
6-BNZ-cAMP	Intracranial (Amygdala-Basolateral Nucleus)	Rat	Enhanced	Tronson, Wiseman, Olausson, & Taylor	2006
AM251	Intracranial (Hippocampus-Dorsal CA1)	Rat	Enhanced	De Oliveira Alvares, Genro, Diehl, Molina, & Quillfeldt	2008
Anandamide	Intracranial (Hippocampus-Dorsal CA1)	Rat	Impaired	Alvares, Genro, Diehl, Molina, & Quillfeldt	2008
Anisomycin	Intracranial (Amygdala-Lateral and Basal Nuclei)	Rat	Impaired	Wang, Ostlund, Nader, & Balleine	2005
Anisomycin	Intracranial (Cerebellum)	Rat	Impaired	Sacchetti, Sacco, & Strata	2007
Anisomycin	Intracranial (Hippocampus-Dorsal CA1)	Rat	Impaired	Rossato, Bevilaqua, Myskiw, Medina, Izquierdo, & Cammarota	2007
Anisomycin	Intracranial (Hippocampus-CA3)	Mouse	Impaired	Artinian, McGauran, De Jaeger, Mouledous, Frances, & Roullet	2008
Anisomycin	Intraperitoneal	Rat Pup	Impaired	Languille, Gruest, Richer, & Hars	2008
Anisomycin	Intraventricular	Rat	Impaired	Nomura & Matsuki	2008
Corticosterone	Intraperitoneal	Rat	Impaired	Abrari, Rashidy-Pour, Semnanian, & Fathollahi	2008
Cycloheximide	Subcutaneous	Rat	Impaired	Flint, Valentine, & Papandrea	2007
D-APV	Intracranial (Amygdala-Basolateral Nucleus)	Rat	Impaired	Milton, Lee, Butler, Gardner, & Everitt	2008
D-Cycloserine	Intraperitoneal; Intracranial (Amygdala)	Rat	Enhanced	Lee, Milton, & Everitt	2006
DRB	Intracranial (Hippocampus-Dorsal CA1)	Rat	Impaired	De Oliveira Alvares, Genro, Diehl, Molina, & Quillfeldt	2008
Ethanol	Intraperitoneal	Rat	Enhanced	Nomura & Matsuki	2008
FN-439	Intracerebroventricular	Rat	Impaired	Brown, Wilson, Cocking, & Sorg	2009
Fructose	Subcutaneous	Rat	Enhanced	Rodriguez, Horne, & Padilla	1999
Glucose	Subcutaneous	Rat	Enhanced	Rodriguez, Horne, & Padilla	1999

Table 4. (*Continued*)

Drug	Route of Administration	Species	Memory Status	Authors	Year
Go6976	Intracranial (Hippocampus-Dorsal CA1)	Rat	Impaired	Bonini, Da Silva, Bevilaqua, Medina, Izquierdo, & Cammarota	2007
Hemicholinium-3	Intracerebroventricular	Mouse	Impaired	Boccia, Acosta, Blake, & Baratti	2004
Ketamine	Intraperitoneal	Rat	Impaired	Zhai, Wu, Chen, Li, Liu, & Lu	2008
L-NAME	Intraperitoneal	Mouse	Impaired	Baratti, Boccia, Blake, & Acosta	2008
Lactacystin	Intracranial (Hippocampus-CA3)	Mouse	Impaired	Artinian, McGauran, De Jaeger, Mouledous, Frances, & Roullet	2008
Midazolam	Intraperitoneal	Rat	Impaired	Bustos, Maldonado, & Molina	2006
Mifepristone	Intracranial (Amygdala-Basolateral Nucleus)	Rat	Impaired	Tronel & Alberini	2007
Mifepristone	Subcutaneous	Rat	Impaired	Taubenfeld, Ricebert, New, & Alberini	2009
MK-801	Intraperitoneal	Rat	Impaired	Lee & Everitt	2008
Nimodipine	Intraperitoneal	Mouse	Reversed Anisomycin	Suzuki, Mukawa, Tsukagoshi, Frankland, & Kida	2008
PD 98059	Intracranial (Ventromedial Prefrontal Cortex)	Rat	Impaired	Maroun & Akirav	2009
Propranolol	Intraperitoneal	Rat	Impaired	Debiec & LeDoux	2004
Propranolol	Intracranial (Amygdala-Lateral & Basal Nuclei)	Rat	Impaired	Debiec & LeDoux	2004
Rapamycin	Intracranial (Hippocampus-Dorsal CA1)	Rat	Impaired	Myskiw, Rossato, Bevilaqua, Medina, Izquierdo, & Cammarota	2008
Rapamycin	Intraperitoneal	Mouse	Impaired	Blundell, Kouser, & Powell	2008
Rimonabant	Intraperitoneal	Mouse	Impaired	Yu et al.	2009
Rp-cAMPS	Intracranial (Amygdala-Basolateral Nucleus)	Rat	Impaired	Tronson, Wiseman, Olausson, & Taylor	2006
SCH 23390	Intracranial (Ventromedial Prefrontal Cortex)	Rat	Impaired	Maroun & Akirav	2009
Scopolamine	Intraperitoneal	Rat	Impaired	Zhai, Wu, Chen, Li, Liu, & Lu	2008
SKF	Intracranial (Ventromedial Prefrontal Cortex)	Rat	Impaired	Maroun & Akirav	2009
SR141716A	Intraperitoneal or Intracranial (Dorsal Hippocampus)	Mouse	Reversed Anisomycin	Suzuki, Mukawa, Tsukagoshi, Frankland, & Kida	2008
Strychnine	Intraperitoneal	Rat	Enhanced	Gordon	1977b
Tetrodotoxin	Intracranial (Amygdala-Basolateral Nucleus)	Rat	Impaired	Baldi, Mariottini, & Bucherelli	2008

Table 4. (*Continued*)

Drug	Route of Administration	Species	Memory Status	Authors	Year
Tetrodotoxin	Intracranial (Cerebellum)	Rat	Impaired	Sacchetti, Sacco, & Strata	2007
Tetrodotoxin	Intracranial (Hippocampus)	Rat	Impaired	Prado-Alcala, Diaz de Guante, Garin-Aguilar, Diaz-Trujillo, Quirarte, & McGaugh	2006
U0126	Intracranial (Amygdala-Lateral Nucleus)	Rat	Impaired	Doyere, Debiec, Monfils, Schafe, & LeDoux	2007
Verapamil	Intracranial (Dorsal Hippocampus)	Mouse	Reversed Anisomycin	Suzuki, Mukawa, Tsukagoshi, Frankland, & Kida	2008
Zif268 Antisense Oligodeoxynucleotides	Intracranial (Amygdala-Basolateral Nucleus)	Rat	Impaired	Lee, Milton, & Everitt	2006a

[6-BNZ-cAMP = specific PKA activator; AM251 = selective CB1 cannabinoid receptor antagonist; Anandamide = CB1 agonist; Anisomycin = protein synthesis inhibitor; Corticosterone = endogenous stress hormone; Cycloheximide = protein synthesis inhibitor; D-APV = specific antagonist of NMDA glutamate receptors; DRB = protein synthesis inhibitor; FN-439 = MMP inhibitor I; Go6976 = PKC and PKCμ inhibitor; Hemicholinium-3 = specific inhibitor of high-affinity choline uptake; Ketamine = noncompetitive NMDA receptor antagonist; L-NAME = non-specific inhibitor of nitric oxide synthase; Lactacystin = protein degradation inhibitor; Midaxolam = GABA agonist; Mifepristone = glucocorticoid receptor antagonist (aka. RU38486); MK-801 = NMDA receptor antagonist; Nimodipine = L-type voltage-gated calcium channels antagonist; PD 98059 = MEK inhibitor; Propranolol = β-adrenergic antagonist; Rapamycin = mTOR inhibitor; Rimonabant = CB1 antagonist; Rp-cAMPS = PKA inhibitor; SCH 23390 = dopamine D1 receptor antagonist; Scopolamine = acetylcholine receptor antagonist; SKF = dopamine D1 receptor agonist; SR141716A = CB1 antagonist; Strychnine = antagonist of the strychnine-sensitive glycine receptor; Tetrodotoxin = neurotoxin that blocks action potentials by binding with voltage-gated Na^+ channels; U0126 = MEK inhibitor; Verapamil = L-type voltage-gated calcium channels antagonist]

The availability of more selective drugs is helping to facilitate our understanding of reconsolidation mechanisms, although this line of research still appears to be in its infancy (see Crowe, Sherry, & Hale, 2008 and Tronson & Taylor, 2007 for detailed reviews). Tables 4 and 5 provide selected references for most of the different pharmacological agents and their routes of administration that have been used to study memory reconsolidation in rodents (Table 4) and non-rodent species (Table 5) thus far.

To summarize some of the work presented in Tables 4 and 5, and other work focused on identifying the specific mechanisms of memory reconsolidation, recent evidence has suggested that hippocampal PKC is required following memory reactivation of a spatial memory trace (Bonni et al., 2007). Using a conditioned fear paradigm, Mamiya et al. (2009) demonstrated that genetic disruption of cAMP-responsive element-binding protein (CREB)-mediated transcription prevented reconsolidation in mice, which was likely associated with the hippocampus and the amygdala. Other studies have demonstrated a potential role for the matrix metalloproteinases (Brown et al., 2007; Brown, Wilson, Cocking, & Sorg, 2009), PKA

Table 5. Some Pharmacological Agents and their Routes of Administration for Modulating Memory Reconsolidation in Non-Rodent Species (alphabetized by drug then route).

Drug	Route of Administration	Species	Memory Status	Authors	Year
Acetoxycycloheximide	Intracranial	Goldfish	Impaired	Davis & Klinger	1969
Anisomycin	Heamocoel Surrounding Central Ganglia	Snail	Impaired	Kemenes, Kemenes, Michel, Papp, & Muller	2006
Anisomycin	Intramuscular (Flight Muscle)	Bee	Impaired	Stollhoff, Menzel, & Eisenhardt	2008
AP5	Intracranial (Forebrain)	Chick	Impaired	Summers, Crowe, & Ng	1997
Bicuculline	Pericardial Sac	Crab	Enhanced	Tano, Molina, Maldonado, & Pedreira	2009
CNQX	Intracranial (Forebrain)	Chick	Impaired	Sherry & Crowe	2008b
Cortisol	Oral	Human	Impaired	Tollenaar, Elzinga, Spinhoven, & Everaerd	2009
Cycloheximide	Intracerebroventricular	Chick	Impaired	Litvin & Anokhin	2000
Cycloheximide	Oral	Drosophila	Impaired	Lagasse, Devaud, & Mery	2009
Cycloheximide	Pericardial Sac	Crab	Impaired	Pedreira & Maldonado	2003
Emetine	Intramuscular (Flight Muscle)	Bee	Impaired	Stollhoff, Menzel, & Eisenhardt	2005
KCl	Intracranial	Goldfish	Impaired	Davis & Klinger	1969
KT5720	Heamocoel Surrounding Central Ganglia	Snail	Impaired	Kemenes, Kemenes, Michel, Papp, & Muller	2006
MS222	Immersion	Medaka	Impaired	Eisenberg & Dudai	2004
Muscimol	Pericardial Sac	Crab	Impaired	Tano, Molina, Maldonado, & Pedeira	2009
Propranolol	Oral	Human	Impaired	Kindt, Soeter, & Vervliet	2009
Puromycin	Intracranial	Goldfish	Impaired	Davis & Klinger	1969
Roscovitine	Intracranial (Forebrain)	Chick	Impaired	Sherry & Crowe	2008a
SCH23390	Subcutaneous	Chick	Impaired	Sherry, Hale, & Crowe	2005

[Acetoxycycloheximide = protein synthesis inhibitor; Anisomycin = protein synthesis inhibitor; AP5 = NMDA receptor antagonist; Bicuculline = comepetitive antagonist of GABA; CNQX = non-NMDA receptor antagonist; Cortisol = stress hormone; Cycloheximide = protein synthesis inhibitor; Emetine = protein synthesis inhibitor; KCl = potassium chloride; KT5720 = selective PKA inhibitor; MS222 = Na^+ channel blocker; Muscimol = GABAergic agonist; Propranolol = β-adrenergic antagonist; Puromycin = protein synthesis inhibitior; Roscovitine = inhibitor of cyclin-dependent kinase 5; SCH23390 = dopamine D1 receptor antagonist]

(Tronson, Wiseman, Olausson, & Taylor, 2006), nitric oxide (Baratti, Boccia, Blake, & Acosta, 2008), mammalian target of rapamycin (Blundell, Kouser, & Powell, 2008; Myskiw et al., 2008), NMDA receptors (Lee & Everitt, 2008; Przybyslawski & Sara, 1997; Summers, Crowe, & Ng, 1997; Torras-Garcia, Lelong, Tronel, & Sara, 2005), ERK1/2 (Duvarcie, Nader, & LeDoux, 2005), the cholinergic system (Boccia, Acosta, Blake, & Baratti, 2004), the serotonergic system (Ogren et al., 2008), the GABAergic system (Carbo Tano, Molina, Maldonado, & Pedreira, 2009; Zhang & Cranney, 2008), and the β-adrenergic system (Przybyslawski, Roullet, & Sara, 1999; Roullet & Sara, 1998).

IMPLICATIONS FOR TREATMENTS OF PSYCHIATRIC DISORDERS

Anxiety Disorders

From an applied perspective, one of the greatest benefits of memory reconsolidation research is its potential to provide treatments for anxiety disorders such as post-traumatic stress disorder (PTSD) and phobias. Characteristic of these disorders is their resistance to extinction, and as a result individuals with PTSD continue to "re-live" the traumatic experience with levels of arousal comparable to those elicited during the original learning (Antony & Stein, 2009; Fanselow, 2008; Pitman & Delahanty, 2007; Shin, Rauch, Pitman & Whalen, 2009; Taylor, Olausson, Quinn, & Torregrossa, 2009). Individuals suffering from phobias may similarly continue to show high levels of arousal and fear to a stimulus in the absence of the US (Cisler, Olatunji, & Lohr, 2009; Shin et al.). Based on memory reconsolidation research, specific treatments may selectively weaken the exaggerated responsiveness demonstrated by patients with PTSD and phobia if administered in conjunction with reactivation of that original memory trace.

Animal models involving variations of fear conditioning have implied that treatments disrupting reconsolidation (i.e., causing amnesia for the original memory) provide good support for treating individuals with certain anxiety disorders. Taubenfeld, Riceberg, New, and Alberini (2009) demonstrated that the glucocorticoid receptor antagonist RU38486 administered at the time of memory retrieval persistently weakened the target memory. Other similar studies have used the mTOR inhibitor rapamycin (Blundell et al., 2008), the GABA agonist midazolam (Zhang & Cranney, 2008), and corticosterone (Cai, Blundell, Han, Greene, & Powell, 2006) to impair fear memory when administered at the time of memory reactivation. Recently, Monfils, Cowansage, Klann, and LeDoux (2009) developed a novel behavioral design for rodents in which the target fear memory was disrupted at the time of retrieval through non-pharmacological means.

A few studies have been conducted with humans to examine the plausibility that impairing reconsolidation of a fear memory might eventually be an effective treatment for anxiety disorders. Tollenaar, Elzinga, Spinhoven, and Everaerd (2008) used a delayed cued recall task, where participants were trained, given a retrieval session with or without stress one day or five weeks later, and then a cued recall test six months following original learning. Results indicated that participants that retrieved the memory under stress at five weeks showed impaired recall at the six month test, suggesting that the neuroendocrine stress response may detrimentally influence the reconsolidation process. In support of these findings, Tollenaar Elzinga, Spinhoven, and Everaerd (2009) have reported that the stress hormone cortisol is able to disrupt reconsolidation for both neutral and emotional information. In this study they failed to find any effect of the β-adrenergic receptor antagonist propranolol on reconsolidation of either type of information. In contrast, Kindt, Soeter, and Vervliet (2009) used propranolol to effectively induce amnesia for fear memory in humans when administered at the time of memory reactivation.

Results such as these from animal models and the few human studies are, indeed, very encouraging. It has yet to be demonstrated that treatments such as cortisol or propranolol at the time of memory retrieval will be able to disrupt the anxiety-provoking target memory in actual patients suffering from anxiety disorders. As mentioned previously, multiple reminder treatments often produce extinction, and treatments that often impair reconsolidation following single reminders have been shown to have little or no effect on the target memory, and instead, apparently produce amnesia for the extinction training (Pedreira & Maldonado, 2003). It is not clear how these issues might be involved in individuals suffering from PTSD, where there is an apparent resistance to extinction. Do the recurrent and disruptive memory-related anxiety responses in patients with PTSD and phobias undergo reconsolidation following their reactivation? Answers to questions such as this are, as yet, unknown, but the potential for benefit from such research is considerable.

Drug Addiction

One of the greatest problems facing the effective treatment of drug addiction is the cue-induced cravings that often occur before and/or co-occur with compulsive drug use (Hernandez & Kelley, 2005; Taylor, Olausson, Quinn, & Torregrossa, 2009). Research on memory reconsolidation provides insight into a potential means of reducing or eliminating these cue-induced cravings. In other words, disrupting the reconsolidation of one or more cues associated with the drug may eliminate the reinforcing properties that lead an individual to drug use. A number of studies using animal models have now demonstrated that Zif286 antisense oligodeoxynucleotides infused into the basolateral amygdala (Hellemans, Everitt, & Lee, 2006; Lee, Milton, & Everitt, 2006a), systemic administration of anisomycin (Bernardi, Lattal, & Berger, 2007; cf. Robinson & Franklin, 2007; Yim, Moraes, Ferreira, & Oliveria, 2006), systemic or intra-amygdala administration of NMDA receptor antagonists (Milton, Lee, Butler, Gardner, & Everitt, 2008; Zhai, Wu, Chen, Li, Liu, & Lu, 2008), and systemic administration of the cholinergic receptor antagonist scopolamine (Zhai et al.) at the time of retrieval of a drug-related memory results in the subsequent amnesia for the original drug memory.

In the only human study of drug addiction-related reconsolidation to date, Zhao, Zhang, Shi, Epstein, and Lu (2009) required abstinent heroin addicts to learn a list comprised of neutral and heroin-related emotional words. The memory for these words was reactivated 24-hours later and followed immediately by a standardized psychosocial laboratory stressor (Trier Social Stress Test) or a control condition. Results of a free recall test 24-hours later indicated that participants were only impaired on the heroin-related emotional words, and not neutral words. In addition to this finding, Zhao et al. reported that the stressor induced a significant increase in salivary free cortisol, providing similar results to Tollenaar et al.

(2009) in that emotional memory was attenuated by an increase in cortisol. These results imply that high cortisol levels decrease memory by impairing memory reconsolidation, and provide implications for the treatment of drug addiction in humans.

Conclusions

The research reviewed in this chapter clearly indicates the existence of a post-retrieval memory reconsolidation process that has been demonstrated in a wide variety of paradigms with many different species, including humans. A number of theories of memory reconsolidation, including a Synaptic Reinforcement-Based Model (Amaral, Osan, Roesler, & Tort, 2008), an Internal Reinforcement Hypothesis (Eisenhardt & Menzel, 2007), and retrieval based explanations (Riccio, Millin, & Bogart, 2006) have been proposed, as well as arguments that reconsolidation activates consolidation-like processes (Nader & Hardt, 2009). Readers interested in the specifics of these arguments should consult the primary sources, as the details of these proposals are beyond the scope of this review. As the behavioral characteristics and biochemical mechanisms of reconsolidation become clear, avenues may evolve providing practitioners with novel treatments for psychiatric conditions such as post-traumatic stress disorder, phobias, and drug addiction.

References

Abrari, K., Rashidy-Pour, A., Semnanian, S. & Fathollahi, Y. (2008). Administration of corticosterone after memory reactivation disrupts subsequent retrieval of a contextual conditioned fear memory: Dependence upon training intensity. *Neurobiology of Learning and Memory*, *89*, 178-184.

Amaral, O. B., Osan, R., Roesler, R. & Tort, A. B. L. (2008). A synaptic reinforcement-based model for transient amnesia following disruptions of memory consolidation and reconsolidation. *Hippocampus*, *18*, 584-601.

Antony, M. M. & Stein, M. B. (Eds.) (2009). *Oxford handbook of anxiety and related disorders.*, New York, NY: Oxford University Press.

Artinian, J., De Jaeger, X., Fellini, L., de Saint Blanquat, P. & Roullet, P. (2007). Reactivation with a simple exposure to the experimental environment is sufficient to induce reconsolidation requiring protein synthesis in the hippocampal CA3 region in mice. *Hippocampus*, *17*, 181-191.

Artinian, J., McGauran, A. M. T., De Jaeger, X., Mouledous, L., Frances, B. & Roullet, P. (2008). Protein degradation, as with protein synthesis, is required during not only long-term spatial memory consolidation but also reconsolidation. *European Journal of Neuroscience*, *27*, 3009-3019.

Bahar, A., Dorfman, N. & Dudai, Y. (2004). Amygdala circuits required for either consolidation or extinction of taste aversion memory are not required for reconsolidation. *European Journal of Neuroscience*, *19*, 1115-1118.

Baldi, E., Mariottini, C. & Bucherelli, C. (2008). Differential roles of the basolateral amygdala and nucleus basalis magnocellularis during post-reactivation contextual fear conditioning reconsolidation in rats. *Neurobiology of Learning and Memory, 90,* 604-609.

Baratti, C. M., Boccia, M. M., Blake, M. G. & Acosta, G. B. (2008). Reactivated memory of an inhibitory avoidance response in mice is sensitive to a nitric oxide synthase inhibitor. *Neurobiology of Learning and Memory, 89,* 426-440.

Berman, D. E. & Dudai, Y. (2001). Memory extinction, learning anew, and learning the new: Dissociations in the molecular machinery of learning in cortex. *Science, 291,* 2417-2419.

Bernardi, R. E., Lattal, K. M. & Berger, S. P. (2007). Anisomycin disrupts a contextual memory following reactivation in a cocaine-induced locomotor activity paradigm. *Behavioral Neuroscience, 121(1),* 156-163.

Blundell, J., Kouser, M. & Powell, C. M. (2008). Systemic inhibition of mammalian target of rapamycin inhibits fear memory reconsolidation. *Neurobiology of Learning and Memory, 90,* 28-35.

Boccia, M. M., Acosta, G. B., Blake, M. G. & Baratti, C. M. (2004). Memory consolidation and reconsolidation of an inhibitiory avoidance response in mice: Effects of I.C.V. injections of hemicholinium-3. *Neuroscience, 124,* 735-741.

Bonini, J. S., Da Silva, W. C., Bevilaqua, L. R. M., Medina, J. H., Izquierdo, I. & Cammarota, M. (2007). On the participation of hippocampal PKC in acquisition, consolidation and reconsolidation of spatial memory. *Neuroscience, 147,* 37-45.

Bregman, N., Nicholas, T. & Lewis, D. J. (1976). Cue-dependent amnesia: Permanence and memory return. *Physiology & Behavior, 17*(2), 276-270.

Brown, T. E., Forquer, M. R., Cocking, D. L., Jansen, H. T., Harding, J. W. & Sorg, B. A. (2007). Role of matric metalloproteinases in the acquisition and reconsolidation of cocaine-induced conditioned place preference. *Learning & Memory, 14,* 214-223.

Brown, T. E., Wilson, A. R., Cocking, D. L. & Sorg, B. A. (2009). Inhibition of matrix metalloproteinase activity disrupts reconsolidation but not consolidation of fear memory. *Neurobiology of Learning and Memory, 91,* 66-72.

Bustos, S. G., Maldonado, H. & Molina, V. A. (2006). Midazolam disrupts fear memory reconsolidation. *Neuroscience, 139,* 831-842.

Cai, W.-H., Blundell, J., Han, J., Greene, R. W. & Powell, C. M. (2006). Postreactivation glucocorticoids impair recall of established fear memory. *The Journal of Neuroscience., 26*(37), 9560-9566.

Carbo Tano, M. C., Molina, V. A., Maldonado, H. & Pedreira, M. E. (2009). Memory consolidation and reconsolidation in an invertebrate model: The role of the GABAergic system. *Neuroscience, 158,* 387-401.

Castellano, C., Cabib, S. & Puglisi-Allegra, S. (1996). Psychopharmacology of memory modulation: Evidence for multiple interaction among neurotransmitters and hormones. *Behavioural Brain Research, 77,* 1-21.

Child, F. M., Epstein, H. T., Kuzirian, A. M. & Alkon, D. L. (2003). Memory reconsolidation in Hermissenda. *Biological Bulletin, 205,* 218-219.

Cisler, J. M., Olatunji, B. O. & Lohr, J. M. (2009). Disgust, fear, and the anxiety disorders: A critical review. *Clinical Psychology Review, 29*(1), 34-46.

Crowe, S. F., Sherry, J. M. & Hale, M. W. (2008). Remembering that things have changed: A review of the cellular mechanisms of memory re-consolidation in the day-old chick. *Brain Research Bulletin, 76,* 192-197.

Davis, R. E. & Klinger, J. D. (1969). Environmental control of amnesia effects of various agents in goldfish. *Physiology & Behavior, 4*, 269-271.

Debiec, J. & LeDoux, L. E. (2004). Disruption of reconsolidation but not consolidation of auditory fear conditioning by noradrenergic blockade in the amygdala. *Neuroscience, 129*, 267-272.

De Oliveira Alvares, L., Genro, B. P., Diehl, F., Molina, V. A. & Quillfeldt, J. A. (2008). Opposite action of hippocampal CB1 receptors in memory reconsolidation and extinction. *Neuroscience, 154*, 1648-1655.

Desgranges, B., Levy, F. & Ferreira, G. (2008). Anisomycin infusion in amygdala impairs consolidation of odor aversion memory. *Brain Research, 1236*, 166-175.

DeVietti, T. L., Conger, G. L. & Kirkpatrick, B. R. (1977). Comparison of the enhancement gradients of retention obtained with stimulation of the mesencephalic reticular formation after training or memory reactivation. *Physiology & Behavior, 19*(4), 549-555.

DeVietti, T. L. & Holliday, J. H. (1972). Retrograde amnesia produced by electroconvulsive shock after reactivation of a consolidated memory trace: A replication. *Psychonomic Science, 29*(3), 137-138.

DeVietti, T. L., Holliday, J. H. & Larson, R. C. (1973). Comparison of amnesias induced by electrovulsive shock administered after training-trial footshock or noncontingent footshock in rats. *Journal of Comparative and Physiological Psychology, 84*(3), 579-585.

DeVietti, T. L. & Kirkpatrick, B. R. (1976). The amnesia gradient: Inadequate as evidence for a memory consolidation process. *Science, 194*(4263), 438-440.

DeVietti, T. L. & Kirkpatrick, B. R. (1977). Stimulation of specific regions of brain in rats modifies retention for newly acquired and old habits. *Journal of Comparative and Physiological Psychology, 91*(3), 562-573.

DeVietti, T. L. & Kirkpatrick, B. R. (1978). Reminder induced by training cues and stimulation of the mesencephalic reticular formation. *Physiological Psychology, 6*(3), 381-386.

Diergaarde, L., Schoffelmeer, A. N. M. & De Vries, T. J. (2006). β-adrenoceptor mediated inhibition of long-term reward-related memory reconsolidation. *Behavioural Brain Research, 170*, 333-336.

Dornelles, A., de Lima, M. N. M., Grazziotin, M., Presti-Torres, J., Garcia, V. A., Scalco, F. S., Roesler, R. & Schroder, N. (2007). Adrenergic enhancement of consolidation of object recognition memory. *Neurobiology of Learning and Memory, 88*(1), 137-142.

Doyere, V., Debiec, J., Monfils, M.-H., Schafe, G. E. & LeDoux, J. E. (2007). Synapse-specific reconsolidation of distinct fear memories in the lateral amygdala. *Nature Neuroscience, 10*(4), 414-416.

Dudai, Y. (2004). The neurobiology of consolidations, or, how stable is the engram? *Annual Review of Psychology, 55*, 51-86.

Dudai, Y. & Morris, R. G. M. (2001). To consolidate or not to consolidate: what are the questions? In J. J. Bolhuis (ed.), *Brain Perception, Memory. Advances in Cognitive Neuroscience* (147-162). Oxford: Oxford University Press.

Duvarci, S., Mamou, C. B. & Nader, K. (2006). Extinction is not a sufficient condition to prevent fear memories from undergoing reconsolidation in the basolateral amygdala. *The European Journal of Neuroscience, 24*(1), 249-260.

Duvarci, S., Nader, K. & LeDoux, J. E. (2005). Activation of extracellular signal-regulated kinase- mitogen-activated protein kinase cascade in the amygdala is required for memory reconsolidation of auditory fear conditioning. *The European Journal of Neuroscience, 21*, 283-289.

Eichenbaum, H. (2003). Memory systems. In M. Gallagher, & R. J. Nelson (Eds.). *Handbook of psychology: Biological psychology* (v 3) (543-559). Hoboken, NJ: John Wiley & Sons, Inc.

Eisenberg, M. & Dudai, Y. (2004). Reconsolidation of fresh, remote, and extinguished fear memory in medaka: Old fears don't die. *European Journal of Neuroscience, 20*, 3397-3403.

Eisenhardt, D. & Menzel, R. (2007). Extinction learning, reconsolidation and the internal reinforcement hypothesis. *Neurobiology of Learning and Memory, 87*, 167-173.

Fanselow, M. S. (2008). The use of conditioning tasks to model fear and anxiety. In R. J. Blanchard, C. D. Blanchard, G. Griebel, & D. Nutt (Eds.). *Handbook of anxiety and fear* (29-48). San Diego, CA: Elsevier Academic Press.

Ferry, B., Roozendaal, B. & McGaugh, J. L. (1999). Role of norepinephrine in mediating stress hormone regulation of long-term memory storage: A critical involvement of the amygdala. *Biological Psychiatry, 46*(9), 1140-1152.

Flint, R. W., Jr. & Marino, C. L. (2007). Cycloheximide impairs reconsolidation of a contextually reactivated memory in a conditioned taste aversion paradigm. *Behavioral Neuroscience, 121*(2), 433-438.

Flint, R. W., Jr. & Riccio, D. C. (1999). Post-training glucose administration attenuates forgetting of passive avoidance conditioning in 18-day-old rats. *Neurobiology of Learning & Memory, 72*(1), 62-67.

Flint, R. W., Jr., Valentine, S. & Papandrea, D., Jr. (2007). Reconsolidation of a long-term spatial memory is impaired by cycloheximide when reactivated with a contextual latent learning trial in male and female rats. *Neuroscience, 148*, 833-844.

Flint, R. W., Jr. & Zak, A. (2002). Memory: A basic overview of systems and neuroanatomy. In R. W. Flint, Jr. (Ed.), *Forget it? Sources, theories, and mechanisms of alterations in mnemonic function* (1-22). North Chelmsford, MA: Courier Custom Publishing.

Forcato, C., Argibay, P. F., Pedreira, M. E. & Maldonado, H. (2009). Human reconsolidation does not always occur when a memory is retrieved: The relevance of the reminder structure. *Neurobiology of Learning and Memory, 91*, 50-57.

Forcato, C., Burgos, V. L., Argibay, P. F., Molina, V. A., Pedreira, M. E. & Maldonado, H. (2007). Reconsolidation of declarative memory in humans. *Learning & Memory, 14*, 295-303.

Frankland, P. W., Ding, H.-K., Takahashi, E., Suzuki, A., Kida, S. & Silva, A. J. (2006). Stability of recent and remote contextual fear memory. *Learning & Memory, 13*, 451-457.

Gainutdinova, T. H., Tagirova, R. R., Ismailova, A. I., Muranova, L. N., Samarova, E. I., Gainutdinov, K. L. & Balaban, P. M. (2005). Reconsolidation of a context long-term memory in the terrestrial snail requires protein synthesis. *Learning & Memory, 12*, 620-625.

Gold, P. E. (1995). Modulation of emotional and nonemotional memories: Same pharmacological systems, different neuroanatomical systems. In J. L. McGaugh, N. M. Weinberger, & G. Lynch (Eds.), *Brain and memory: Modulation and mediation of neuroplasticity* (41-74). New York, NY: Oxford University.

Gold, P. E. (1986). Glucose modulation of memory storage processing. *Behavioral & Neural Biology*, *45*(3), 342-349.

Gold, P. E. & van Buskirk, R. B. (1975). Facilitation of time-dependent memory processes with posttrial epinephrine injections. *Behavioral Biology*, *13*(2), 145-153.

Gordon, W. C. (1977a). Similarities of recently acquired and reactivated memories in interference. *American Journal of Psychology*, *90*(2), 231-242.

Gordon, W. C. (1977b). Susceptibility of reactivated memory to the effects of strychnine: A time-dependent phenomenon. *Physiology & Behavior*, *18*(1), 95-99.

Gordon, W. C. & Spear, N. E. (1977a). Effect of reactivation of a previously acquired memory on the interaction between memories in the rat. *Journal of Experimental Psychology*, *99*(3), 349-355.

Gordon, W. C. & Spear, N. E. (1977b). The effects of strychnine on recently acquired and reactivated passive avoidance memories. *Physiology & Behavior*, *10*(6), 1071-1075.

Harrod, S. B., Metzger, M. M. & Riccio, D. C. (1996). Does induced recovery from amnesia represent a disinhibition effect? *Physiology & Behavior*, *60*(5), 1375-1378.

Hellemans, K. G. C., Everitt, B. J. & Lee, J. L. C. (2006). Disrupting reconsolidation of conditioned withdrawal memories in the basolateral amygdala reduces suppression of heroin seeking rats. *The Journal of Neuroscience*, *26*(49), 12694-12699.

Hernandez, P. J. & Kelley, A. E. (2005). Cracking addiction the second time around: reconsolidation of drug-related memories. *Neuron*, *47*(6), 772-775.

Hernandez, P. J. & Kelley, A. E. (2004). Long-term memory for instrumental responses does not undergo protein synthesis-dependent reconsolidation upon retrieval. *Learning & Memory*, *11*(6), 748-754.

Houpt, T. A. & Berlin, R. (1999). Rapid, labile, and protein synthesis-independent short-term memory in conditioned taste aversion. *Learning & Memory*, *6*(1), 37-46.

Howard, R. L. & Meyer, D. R. (1971). Motivational control of retrograde amnesia in rats: a replication and extension. *Journal of Comparative and Physiological Psychology*, *74*(1), 37-40.

Hupbach, A., Gomez, R., Hardt, O. & Nadel, L. (2007). Reconsolidation of episodic memories: A subtle reminder triggers integration of new information. *Learning & Memory*, *14*, 47-53.

Inda, M. C., Delgado-Garcia, J. M. & Carrion, A. M. (2005). Acquisition, consolidation, reconsolidation and extinction of eyelid conditioning responses require de novo protein synthesis. *The Journal of Neuroscience*, *25*, 2070-2080.

Izquierdo, I., Bevilaqua, L. R., Rossato, J. I., Bonini, J. S., Da Silva, W. C., Medina, J. H. & Cammarota, M. (2006). The connection between the hippocampal and the striatal memory systems of the brain: a review of recent findings. *Neurotoxicity Research*, *10*(2), 113-121.

Judge, M. E. & Quartermain, D. (1982). Characteristics of retrograde amnesia following reactivation of memory in mice. *Physiology & Behavior*, *28*, 585-590.

Kemenes, G., Kemenes, I., Michel, M., Papp, A. & Muller, U. (2006). Phase-dependent molecular requirements for memory reconsolidation: differential roles for protein synthesis and protein kinase A activity. *The Journal of Neuroscience*, *26*(23), 6298-6302.

Kindt, M., Soeter, M. & Vervliet, B. (2009). Beyond extinction: erasing human fear responses and preventing the return of fear. *Nature Neuroscience*, *12*(3), 256-258.

Lagasse, F., Devaud, J.-M. & Mery, F. (2009). A switch from cycloheximide-resistant consolidated memory to cycloheximide-sensitive reconsolidation and extinction in *Drosophila. The Journal of Neuroscience, 29*(7), 2225-2230.

Land, C., Bunsey, M. & Riccio, D. C. (2000). Anomalous properties of hippocampal lesion-induced retrograde amnesia. *Psychobiology, 28*(4), 476-485.

Languille, S., Gruest, N., Richer, P. & Hars, B. (2008). The temporal dynamics of consolidation and reconsolidation decrease during postnatal development. *Learning & Memory, 15*, 434-442.

Lattal, K. M., Honarvar, S. & Abel, T. (2004). Effects of post-session injections of anisomycin on the extinction of a spatial preference and on the acquisition of a spatial reversal preference. *Behavioural Brain Research, 153*, 327-339.

Lee, J. L. C., Milton, A. L. & Everitt, B. J. (2006a). Cue-induced cocaine seeking and relapse are reduced by disruption of drug memory reconsolidation. *The Journal of Neuroscience, 26*(22), 5881-5887.

Lee, J. L. C., Milton, A. L. & Everitt, B. J. (2006b). Reconsolidation and extinction of conditioned fear: inhibition and potentiation. *The Journal of Neuroscience, 26*, 10051-10056.

Lee, J. L. C. & Everitt, B. J. (2008). Appetitive memory reconsolidation depends upon NMDA receptor-mediated neurotransmission. *Neurobiology of Learning and Memory, 90*, 147-154.

Levesque, M., Bedard, M. A., Courtemanche, R., Tremblay, P. L., Scherzer, P. & Blanchet, P. J. (2007). Raclopride-induced motor consolidation impairment in primates: role of the dopamine type-2 receptor in movement chunking into integrated sequences. *Experimental Brain Research, 182*(4), 499-508.

Lewis, D. J. (1979). Psychobiology of active and inactive memory. *Psychological Bulletin, 86*(5), 1054-1083.

Lewis, D. J., Bregman, N. J. & Mahan, J. J., Jr. (1972). Cue-dependent amnesia in rats. *Journal of Comparative and Physiological Psychology, 81*(2), 243-247.

Lewis, D. J. & Bregman, N. J. (1973). Source of cues for cue-dependent amnesia in rats. *Journal of Comparative and Physiological Psychology, 85*(2), 421-426.

Lima, R. H., Rossato, J. I., Furini, C. R., Bevilaqua, L. R., Izquierdo, I. & Cammarota, M. (2009). Infusion of protein synthesis inhibitors in the entorhinal cortex blocks consolidation but not reconsolidation of object recognition memory. *Neurobiology of Learning and Memory, 91*, 466-472.

Litvin, O. O. & Anokhin, K. V. (2000). Mechanisms of memory reorganization during retrieval of acquired behavioral experience in chicks: the effects of protein synthesis inhibition in the brain. *Neuroscience and Behavioral Physiology, 30*(6), 671-678.

Mactutus, C. F., Riccio, D. C. & Ferek, J. M. (1979). Retrograde amnesia for old (reactivated) memory: Some anomalous characteristics. *Science, 204*, 1319-1320.

Madsen, M. C. & McGaugh, J. L. (1961). The effect of ECS on one-trial avoidance learning. *Journal of Comparative and Physiological Psychology, 54*(5), 522-523.

Mamiya, N., Fukushima, H., Suzuki, A., Matsuyama, Z., Homma, S., Frankland, P. W. & Kida, S. (2009). Brain region-specific gene expression activation required for reconsolidation and extinction of contextual fear memory. *The Journal of Neuroscience, 29*(2), 402-413.

Maroun, M. & Akirav, I. (2009). Differential involvement of dopamine D1 receptor and MEK signaling pathway in the ventromedial prefrontal cortex in consolidation and reconsolidation of recognition memory. *Learning & Memory, 16*, 243-247.

McGaugh, J. L. (1989). Involvement of hormonal and neuromodulatory systems in the regulation of memory storage. *Annual Review of Neuroscience, 12*, 255-287.

McGaugh, J. L. (1966). Time-dependent processes in memory storage. *Science, 153*, 1351-1358.

McGaugh, J. L. & Alpern, H. P. (1966). Effects of electroshock on memory: Amnesia without convulsions. *Science, 152*(3722), 665-666.

Medina, J. H., Bekinschtein, P., Cammarota, M. & Izquierdo, I. (2008). Do memories consolidate to persist or do they persist to consolidate? *Behavioural Brain Research, 192*(1), 61-69.

Milton, A. L., Lee, J. L. C., Butler, V. J., Gardner, R. & Everitt, B. J. (2008). Intra-amygdala and systemic antagonism of NMDA receptors prevents the reconsolidation of drug-associated memory and impairs subsequently both novel and previously acquired drug-seeking behaviors. *The Journal of Neuroscience, 28*(33), 8230-8237.

Misanin, J. R., Miller, R. R. & Lewis, D. J. (1968). Retrograde amnesia produced by electroconvulsive shock after reactivation of a consolidated memory trace. *Science, 160*, 554-555.

Mohanty, A. & Flint, R. W., Jr. (2001). Differential effects of glucose on modulation of emotional and nonemotional spatial memory tasks. *Cognitive, Affective, & Behavioral Neuroscience, 1*(1), 90-95.

Monfils, M.-H., Cowansage, K. K., Klann, E. & LeDoux, J. E. (2009). Extinction-reconsolidation boundaries: Key to persisten attenuation of fear memories. *Science, 324*, 951-955.

Morgan, R. E., Flint, R. W., Jr. & Riccio, D. C. (1998). Time-dependent changes in inaccessible memory. *Psychonomic Bulletin & Review, 5*(3), 523-527.

Morris, R. G. M., Inglis, J., Ainge, J. A., Olverman, H. J., Tulloch, J., Dudai, Y. & Kelly, P. A. T. (2006). Memory reconsolidation: Sensitivity of spatial memory to inhibition of protein synthesis in dorsal hippocampus during encoding and retrieval. *Neuron, 50*, 479-489.

Myskiw, J. C., Rossato, J. I., Bevilaqua, L. R. M., Medina, J. H., Izquierdo, I. & Cammarota, M. (2008). On the participation of mTOR in recognition memory. *Neurobiology of Learning and Memory, 89*, 338-351.

Nader, K. & Hardt, O. (2009). A single standard for memory: the case for reconsolidation. *Nature Reviews Neuroscience, 10*(3), 224-234.

Nader, K., Schafe, G. E. & Le Doux, J. E. (2000). Fear memories require protein synthesis in the amygdala for reconsolidation after retrieval. Nature, 406, 722-726.

Nomura, H. & Matsuki, N. (2008). Ethanol enhances reactivated fear memories. *Neuropsychopharmacology, 33*, 2912-2921.

Ogren, S. O., Eriksson, T. M., Elvander-Tottie, E., D'Addario, C., Ekstrom, J. C., Svenningsson, P., Meister, B., Kehr, J. & Stiedl, O. (2008). The role of 5-HT_{1A} receptors in learning and memory. *Behavioural Brain Research, 195*, 54-77.

Pedreira, M. E. & Maldonado, H. (2003). Protein synthesis subserves reconsolidation or extinction depending on reminder duration. *Neuron, 38*, 863-869.

Pedreira, M. E., Perez-Cuesta, L. M. & Maldonado, H. (2002). Reactivation and reconsolidation of long-term memory in the crab Chasmagnathus: Protein synthesis requirement and mediation by NMDA-type glutamatergic receptors. *Journal of Neuroscience*, *22*, 8305-8311.

Perrin, G., Ferreira, G., Meurisse, M., Verdin, S., Mouly, A.-M. & Levy, F. (2007). Social recognition memory requires protein synthesis after reactivation. *Behavioral Neuroscience*, *121*(1), 148-155.

Pitman, R. K. & Delahanty, D. L. (2007). Conceptually driven pharmacological approaches to acute trauma. In M. T. Tsuang, W. S. Stone, & M. J. Lyons (Eds.). *Recognition and prevention of major mental and substance use disorders* (371-387). Arlington, VA: American Psychiatric Publishing, Inc.

Power, A. E., Berlau, D. J., McGaugh, J. L. & Steward, O. (2006). Anisomycin infused into the hippocampus fails to block "reconsolidation" but impairs extinction: The role of re-exposure duration. *Learning & Memory*, *13*, 27-34.

Prado-Alcala, R. A., Diaz del Guante, M. A., Garin-Aguilar, M. E., Diaz-Trujillo, A., Quirarte, G. L. & McGaugh, J. L. (2006). Amygdala or hippocampus inactivation after retrieval induces temporary memory deficit. *Neurobiology of Learning and Memory*, *86*, 144-149.

Przybyslawski, J., Roullet, P. & Sara, S. J. (1999). Attenuation of emotional and non-emotional memories after their reactivation: Role of beta adrenergic receptors. *The Journal of Neuroscience*, *19*, 6623-6628.

Przybyslawski, J. & Sara, S. J. (1997). Reconsolidation of memory after its reactivation. *Behavioural Brain Research*, *84*, 241-246.

Quartermain, D., McEwen, B. S. & Azmitia, E. C., Jr. (1972). Recovery of memory following amnesia in the rat and mouse. *Journal of Comparative and Physiological Psychology*, *79*(3), 360-370.

Rasch, B. & Born, J. (2007). Maintaining memories by reactivation. *Current Opinion in Neurobiology*, *17*(6), 698-703.

Riccio, D. C., Gaebelein, C. & Cohen, P. (1968). Some behavioral aspects of retrograde amnesia produced by hypothermia. *Physiology & Behavior*, *3*(6), 973-976.

Riccio, D. C., Hodges, L. A. & Randall, P. K. (1968). Retrograde amnesia produced by hypothermia in rats. *Journal of Comparative and Physiological Psychology*, *66*(3, Pt. 1), 618-622.

Riccio, D. C., Millin, P. M. & Bogart, A. R. (2006). Reconsolidation: A brief history, a retrieval view, and some recent issues. *Learning & Memory*, *13*(5), 536-544.

Riccio, D. C., Millin, P. M. & Gisquet-Verrier, P. (2003). Retrograde amnesia: Forgetting back. *Current Directions in Psychological Science*, *12*(2), 41-44.

Riccio, D. C. & Richardson, R. (1984). The status of memory following experimentally induced amnesias: Gone, but not forgotten. *Physiological Psychology*, *12*(2), 59-72.

Robbins, M. J. & Meyer, D. R. (1970). Motivational control of retrograde amnesia. *Journal of Experimental Psychology*, *84*(2), 220-225.

Robinson, M. J., F. & Franklin, K. B. J. (2007). Effects of anisomycin on consolidation and reconsolidation of a morphine-conditioned place preference. *Behvioural Brain Research*, *178*, 146-153.

Rodriguez, W. A., Horne, C. A., Haas, B. H. & Padilla, J. L. (2000). Effects of reactivation context on glucose modulation of reactivated memories. *Psychobiology*, *28*(4), 525-531.

Rodriguez, W. A., Horne, C. A. & Padilla, J. L. (1999). Effects of glucose and fructose on recently reactivated and recently acquired memories. *Progress in Neuro-Psychopharmacology & Biological Psychiatry*, *23*, 1285-1317.

Rodriguez, W. A., Van Ausdle, L. R., Dhanens, K. & Mondragon, A. N. (1993). Glucose modulates recently reactivated memories. *Psychobiology*, *21*(2), 93-100.

Rodriguez-Ortiz, C. J., Garcia-DeLaTorre, P., Benavidez, E., Ballesteros, M. A. & Bermudez-Rattoni, F. (2008). Intrahippocampal anisomycin infusions disrupt previously consolidated spatial memory only when memory is updated. *Neurobiology of Learning and Memory*, *89*, 352-359.

Roediger, H. L., Dudai, Y. & Fitzpatrick, S. M. (2007). *Science of memory: concepts*. New York, NY: Oxford University Press.

Rose, J. K. & Rankin, C. H. (2006). Blocking memory reconsolidation reverses memory-associated changes in glutamate receptor expression. *Journal of Neuroscience*, *26*, 11582-11587.

Rossato, J. I., Bevilaqua, L. R. M., Myskiw, J. C., Medina, J. H., Izquierdo, I. & Cammarota, M. (2007). On the role of hippocampal protein synthesis in the consolidation and reconsolidation of object recognition memory. *Learning & Memory*, *14*, 36-46.

Sacchetti, B., Sacco, T. & Strata, P. (2007). Reversible inactivation of amygdala and cerebellum but not perirhinal cortex impairs reactivated fear memories. *European Journal of Neuroscience*, *25*, 2875-2884.

Schneider, A. M. & Sherman, W. (1968). Amnesia: a function of the temporal relation of footshock to electroconvulsive shock. *Science*, *159*(3811), 219-221.

Sherry, J. M. & Crowe, S. F. (2008a). Inhibition of cyclin-dependent kinase 5 by roscovitine impairs memory consolidation and reconsolidation in the day-old-chick. *Pharmacology, Biochemistry, and Behavior*, *91*, 59-66.

Sherry, J. M. & Crowe, S. F. (2008b). The non-NMDA receptor antagonist 6-cyano-7-nitroquinoxaline-2,3-dione (CNQX) impairs later reconsolidation of passive avoidance learning in the day-old chick. *Neuroscience Letters*, *442*, 244-248.

Sherry, J. M., Hale, M. W. & Crowe, S. F. (2005). The effects of the dopamine D1 receptor antagonist SCH23390 on memory reconsolidation following reminder-activated retrieval in day-old chicks. *Neurobiology of Learning and Memory*, *83*, 104-112.

Shin, L. M., Rauch, S. L., Pitman, R. K. & Whalen, P. J. (2009). The human amygdala in anxiety disorders. In P. J. Whalen & E. A. Phelps (Eds.). *The human amygdala* (321-343). New York, NY: Guilford Press.

Soriano-Mas, C., Redolar-Ripoll, D., Guillazo-Blanch, G., Morgado-Bernal, I. & Segura-Torres, P. (2007). Intracranial self-stimulation after memory reactivation: Immediate and late effects. *Brain Research Bulletin*, *74*, 51-57.

Squire, L. R., Stark, C. E. L. & Clark, R. E. (2004). The medial temporal lobe. *Annual Review of Neuroscience*, *27*, 279-306.

Squire, L. R. & Zola, S. M. (1998). Episodic memory, semantic memory, and amnesia. *Hippocampus*, *8*(3), 205-211.

Stollhoff, N., Menzel, R. & Eisenhardt, D. (2005). Spontaneous recovery from extinction depends on the reconsolidation of the acquisition memory in an appetitive learning paradigm in the honeybee (Apis mellifera). *The Journal of Neuroscience*, *25*, 4485-4492.

Summers, M. J., Crowe, S. F. & Ng, K. T. (1997). Administration of DL-2-amino-5-phosphonovaleric acid (AP5) induces transient inhibition of reminder-activated memory retrieval in day-old chicks. *Cognitive Brain Research*, *5*, 311-321.

Suzuki, A., Josselyn, S. A., Frankland, P. W., Masushige, S., Silva, A. J. & Kida, S. (2004). Memory reconsolidation and extinction have distinct temporal biochemical signatures. *The Journal of Neuroscience*, *24*(20), 4787-4795.

Suzuki, A., Mukawa, T., Tsukagoshi, A., Frankland, P. W. & Kida, S. (2008). Activation of LVGCCs and CB1 receptors required for destabilization of reactivated contextual fear memories. *Learning & Memory*, *15*, 426-433.

Taubenfeld, S. M., Riceberg, J. S., New, A. S. & Alberini, C. M. (2009). Preclinical assessment for selectively disrupting a traumatic memory via postretrieval inhibition of glucocorticoid receptors. *Biological Psychiatry*, *65*, 249-257.

Taylor, J. R., Olausson, P., Quinn, J. J. & Torregrossa, M. M. (2009). Targeting extinction and reconsolidation mechanisms to combat the impact of drug cues on addiction. *Neuropharmacology*, *56*, 186-195.

Tollenaar, M. S., Elzinga, B. M., Spinhoven, P. & Everaerd, W. (2009). Immediate and prolonged effects of cortisol, but not propranolol, on memory retrieval in healthy young men. *Neurobiology of Learning and Memory*, *91*, 23-31.

Tollenaar, M. S., Elzinga, B. M., Spinhoven, P. & Everaerd, W. (2008). Long-term outcomes of memory retrieval under stress. *Behavioral Neuroscience*, *122*(3), 697-703.

Torras-Garcia, M., Lelong, J., Tronel, S. & Sara, S. J. (2005). Reconsolidation after remembering an odor-reward association requires NMDA receptors. *Learning & Memory*, *12*, 18-22.

Trifilieff, P., Calandreau, L., Herry, C., Mons, N., Micheau, J. (2007). Biphasic ERK1/2 activation in both the hippocampus and amygdala may reveal a system consolidation of contextual fear memory. *Neurobiology of Learning and Memory*, *88*(4), 424-434.

Tronel, S. & Alberini, C. M. (2007). Persistent disruption of a traumatic memory by postretrieval inactivation of glucocorticoid receptors in the amygdala. *Biological Psychiatry*, *62*, 33-39.

Tronson, N. C. & Taylor, J. R. (2007). Molecular mechanisms of memory reconsolidation. *Nature Reviews Neuroscience*, *8*, 262-275.

Tronson, N. C., Wiseman, S. L., Olausson, P. & Taylor, J. R. (2006). Bidirectional behavioral plasticity of memory reconsolidation depends on amygdalar protein kinase A. *Nature Neuroscience*, *9*(2), 167-169.

van der Staay, F. J., Rutten, K., Barfacker, L., DeVry, J., Erb, C., Heckroth, H., et al., (2008). The novel selective PDE9 inhibitor BAY 73-6691 improves learning and memory in rodents. *Neuropharmacology*, *55*(5), 908-918.

Walker, M. P., Brakefield, T., Hobson, J. A. & Stickgold, R. (2003). Dissociable stages of human memory consolidation and reconsolidation. *Nature*, *425*, 616-620.

Walker, M. P., Brakefield, T., Morgan, A., Hobson, J. A. & Stickgold, R. (2002). Practice with sleep makes perfect: Sleep-dependent motor skill learning. *Neuron*, *35*, 205-211.

Wang, S.-H., Ostlund, S. B., Nader, K. & Balleine, B. W. (2005). Consolidation and reconsolidation of incentive learning in the amygdala. *The Journal of Neuroscience*, *25*(4), 830-835.

Yim, A. J., Moraes, C. R. G., Ferreira, T. L. & Oliveira, M. G. M. (2006). Protein synthesis inhibition in the basolateral amygdala following retrieval does not impair expression of morphine-associated conditioned place preference. *Behavioural Brain Research, 171*, 162-169.

Yu, L.-l., Wang, X.-y., Zhao, M., Liu, Y., Li, Y.-q., Li, F.-q., Wang, X., Xue, Y.-x. & Lu, L. (2009). Effects of cannabinoid CB1 receptor antagonist rimonabant in consolidation and reconsolidation of methamphetamine reward memory in mice. *Psychopharmacology, 204*, 203-211.

Zamecnik, A. E., Bengsz, K. H. & Flint, R. W., Jr. (2009). *Human memory reconsolidation: Effects of delayed or distributed trials on susceptibility to disruption of a reactivated motor memory task.* Presentation at the 80th annual Eastern Psychological Association meeting, Pittsburgh, PA.

Zhai, H., Wu, P., Chen, S., Li, F., Liu, Y. & Lu, L. (2008). Effects of scopolamine and ketamine on reconsolidation of morphine conditioned place preference in rats. *Behavioural Pharmacology, 19*, 211-216.

Zhang, S. & Cranney, J. (2008). The role of GABA and anxiety in the reconsolidation of conditioned fear. *Behavioral Neuroscience, 122*(6), 1295-1305.

Zhao, L-Y., Zhang, X-L., Shi, J., Epstein, D. H. & Lu, L. (2009). Psychosocial stress after reactivation of drug-related memory impairs later recall in abstinent heroin addicts. *Psychopharmacology, 203*, 599-608.

In: Learning and Memory Developments...
Editors: L. C. Eklund, A. S. Nyman, pp. 155-172
ISBN: 978-1-60876-397-9

Chapter 6

INTELLECTUAL DISABILITY: BEYOND IQ SCORES

Nahal Goharpey[2], David P. Crewther[2] and Sheila G. Crewther[1*]

[1]School of Psychological Science, La Trobe University, Victoria, Australia, 3086.
[2]Brain Sciences Institute, Swinburne University of Technology, Hawthorn, Australia, 3122.

ABSTRACT

Currently Intellectual Disability (ID) is classified as a Wechsler Intelligence Scale for Children - Fourth Edition (WISC-IV) Intelligence Quotient (IQ) below 70 and an impairment in adaptive skills during the developmental period. We suggest that the the non-verbal visual matching Raven's Coloured Porgressive Matrices (RCPM) should replace the commonly used WISC-IV measure of intelligence, as a means of matching groups of ID to a Typically Developing (TD) group according to their mental age, as it is a better measure of reasoning ability in children with ID who invariably have verbally based deficits. In addition, we present evidence that RCPM mental aged matched children with Low Functioning (LF) Autism, Down Syndrome (DS) and Idiopathic ID use different problem solving strategies than TD children, to achieve the same overall performance on the RCPM. This is presumably due to group differences in brain impairments as evidenced by brain imaging studies. We also present evidence from the literature that working memory is a major component of successful performance on an IQ test and that impairment in working memory in ID could affect problem solving abilities on the RCPM. The theoretical and educational implications of the discrepancy between similar overall performance level on an intelligence test, but different use of problem solving strategies are also explored.

Keywords: Intellectual Disability, Autism Spectrum Disorder, Down Syndrome, Idiopathic Intellectual Disability, working memory, Ravens Coloured Progressive Matrices, WISC-IV.

---

* Corresponding author: 400 Burwood Rd., Bundoora, Victoria , Australia 3086, screwther@latrobe.edu.au, t +613 9214 5877, f +6139214 5525

Intellectual Disability (ID) is commonly defined by three criteria: (1) a Wechsler Intelligence Sale for Children Intelligence Quotient (IQ) 2 SD below the norm of 100 (i.e. <70), (2) impairment in adaptive behaviour and (3) manifested developmental delay identified early in and persisting through childhood (birth to age 18 years; Katz & Lazcano-Ponce, 2008; Leonard, Petterson, Bower & Sanders, 2003; Pratt & Greydanus, 2007; Salvador-Carulla & Bertelli, 2008; Shevell, 2008; WHO, 1993). As well as informing the classification of an individual with ID, IQ test scores are used in research settings to to co-vary intellectual ability and in clinical settings to help inform educational goals and evaluate therapeutic interventions (Dawson, Soulières, Gernsbacher & Mottron, 2007).

We will briefly present the argument for mental age (MA) and chronological age (CA) matching from the developmentalist and difference theorists. We will then argue that when matching children with ID and TD on MA using the Raven's Coloured Progressive Matrices (RCPM) should replace the more commonly used Wechsler Intelligence Scale for Children-Fourth Edition (WISC-IV), as the RCPM is a more valid measure of reasoning ability in children with an ID. We provide evidence that MA matched children with Low Functioning (LF) Autism, Down Syndrome (DS) and Idiopathic ID use different problem solving strategies compared to TD children when completing the RCPM, despite comparable overall performance. We argue that this is presumably due to different brain impairments in ID, as evidenced by brain imaging studies. We also present evidence from the literature that working memory is a major component of successful performance on an IQ test as it presumably provides the opportunity for the use of higher order problem solving strategies. In order to enhance the education of children with ID, it is important to further explore the problem solving strategies utilised and implement understanding to drive personalized programs of education for each child. We also propose a revised position on the developmental/ difference debate and further explore the educational implications of the discrepancy between similar overall performance level on an intelligence test, but use of different problem solving strategies.

1. What is Intellectual Disability?

Understanding the etiology and prevalence of the ID affecting individuals will inform the management, prognosis and educational and support resources available to assist each in their day to day living (Soto-Ares, Joyes, Lemaître, Vallée & Pruvo, 2003). According to the American Association on Intellectual and Developmental Disabilities (AAIDD), more than 350 causes of ID were reported to exist in 1992 (King, State, Shah, Davanzo & Dykens, 1997 ; Luckasson et al., 1992). There are many different causes of ID, however, in 30-50% cases of ID, a genetic etiology has not yet been identified (Soto-Ares et al). ID of known etiology is classified as either genetic in origin or acquired (i.e. congenital or developmental; Katz & Lazcano-Ponce, 2008; Pratt & Greydanus, 2007).. Research suggests that currently the most common hereditary form of ID is DS, which occurs in 15 of every 10,000 births due to an extra (partial or full) chromosome 21 or the translocation of chromosome 21 and 15. Other ID conditions that have a genetic origin include Fragile X, Prader-Willi syndrome, Rett syndrome and neurofibromatosis (Katz & Lazcano-Ponce), to name just a few. In fact, according to Harris (1995; King et al.) there are more than 500 different genetic causes of ID and Feldman (1996; King et al.) suggests that at least 95 ID conditions have been linked to abnormalities of the X chromosome. This link with the X chromosome explains the prevalence ratio of 4:1 males to females with ID (Steyaert & De La Marche, 2008). In addition, there is a greater prevalence of mental illness in individuals with ID than those with TD (King et al.).

Accurate estimates of prevalence rates of ID are important for the planning and provision of services, such as educational and family support services (Leonard et al., 2003). However, prevalence rates vary widely depending on the classifications of ID used, method of data collection and study location. Prevalence of ID in developed countries has been estimated at 1-3% in 1996 (Hodapp & Dykens, 1996; King et al., 1997).

The Australian Bureau of Statistics estimate in 1997 was that 1% of the Australian population had an ID which required assistance in self-care, mobility and communication (Bower, Leonard & Petterson, 2000). Prevalence studies carried out in Western Australia indicated a gradual rise in ID diagnoses in the past 20 years, which included an estimated 7.6 per 1000 individuals between the ages of 6 and 16 years being categorized as having an ID between the years 1967-1976 alone (Bower et al; Leonard et al., 2003; Wellesley, Hockey, Montgomery & Stanley, 1992). This rate had risen to 8.3 per 1000 individuals approximately a decade later (between 1980-1990; Alessandri, Leonard, Blum & Bower, 1996; Bower,et al; Leonard et al.). A further study in Western Australia reported the prevalence of ID in the period between 1983-1992 to be 14.3 per 1000 individuals, with 10.6 per 1000 of those individuals classified as having ID of mild to moderate level of severity1.4 per 1000 were classified as severe ID and the classification of the remaining 2.3 per 1000 was unspecified. In addition, the prevalence of ID in Aboriginal mothers was 30.8 per 1000 live births, which was double the prevalence rate of ID children for Caucasian mothers in the region (Leonard et al.).

1.1. Autism

Autism is the most severe neurodevelopmental disorder on the Autism Spectrum and is characterized by impaired social and communication development and the presence of repetitive behaviours and fixed interests (American Psychiatric Association, 2000; WHO, 1993). It affects males four times more often than females (Steyaert & De La Marche, 2008) suggesting an X-linked inheritance pattern. Approximately 50-70% of individuals with Autism Spectrum Disorder are also diagnosed with ID (Matson & Shoemaker, 2009). Autism has a strong genetic and biological component, but it is still diagnosed behaviourally as distinctive biological and genetic markers have yet to be established (Glessner et al., 2009; Happé, 1999). Research suggests that the prevalence of Autism is rising. Crewther et al. (2003) estimated 27 out of 10,000 children in Victoria, Australia, had severe Autism (as children diagnosed by age 6 years are predominantly those with extreme behavioural impairments). This increase in diagnosis is likely to be partially due to a broader interpretation of the diagnostic criterion (Steyaert & De La Marche). Most research is performed on Higher Functioning (HF) children with Autism (who do not qualify as ID) and very little research on children with Lower Functioning (LF) and severe Autism (who do qualify as ID). Therefore, our understanding of the nature of Autism currently remains limited and skewed.

1.2. Down Syndrome

Down Syndrome (DS) is the most common cause of ID. In 95% of cases DS is caused by an extra chromosome 21 (or a region of it; Pinter, Eliez, Schmitt, Capone & Reiss, 2001). The replication of this chromosome results in specific facial features that are characteristic of those with DS. Though ID is a common feature of DS, its severity varies widely between individuals (Catalano, 1990; Filder & Nadel, 2007; Sherman, Allen, Bean & Freeman, 2007; Silverman, 2007). A recent study reported the prevalence of DS to be one in every 732 infants in the United States (Sherman et al.) and its incidence as 1 in 800 live births (Pinter et al.).

In order to accurately determine the causality and treatment options for ID it is vital for international classification bodies to agree upon a universal definition of ID. Currently, one of the major discrepancies between the various classifications of ID is whether IQ or adaptive functioning should be the central defining characteristic .The classification of ID according to the American Association of Intellectual Disability (AAID) places more weight on the adaptive functioning criterion rather than the severity of IQ score. More specifically, the AAID definition requires that the individual be deficient in two of ten adaptive functioning domains. These domains were not empirically selected and reflect how much day to day support an individual with ID rather then their level of cognitive impairment compared to a large normative population as determined by a standardized IQ score (Luckasson et al., 1992; King et al., 1997). However, if the definition of ID placed more weight on the individual's IQ level than their adaptive functioning, a universal IQ test would be required to ensure comparability of results. In addition, the IQ test would have to be a valid and reliable measure of intelligence for children from 0 to 100th percentile. Currently the appropriateness of the WISC-IV as an IQ test of children with ID is questionable and the meaning of an IQ score has remained unexplored.

2. Mental Age Versus Chronological Age Matching: The Developmental Origins of Intellectual Disability

The developmental/difference debate surrounds the question of whether development is delayed (developmental perspective) or impaired (difference perspective) in ID. According to the developmental perspective, individuals with ID of a known etiology are developmentally deviant from the norm, as a result of neurological impairments, where as individuals with ID of unknown etiology are only developmentally delayed and functioning on the lower end of the normal distribution of intelligence. These predictions are also known as the similar structure and similar sequence hypothesis (Zigler & Hodapp, 1986). The difference model on the other hand, which was initially proposed by Lewin (1936) and revised by Kounin (1941) claims that individuals with ID (regardless of the etiology) develop differently to TD individuals because of their neurological deficiencies.

Although the relatively recent advent of understanding of the interacting genetic and neuroanatomical bases of many types of ID has largely made this debate anachronistic, the distinction between the developmental and difference theorists with regard to methods of matching of ID and TD groups on cognitive ability in research studies remains important. The developmentalists usually matched groups on MA and the difference theorists match groups on CA. Indeed according to the developmentalists, MA provides an estimate of cognitive development and a means of testing whether individuals with ID are developmentally delayed or deviant whereas the use of CA only confirms the differences in developmental level between ID and TD individuals. On the other hand, according to the difference theorists, ID and TD groups show qualitative and quantitative differences in cognition. Therefore, MA only reflects similarities in overall performance between ID and TD groups and does not indicate differences in problem solving strategies used between groups (Bennett-Gates & Zigler, 1998). Difference theorists prefer to match on CA as this demonstrates how individuals with ID differ compared to individuals who have developed typically. This debate is relevant and important both in the research and clinical settings. Matching strategies in research effect conclusions from research findings that are drawn as a result, which in in turn effects the conceptualization of ID and intelligence. In addition, understanding CA and MA differences between groups of ID and TD informs how we educate children with ID individually and alongside TD children.

3. Psychometric Measures Of Mental age: the Meaning of an IQ Score

3.1. WISC-IV Versus the Raven's Coloured Progressive Matrices as a Valid Measure of Intelligence in Children with Intellectual Disability

Tests of intelligence are often a measure of crystallized intelligence, fluid intelligence, or both (Kluever, Smith, Green, Holm & Dimson, 1995; Prabhakaran, Smith, Desmond, Glover & Gabrieli, 1997). Crystallized intelligence refers to long term knowledge, such as knowing the capital city or the population of a country, whereas fluid intelligence refers to the ability to solve a novel problem with the use of analytical reasoning (Prabhakaran et al.). In many research studies individuals with an ID are matched to other ID groups or to a TD group based on their performance on a fluid intelligence test. Thus, it is vital to base this matching on a valid measure of intelligence. In the low IQ range, inability to successfully complete items may be attributable to a number of causes, such as difficulty resulting in lack of motivation. What a test does though is shed light on which items were completed purposefully using a strategy of some sort and estimates the probability of how many answers to items were guesses. In order to obtain a valid estimate of an individual with ID's IQ score, an intelligence test that reduces the probability of guessing is to be favoured.

The Wechsler Intelligence Scale for Children is the "gold standard" for intelligence testing and the most commonly used test of intelligence in children (Hale, Fiorello, Kavanagh, Hoeppner & Gaither, 2001; Kaufman, Flanagan, Alfanso & Mascolo, 2006; Keith, Fine, Taub, Reynolds & Kranzler, 2006; Wilson & Reschly, 1996). The most recent edition is the Wechsler Intelligence Scale for Children- Fourth Edition (WISC-IV) which is a revision of the Wechsler Intelligence Scale for Children- Third Edition (WISC-III). David Wechsler devised the first of series of Wechsler tests known as the Wechsler-Bellevue Intelligence Scale in 1939 (Wechsler, 1939), which was followed by the development of Form II of the Wechsler-Belleve test in 1946. In 1949 the Wechsler Intelligence Scale for Children was published (Wechsler, 1949) and revised three times in 1974, 1991 and 2003 (Wechsler, 1974, 1991, 2003), each applicable to a 6-16 year old age range. The current revision, WISC-IV gives 4 measures: Verbal Comprehension Index (VCI), Perceptual Reasoning Index (PRI), Working Memory Index (MRI) and Processing Speed Index (PSI) which are considered measures of crystallized intelligence, visual processing, fluid reasoning, short-term memory and processing speed (Keith et al.). WISC-IV has changed in some fundamental ways from the WISC-III. Firstly, it does not produce an overall Verbal IQ and Performance IQ and there is an increased emphasis on measuring fluid reasoning skills, with the addition of the Matrix Reasoning and Picture Concepts subsets. In addition, easier items have been included to improve the test for lower functioning children as well as chronologically young children (Keith et al.).

Despite these changes, Wechsler scales are still likely to be inappropriate IQ measures for children suspected of an ID because they are lengthy to administer and require verbal comprehension and expression from a population typically characterized by low verbal skills and comprehension. The scales do not accommodate low functioning children's deficit in attention and communication and therefore do not motivate or sustain performance. Thus, performance on these scales could be more reflective of lack of motivation than level of mental maturation (Bello, Goharpey, Crewther & Crewther, 2008). Indeed, David Wechsler views his scales as meant for people with average intelligence, not those of IQ above 130 or below 70. When told that most clinicians use his tests to identify the extreme populations, he stated "It's not what I tell them to do, and it's not what a good clinician ought to do. They should know better" (Kaufman, 1994). Bello et al. suggest that a more suitable measure of mental maturation in lower functioning children is the Ravens Coloured Progressive Matrices (RCPM; Raven, 1965a) as it is an un-timed, non-verbal measure of reasoning ability (Carpenter, Just & Shell, 1990; Cotton et al., 2005; Sattler, 2001), requires minimum language to explain the task and requires no verbal response for completion. This increases the probability that attention and motivation will be sustained throughout the time of testing and performance will be reflective of ability then guessing coming from a lack of motivation.

The RCPM is one of three non-verbal measures of fluid reasoning ability devised by Raven, Raven & Court in 1949 (Kluever et al., 1995). The Raven's progressive matrices include the RCPM used for children aged between 5-12 years, the elderly and individuals with ID (Green & Kluever, 1991), the Raven's Standard Progressive Matrices (used with adolescents and adults; RSPM; Raven, 1956) and the Raven's Advanced Progressive Matrices (used with adults; RAPM; Raven, 1965b). The Ravens Progressive Matrices are widely used as culture free measures of fluid intelligence that do not require any crystallized knowledge for successful completion (Prabhakaran et al., 1997). The RCPM has been utilized with children with severe ID, including those with Autism (Clark & Rutter, 1979; Koegel, Koegel & Smith, 1997) in research settings to control for non-verbal mentation (Cotton et al., 2005; Crewther, Lawson, Bello & Crewther, 2007; Barnard, Crewther & Crewther, 1998) and in educational settings to determine their level of functioning and treatment progress as part of a battery of tests (Anderson, Kern, & Cook, 1968; Budoff & Corman, 1976).

The RCPM is made up of 36 coloured multiple choice matrices (although colour is irrelevant to the completion of the task), organized in three increasingly complex sets, Sets A, Ab and B (Raven, Raven & Court, 1998; Raven, Court & Raven, 1992). Each item consists of a matrix of geometric designs that is presented as the problem, with one design removed from the sequence. Beneath each pattern are six separate pieces, with one piece correctly completing the pattern. The goal is to deduce the theme of relations expressed among the designs and choose the missing figure from among the alternative set of six. Items can be solved using visuospatial analysis such as pattern matching or analytical or abstract reasoning. The RCPM is made up of more visuospatial items than analytical items in comparison to the RAPM and the RSPM (Prabhakaran et al., 1997; Villardita, 1985).

The RCPM board form is another version of the RCPM standard form designed for greater appeal to the lower functioning population, due to it's movable pieces. It has a test retest reliability of 0.8, however evidence of its validity are limited (Raven et al., 1992). The board form is also limited in that it's 36 separate wooden board pieces tend to become disorganized easily and the administration process can be time consuming (Raven et al.). These limitations are potentially a problem for children with ID who often have difficulty sustaining their motivation and attention during testing. Therefore, in order to address the limitations of the RCPM board form, Bello et al. devised a velcro version (i.e. a tactile puzzle form) of the standard RCPM (i.e. RCPM puzzle form), particularly designed to sustain the motivation and attention of lower functioning children. Each response option was laminated and then velcroed in place. Items were completed by physically removing a response option and placing this velco compatible piece in the section of the item that was vacant. In the first study, the validity of the RCPM puzzle version was tested by comparing TD children's performance on the puzzle form to the standard book form of the RCPM test. Seventy six TD aged between 5 and 11 years old (*M*=8.57 years, *SD*=2.06 years) were split into two groups. Half the children attempted the book form first while the other half attempted the puzzle form. The two groups were comparable on CA. The alternate form of the RCPM was administered after three weeks to each group, in order to minimize the impact of maturation in learning and memory or practice effects on performance. Results of the study showed a comparable performance between the RCPM puzzle and book forms in the TD school-aged children, regardless of order of completion and a strong correlation between first and second performance of the RCPM suggesting that RCPM puzzle and standard forms measure the same construct/s.

In the second study, 164 children with an ID, including 101 children with Autism, 20 with DS and 43 with Idiopathic ID were either administered the RCPM puzzle form or the standard form in order to determine which version of the RCPM would result in better performance and higher completion rate in children with ID Results showed a significantly higher performance and completion rate for the puzzle form (76.2%) than for the standard form (40%), regardless of clinical group. Fifty five per cent of children with Autism, 68% of children with DS, and 67% of children with Idiopathic ID were unable to complete the standard form but were able to complete the entire puzzle form,. The authors suggested that the puzzle form produced a performance and completion rate advantage in test takers with ID, possibly because the motor aspect of moving responses onto the item to complete the pattern served to engage test takers attention and interest longer than the standard version. Findings of this study suggest that the RCPM puzzle form is a valid measure of reasoning ability in children with TD and ID and thus should replace the Wechsler scales as a measure of intelligence in children with ID. This ensures that test performance of children with ID is an accurate reflection of their reasoning ability, which enables researchers to better understand their capacity and clinicians to provide more suitable treatment options for them.

3.2. Similar Mental age on the Raven's Coloured Progressive Matrices Does Not Mean the Use of Similar Problem Solving Strategies

Overall performance score on tests of ability such as the RCPM is commonly used as a measure of MA. However, similar MA on an IQ test does not necessarily equate to similar problem solving strategies used to solve the items. Investigating how different groups of ID solve problems on the RCPM can provide an insight into learning styles associated with different etiologies of ID as well as highlight the abilities and skills that are commonly associated with intellectual functioning.

One attempt to explore the problem solving strategies used on the RCPM has been by assessing the type of erroneous responses made on the RCPM. According to Raven et al. (1998), after completion of the test, incorrect responses can be categorized into one of four error categories which indicate different problem solving strategies and correlate with intellectual development. The error types were: a) Difference error, when the chosen piece has either no pattern of any kind or one of direct relevance to the target pattern; b) Figure Repetition error, when the chosen piece has either part of the pattern immediately above or beside the target gap in the pattern; c) Inadequate Individuation error, when the chosen piece is contaminated by irrelevancies, distortions or incomplete patterns; and d) Incomplete Correlate error, when the chosen piece correctly identifies part of the target pattern though the figure may be wrongly oriented or incomplete. Although Raven et al. were not clear as to what cognitive abilities are being used when certain errors are made, they did associate the errors with stages of cognitive development. For example, some errors such as Difference error were found to be made earlier in development before pattern differentiation matured, rather than later in development when abstract reasoning begins to appear.

Gunn and Jarrold (2004) explored the pattern of errors made on the RCPM task of children with DS matched on overall performance to children with moderate learning disability and TD. They found that TD and DS children made different error types on the RCPM even when their overall performance was comparable. They also found that overall RCPM performance showed a significant positive correlation with CA for both TD and DS groups, which suggests that individuals with DS perform better as they get older but continue to make the same types of errors. A study by Goharpey, Bello, Crewther & Crewther (under review) examined patterns of error types on the RCPM in children of similar MA (assessed on the RCPM), which included 38 children with LF Autism (*M*=7.44 years, *SD*=2.60 years), 17 with DS (*M*=6.59 years, *SD*=0.77 years), 32 with Idiopathic ID (*M*=6.73 years, *SD*=1.71 years) and 46 TD children (*M*=7.76 years, *SD*=2.21 years), as the basis for understanding strategies of problem solving ability in ID.

All clinical groups showed a similar spread of error types, but the TD group showed a different pattern of errors to the clinical groups. Verbal reasoning ability and working memory (the capacity to store and manipulate information for a brief length of time) has been consistently associated with successful performance on the Ravens matrices (Carpenter et al.,

1990; Fry & Hale, 1996; Prabhakaran et al., 1997). Therefore, in attempting to explore possible strategies that may be associated with different error types, working memory capacity (as measured by visual forward digit span and backward digit span) and receptive language capacity (as measured by the PPVT), were correlated with error types and overall RCPM performance and compared between groups. Performance of the TD group on the RCPM increased with the ability to correctly recall information forward and backwards (short term working memory) and with a greater receptive language capacity. However, in the clinical groups, performance on the RCPM increased only with forward but not backwards working memory performance and receptive language ability was associated with better performance in some but not all ID groups. The findings suggest that differences in problem solving strategy in children with LF Autism, DS and Idiopathic ID in comparison to TD children is partially indicative of an inability to use language to solve problems and an inability to manipulate information in short term working memory.

4. The Role of Working Memory in IQ Performance of Individuals with Intellectual Disability

The activities of the fronto-parietal regions of the brain that have been consistently associated with working memory have also been shown to be associated with attention function (Cabeza & Nyberg, 2000; Naghavi & Nyberg, 2005; Kane & Engle, 2002; Pessoa, Kastner & Ungerleider, 2003). Naghavi and Nyberg who reviewed studies using functional magnetic resonance imaging (fMRI) and positron emission tomography (PET) found attention and memory functions have a common activation in the dorsolateral prefrontal and parietal cortex. It is conceptually logical that areas of the brain involved in working memory are also involved in attention function as attention can not be sustained unless there is a memory of relevant previous information with which to compare incoming information.

Working memory has also been shown to be a major component of intelligence. Colm, Jung and Haier (2007) conducted a study in order to find the brain regions common to working memory and general intelligence ("g"). Vocabulary and block design performance of 48 adults on the Wechsler Adult Intelligence Scale (WAIS) were used to measure "g" and forward and backward digit span components of the WAIS were used to measure working memory. Correlation of magnetic resonance imaging (MRI) with these performances showed BA 10 (right superior gyrus and left middle frontal gyrus) in the frontal lobe and BA 40 (right inferior parietal lobule) in the parietal lobe to be common regions associated with working memory and "g".

A recent study by Alloway (2009) used a regression analysis to show that working memory (as measured by the Working Memory Test Battery for Children; Pickering & Gathercole, 2001) and not IQ (as measured by WISC-III; Wechsler, 1992) was a significant predictor of learning outcomes (as measured by The Wechsler Objective Reading Dimensions; Wechsler, 1993 and The Wechsler Objective Numerical Dimensions; Wechsler, 1996) in a group of 64 children with mild to moderate learning disability aged 7 to 11 year (*M*=9.0 years, *SD*=1.2 years). However, in this study IQ was measured using the WISC-III, which includes only a small subset of tests that measure working memory, which is perhaps why IQ did not predict learning outcomes. If an IQ measure that was strongly associated with working memory (e.g. RSPM and RAPM; Borella, Carretti & Mammarella, 2006; Carpenter et al., 1990; Colom, Flores- Mendoza & Rebollo, 2003; Prabhakaran et al., 1997) was used in the study, it may have in fact been a significant predictor of learning outcome.

Over the last decade, in an attempt to understand the nature of intelligence in the brain, Jung and Haier (2007) reviewed 37 studies that had imaged the brains of individuals using various techniques such as fMRI and PET as they completed items from measures of intelligence, such as the RSPM and the RAPM (Prabhakaran et al., 1997). They found a common overlap of individual differences in the activation of the frontal and parietal regions of the brain. Frontal lobe regions included Brodmann area (BA) 9, 46, 45 and 47 and parietal lobes regions included Brodmann Area (BA) 40, 39 and 7. Some regions in the temporal (BAs 21, 22 and 37) and occipital lobes (BA 18 and 19) were also identified. The authors used the evidence to propose a model of the biology of intelligence, known as the Parietal-Frontal Integration Theory (P-FIT). The model suggests that intellectual ability is underpinned by the interaction between certain areas of the frontal and parietal brain regions when effectively linked by white matter structures. According to the P-FIT model, Wernicke's area (BA 22) processes incoming auditory information and the extrastriate cortex (BA 18 and 19) and fusiform gyrus (BA 37) of the occipital lobe process incoming visual information. This information is then integrated by the parietal brain regions, predominately the supramarginal (BA 40), superior parietal (BA 7) and angular (BA 39) gyri. The problem is then evaluated by interaction of these parietal and frontal regions (BA 6, 9, 10, 45-47). The anterior cingulate (BA 32) then acts to select the best response and inhibit alternating choices. The white matter was considered to ensure that information is reliably transferred from one brain region to another (Jung & Haier) but no consideration was given to the possibility that there could be white matter complications.

In an open peer commentary, Cohen, Walsh and Henik indicated that BA 10 in the frontal lobe and BA 39 and 40 in the parietal lobe were the only regions in the P-FIT that were strongly supported by the structural data in the literature, providing little evidence to support for the P-FIT model (Jung & Haier, 2007). In addition, Cohen et al argumed that parietal-frontal regions related to attention are only one component of intelligence and do not define intelligence as a whole construct. One main reason for the inconsistent evidence in the literature in support of the P-FIT is that results from brain imaging studies are limited in that they do not provide information on whether participants completed items correctly during the imaging and what strategies they used to come up with their responses. These factors can result in different regions of the brain being activated during completion of an IQ measure.

Research shows that accuracy does make a difference in brain imaging results. In a series of studies, Haier and colleagues (1988) found an inverse correlation between regional glucose metabolic rate (GMR) and performance on the RAPM in 8 young males. Essentially, the brains of individuals who had high scores on the RAPM utilized less glucose when completing the task that those with low scores. It was not clear from the study how low and high performers were defined but never the less, this same pattern was also shown in a PET study of 16 individuals completing a high g-loaded verbal fluency test (Parks et al., 1988). Such observations support a model of neural efficiency (Kwan & Reiss, 2006)
Interestingly, the opposite pattern was shown for individuals with an ID. Higher rate of glucose metabolism was found throughout the brain of adults with Autism (Rumsey et al., 1985), DS (Haier et al., 1995; Schwartz, Duara, Haxby & Grady, 1983) and Idiopathic ID compared to TD individuals during task performance (Haier et al.). This suggests that a more

intelligent brain uses its glucose more efficiently than a less intelligent brain. It also suggests that different levels of accuracy on a test of intelligence in TD can result in different activation patterns, making it difficult to separate the activations sites associated with high performers and those associated with low performers.

In addition, use of different strategies to complete the same items on the RCPM results in activation of different regions of the brain. In a study by Prabhakaran and colleagues (1997), young adults (Mean age of 26 years) attempted three different types of problems on the RSPM and the RAPM, whilst their brain activation was being measured by fMRI. The three problems involved (1) analytical reasoning, (2) figural or visuospatial reasoning; or (3) simple pattern matching which served as a control for the motor and perceptual activation involved in completing each item. Results showed that different regions of the brain associated with working memory were activated when each question type was attempted. Bilateral frontal and left parietal, occipital and temporal regions were activated more by analytical problems than pattern matching problems. Thus, if test takers use other strategies such as verbal abilities to problem solve or simply guessing, different regions of the brain would be expected to be activated as a result.

According to the literature, working memory is a major component of intelligence and we speculate that this may be because working memory capacity allows information to be available for inspection and manipulation longer and therefore provides an opportunity for information to be manipulated using higher order problem strategies such as reasoning by analogy. Thus, an individual with ID who has a lower working memory capacity may not be able to retain information long enough to apply principles of analogy to successfully solve more difficult problems. Therefore, they may have to rely on using lower level abilities such as pattern matching or guessing as a strategy to solve problems that require reasoning by analogy for successful completion.

This explanation is supported by research which shows that individuals with an ID generally have deficits in working memory and attention. For example, individuals with Autism have been consistently shown to have difficulties with executive functions associated with a fronto-parietal connectivity deficit (Just, Cherkassky, Keller, Kana & Minshew, 2007; Kana, Keller, Minshew & Just, 2007; Solomon et al., 2009). In a recent study by Solomon and colleagues, 22 adolescents with HF Autism and 23 age, gender and IQ matched TD adolescents performed a visual response task that had previously been shown to activate fronto-parietal regions associated with executive functions, such as dorsolateral prefrontal cortex (DLPC; BA 9), anterior frontal (BA 10), parietal cortex (BA 7 and 40) and anterior cingulate cortex (ACC; BA 32). Results showed less activation in these regions in the Autism group compared to the TD group. Future research will need to conduct brain imaging studies using both HF and LF children with Autism in order to determine whether a deficit in frontal-parietal regions of the brain are associated with the Autism diagnosis or only children with Autism who do not have an ID. Unlike individuals with Autism, research shows a preservation of the parietal lobe in individuals with DS despite impaired language ability including verbal working memory (Pinter et al., 2001). Using an fMRI procedure, Pinter and colleagues showed that consistent with behavioural evidence of typical parietal functioning in DS, there was also preservation of prefrontal lobe grey matter in the sample of 16 individuals with DS (mean age= 11.3 years). This preservation in the prefrontal lobe was also shown in a study by Jernigan, Bellugi, Sowell, Doherty and Hesselink (1993) who found typical parietal and occipital gray matter in fMRI study on 6 children with DS. Findings suggests that areas of working memory maybe effected differently depending on the etiology of the ID.

Impairments in other brain regions in individuals with ID may also be associated with differences in problem solving strategies used to complete tests of intelligence, such as the RCPM (Goharpey et al., under review). Lawrence, Lott and Haier (2005) reviewed structural and brain function studies and found six brain areas that were commonly affected in Autism, DS and Idiopathic ID, but not always in the same way. These brain areas included the cerebellum volume, brain stem volume, hippocampus volume, abnormal dendritic development, whole brain volume and whole brain metabolism. Studies have consistently shown a smaller cerebellum, brain stem and hippocampal volume as well as abnormal dendrites in Autism, DS and Idiopathic ID groups in comparison to TD individuals. In addition, a larger brain size has been related to increased intelligence in Autism. Individuals with DS or Idiopathic ID also show smaller brain size in comparison to TD individuals and a high brain metabolism in resting state, which suggests that a less intelligent brain needs to work harder (Lawrence et al.).

Working memory and attention are a significant component of intelligence. However the use of other cognitive abilities to solve problems on measures of intelligence in children with ID needs to be further explored in future studies. This will highlight cognitive abilities associated with intelligence as well as inform educational interventions for children with ID.

5. IMPLICATIONS FOR WORKING WITH CHILDREN WITH INTELLECTUAL DISABILITY

5.1. Theoretical Implications: the Developmental/Difference Debate Revised

The main issue in the developmental/ difference debate centering on whether there is any neurological impairment in individuals with Idiopathic ID that correlates with their cognitive ability is now considered less relevant. Indeed if brain imaging studies identified clear brain areas that were anatomically different in children with Idiopathic ID compared to TD children, then the debate will cease to be an issue. Though more research is required, we believe that the evidence in the literature on the pathological impairments in individual with Idiopathic ID is sufficient to demonstrate that it involves neurological impairments that result in developmental deviance and not just developmental delay *per se* (Lawrence et al., 2005; Soto-Ares et al., 2003). In a study by Soto-Ares and colleagues, thirty children with ID of unknown etiology (*M*= 5.2 years) underwent an MRI in order to determine the neuroanatomical abnormalities associated with ID. The study found subtle brain abnormalities of the cerebral cortex or ventricles, midline structures (corpus callosum and septum pellucidum) and the posterior fossa (cerebellar hemisphere or vermis) in the brain of participants. However more research is required to understand the origins and implications of these brain abnormalities and their relationship to behavioural phenotypes in children with ID of unknown etiology.

Although we agree with the difference theorists that ID of unknown etiology involves brain impairments that, like other forms of ID, result in deviant development of cognitive ability, we do not agree with them in using CA as a means of matching ID and TD children in research studies. We hold the position that MA is a more meaningful method of matching children with an ID and TD as it allows us to explore the developmental profile of different groups of ID in comparison to one another and to TD with out introducing additional variance between groups such as learning opportunity and life experience, that would occur with CA matching.

5.2. Educational Implications: how do we teach Children with Intellectual Disability?

The evidence in the literature suggests that there is no single profile of ID. Different groups of ID show different brain impairments that vary due to the severity of ID and etiology. However, when educating children with ID of varying etiologies, it is important to note that even though their performance on certain tasks may be comparable, problem solving strategies used to achieve that performance may not be. This is presumably due to differences in brain structure and function in different groups of ID. The type of problem solving strategies used by children with ID, whether it be visual, auditory or audiovisual in naturel needs to be further investigated. Educational tasks and curriculums need to be designed so that they engage visual, auditory and motor as well as audiovisual abilities of children with ID. Educational approaches should be selected based on what a child with ID finds motivating and engaging. Thus, strategies that engage and try to maintain a child's attention are likely to provide the best opportunity for learning. as few would despute that, a child can not begin to learn or solve a problem unless their attention and working memory are activated. The next step is to discover through research, how the child is engaging with this information so that we can then understand how to facilitate this engagement and begin to increase educational outcomes for children with ID.

REFERENCES

Alessandri, L. M., Leonard, H., Blum, L. M., & Bower, C. (1996). *Disability counts: A profile of disability in Western Australia.* Perth: Disability Services Commission.

Alloway, T. P. (2009). Working Memory, but not IQ predicts subsequent learning in children with learning difficulties. *European Journal of Psychological Assessment, 25*(2), 92-98.

American Psychiatric Association. Diagnostic and statistical manual of mental disorders (4th ed.) (2000). Text revision: DSM IV-TR. 4th edition. Washington, DC: American Psychiatric Association.

Anderson, H. E., Kern, F. E., & Cook, C. (1968). Sex, brain damage, and race effects in the progressive matrices with retarded populations. *Journal of Social Psychology, 76*(2), 207-211.

Barnard, N., Crewther, S. G., & Crewther, D. P. (1998) Development of a magnocellular function in good and poor primary school-age readers. *Optometry and Visual Science, 75*(1), 62-8.

Bello, K. D., Goharpey, N., Crewther, S. G., & Crewther, D. P. (2008). A puzzle form of a non-verbal intelligence test gives significantly higher performance measures in children with severe intellectual disability. *BMC Pediatrics, 8,* 1-8.

Bennett-Gates, D., & Zigler, E. (1998). Resolving the developmental-difference debate: An evaluation of the triarchic and systems theory models. In J. A. Burack, R. M. Hodapp & E. Zigler (Eds.), *Handbook of mental retardation and development* (pp. 115-131). New York: Cambridge University Press.

Borella, E., Carretti, B., & Mammarella, I. C. (2006). Do working memory and susceptibility to interference predict individual differences in fluid intelligence? *European Journal of Cognitive Psychology, 18,* 51-69.

Bower, C., Leonard, H., & Petterson, B. (2000). Intellectual disability in Western Australia. *Journal of Paediatrics and Child Health, 36,* 213-215.

Budoff, M., & Corman, L. (1976). Effectiveness of a learning potential procedure in improving problem-solving skills of retarded and nonretarded children. ***American Journal of Mental Deficiency, 81***(3), 260-264.

Cabeza, R., & Nyberg, L. (2000). Imaging cognition II: An empirical review of 275 PET and fMRI studies. *Journal of Cognitive Neuroscience, 12,* 1-47.

Carpenter, P. A., Just, M. A., & Shell, P. (1990). What one intelligence test measures: A theoretical account of the processing in the Raven Progressive Matrices Test. *Psychological Review, 97*(3), 404-431.

Catalano, R. A. (1990). Down Syndrome. *Reviews in Medicine, 34 (5),* 385-398.

Clark, P., & Rutter, M. (1979). Task difficulty and task performance in autistic children. ***Journal of Child Psychology and Psychiatry, 20***(4), 271-285.

Colom, R., Flores-Mendoza, C., & Rebollo, I. (2003). Working memory and intelligence. *Personality and Individual Differences, 34,* 33-39.

Colom, R., Jung, R. E., & Haier, R. J. (2007). General intelligence and memory span: Evidence for a common neuroanatomic framework. *Cognitive Neuropsychology, 24***(8),** 867-878.

Cotton, S. M., Kiely, P. M., Crewther, D. P., Thomson, B., Laycock, R., & Crewther, S. G. (2005). A normative and reliability study of the Raven's Coloured Progressive Matrices for primary school aged children from Victoria, *Australia. Personality and Individual Differences, 39*(3), 647-659.

Crewther, S. G., Goodyear, M. J., Bavin, E. L., Lawson, M. L., Wingenfield, S. A., & Crewther, D. P. (2003). *Autism in Victoria: An investigation of prevalence and service delivery for children aged 0-6 years.* Victorian Government Department of Human Services, Melbourne, Victoria.

Crewther, S. G., Lawson, M. L., Bello, K. D., & Crewther, D. P. (2007). The visual attentional blink reflects constraints on temporal visual processing, not just a lapse of visual memory . *Clinical and Experimental Optometry, 90*(4), 282-289.

Dawson, M., Soulières, I., Gernsbacher, M. A., & Mottron, L. (2007). The level and nature of autistic intelligence. *Psychological Science, 18*(8), 657-662.

Feldman, E. J. (1996). The recognition and investigation of X-linked learning disability syndromes. *Journal of Intellectual Disability Research, 40,* 400-411.

Fidler, E. J., & Nadel, L. (2007). Education and children with Down syndrome: Neuroscience, development, and intervention. *Mental Retardation and Developmental Disabilities, 13,* 262-271.

Fry, A. F., & Hale, S. (1996). Processing speed, working memory, and fluid intelligence: evidence for a developmental cascade. *Psychological Science, 7,* 237-241.

Glessner, J. T., Wang, K., Cai, G., Korvatska, o., Kim, C. E., Wood, S., et al. (2009). Autism genome-wide copy number variation reveals ubiquitin and neuronal genes. *Nature, 459,* 569-573.

Goharpey, N., Bello, K., Crewther, S., & Crewther, D. (under review). Similar mental age does not mean similar problem solving strategy in children with intellectual disability and typical development.

Green, K. E., & Kluever, R. C. (1991). Structural properties of Raven's Coloured Progressive Matrices for a sample of gifted children. *Perceptual and Motor Skills, 72,* 59-64.

Gunn, D. M., & Jarrold, C. (2004). Raven's Matrices performance in Down syndrome: Evidence of unusual errors. ***Research in Developmental Disabilities, 25***(5), 443-457.

Haier, R. J., Chueh, D., Touchette, P., Lott, I., Buchsbaum, M. S., Macmillan, D., et al. (1995). Brain size and cerebral glucose metabolic rate in nonspecific mental retardation and Down syndrome. *Intelligence, 20***(2),** 191-210.

Haier, R. J., Siegel, B. V., Nuechterlein, K. H., Hazlett, E., Wu, J. C., Paek, J., Browning, H., et al. (1988). Cortical glucose metabolic rate correlates of abstract reasoning and attention studied with positron emission tomography. *Intelligence, 12***(2),** 199-217.

Hale, J. B., Fiorello, C. A., Kavanagh, J. A., Hoeppner, J. B., & Gaither, R. A. (2001). WISC-III predictors for academic achievement for children with learning disabilities: Are global and factor scores comparable? *School Psychology Quarterly, 16,* 31-55.

Happé, F. (1999). Autism: cognitive deficit or cognitive style? *Trends in Cognitive Sciences, 3***(6),** 216-222.

Harris, J. C. (1995). *Developmental Neuropsychiatry, Vol 2.* Oxford, England: Oxford University Press, *103.*

Hodapp, R. M., & Dykens, E. M. (1996). Mental retardation. In E. J. Mash, & Barkley, R. A (Eds.), *Child psychopathology* (pp. 362-389). New York: Guildford Press.

Jernigan, T. L., Bellugi, U., Sowell, E., Doherty, S., & Hesselink, J. R. (1993). Cerebral morphologic distinctions between Williams and Down syndromes. *Archives of Neurology, 50,* 186-191.

Jung, R. E., & Haier, R. J. (2007). The Parietal-Frontal Integration Theory (P-FIT) of intelligence: Converging neuroscience evidence. *Behavioral and Brain Sciences, 30*(2), 135-187.

Just, M., Cherkassky, V., Keller, T., Kana, R., & Minshew, N. (2007). Functional and anatomical cortical underconnectivity in autism: Evidence from an fMRI study of an executive function task and corpus collosum morphometry. *Cerebral Cortex, 17,* 951-961.

Kane, M. J., & Engle, R. W. (2002). The role of prefrontal cortex in working memory capacity, executive attention, and general fluid intelligence: An individual-difference perspective. *Psychonomic Bulletin & Review, 9*(4), 637-671.

Kana, R. K., Keller, T. A., Minshew, N. J., & Just, M. A. (2007). Inhibitory control in high-functioning autism: Decreased activation and underconnectivity in inhibition networks. *Biological Psychiatry, 62*(3), 198-206.

Katz, G., & Lazcano-Ponce, E. (2008). Intellectual disability: definition, etiological factors, classification, diagnosis, treatment and prognosis. *Salud pública de México, 50 suppl (2),* 132-141.

Kaufman, A. S. (1994). Intelligence testing with the WISC-III. New York, Wiley.

Kaufman, A. S., Flanagan, D. P., Alfonso, V. C. & Mascolo, J. T. (2006). Test review: Wechsler Intelligence Scale for Children Fourth Edition (WISC-IV). *Journal of Psychoeducational Assessments, 24,* 278-295.

Keith, T. Z., Fine, J. G., Taub, G. E., Reynolds, M. R., & Kranzler, J. H. (2006). Higher order, multisample, confirmatory factor analysis of the Wechsler Intelligence Scale for Children-Fourth Edition: What does it measure? *School Psychology Review, 35,* 108-127.

King, B. H., State, M. W., Shah, B., Davanzo, P., & Dykens, E. (1997). Mental retardation: A review of the past 10 years. Part I. *Journal of the American Academy of Child and Adolescent Psychiatry, 36*(**12**)**,** 1656-1663.

Kluever, R. C., Smith, D. K., Green, K. E., Hom, C. B., & Dimson, C. (1995). The WISC-III and Raven Coloured Progressive Matrices Test: A pilot study of relationships. Paper presented at the Annual Meeting of the American Educational Research Association (San Francisco, CA, April 18-22, 1995).

Koegel, L. K., Koegel, R. L., & Smith, A. (1997). Variables related to differences in standardized test outcomes for children with autism. *Journal of Autism and Developmental Disorders, 27*(3), 233-243.

Kounin, J. (1941). Experimental studies of rigidity: I. The measurement of rigidity in normal and feebleminded persons. *Character and Personality, 9,* 251-272.

Kwan, H., & Reiss, A. (2006). Neurobiology of mental retardation. In D. S. Charney & E. J. Nestler (Eds.), *Neurobiology of mental illness* (pp. 944-951). New York: Oxford University Press.

Lawrence, C. J., Lott, I., & Haier, R. J. (2005). Neurobiology of autism, mental retardation, and down syndrome. In C. Stough (Ed.), ***Neurobiology of Exceptionality*** (pp. 125-145). New York: Kluwer Academic/ Plenum.

Leonard, H., Petterson, B., Bower, C., & Sanders, R. (2003). Prevalence of intellectual disability in Western Australia. *Paediatric and Prenatal Epidemiology, 17,* 58-67.

Lewin, K. (1936). ***A dynamic theory of personality.*** New York: McGraw-Hill.

Luckasson, R., Coulter, D., Polloway, E. A., Reiss, S., Schalock, R. L., Snell, M. E., et al. (Eds.). (1992). *Mental Retardation: Definition, classification, and systems of support* (9th ed.). Washington, DC: American Association on Mental Retardation.

Matson, J. L., & Shoemaker, M. (2009). Intellectual disability and its relationship to autism spectrum disorders. ***Research in Developmental Disabilities, 30,*** 1107-1114,

Naghavi, H. R., & Nyberg, L. (2005). Common fronto-parietal activity in attention, memory, and consciousness: Shared demands on integration? *Consciousness and Cognition, 14*(**2**)**,** 390-425.

Parks, R., Loewenstein, D., Dodrill, K., Baker, W., Yoshii, F., Chang, I., et al. (1988). Cerebral metabolic effects of a verbal fluency test: A PET scan study. ***Journal of Clinical and Experimental Neuropsychology (Neuropsychology, Development and Cognition: Section A), 10***(5), 565-575.

Pessoa, L., Kastner, S., & Ungerleider, L. G. (2003). Neuroimaging studies of attention: From modulation of sensory processing to top-down control. *The Journal of Neuroscience, 23*(**10**)**,** 3990-3998.

Pickering, S. J., & Gathercole, S. E. (2001). *Working memory test battery for children.* London: Harcourt Assessment.

Pinter, J. D., Eliez, S., Schmitt, J. E., Capone, G. T., & Reiss, A. L. (2001). Neuroanatomy of Down's syndrome: A high-resolution MRI study. *American Journal of Psychiatry, 158*(**10**), 1659-1665.

Prabhakaran, V., Smith, J. A. L., Desmond, J. E., Glover, G. H., & Gabrieli, J. D. E. (1997). Neural substrates of fluid reasoning: An fMRI study of neocortical activation during performance of the Raven's Progressive Matrices Test. *Cognitive Psychology, 33,* 43-63.

Pratt, H. D., & Greydanus, D. E. (2007). Intellectual disability (mental retardation) in children and adolescents. *Primary Clinics in Office Practice, 34,* 375-386.

Raven, J. C. (1956). *Guide to the Standard Progressive Matrices, Sets A, B, C, D and E.* London: H. K. Lewis & Co.

Raven, J. C. (1965a). *Guide to using the Coloured Progressive Matrices Sets A, Ab, B.* Dumfries, Scotland: Grieve.

Raven, J. C. (1965b). *Advanced Progressive Matrices: Sets I and II.* London: Lewis.

Raven, J. C., Court, J. H., & Raven, J. (1992). *Manual for Raven's Progressive Matrices.* Oxford: Oxford Psychologist Press.

Raven, J., Raven, J., & Court, J. (1998). *Manual for Raven's progressive matrices and vocabulary scales.* Oxford: Oxford Psychologists Press.

Rumsey, J. M., Duara, R., Grady, C., Rapoport, J. L., Margolin, R. A., Rapoport, S. I., et al. (1985). Brain metabolism in autism (resting cerebral glucose utilization rates as measured with positron emission tomography). *Archives of General Psychiatry, 42,* 448-455.

Salvador-Carulla, L., & Bertelli, M. (2008). 'Mental Retardation' or 'Intellectual Disability': time for a conceptual change. *Psychopathology, 41,* 10-16.

Sattler, J. M. (Ed.). (2001). *Assessment of Children: Behavioural and Clinical* Application (4th ed.). San Diego, CA: Jerome M. Sattler Publishing, Inc.

Schwartz, M., Duara, R., Haxby, J., & Grady, C. (1983). Down's syndrome in adults: Brain metabolism. *Science, 221,* 781-783.

Sherman, S. L., Allen, E. G., Bean, L. H., & Freeman, S. B. (2007). Epidemiology of Down syndrome. *Mental Retardation and Developmental Disabilities, 13,* 221-227.

Shevell, M. (2008). Global developmental delay and mental retardation or intellectual disability: Conceptualization, evaluation, and etiology. *Pediatric Clinics of North America, 55,* 1071-1084.

Silverman, W. (2007). Down syndrome: cognitive phenotype. *Mental Retardation and Developmental Disabilities, 13,* 228-236.

Solomon, M., Ozonoff, S., Ursu, S., Ravizza, S., Cummings, N., Stanford, L., & Carter, C. (2009). The neural substrates of cognitive control deficits in autism spectrum disorders *Neuropsychologia, 47*(12), 2515-2526.

Soto-Ares, G., Joyes, B., Lemaître, M., Vallée, L., & Pruvo, J. (2003). MRI in children with mental retardation. *Pediatric radiology, 33,* 334-345.

Steyaert, J. G., & De la Marche, W. (2008). What's new in autism? *European Journal of Pediatrics, 167*(10), 1091-1101.

Villardita, C. (1985). Raven's Colored Progressive Matrices and intellectual impairments in patients with focal brain damage. *Cortex, 21,* 627-634.

Wechsler, D. (1939). *Wechsler- Bellevue Intelligence Scale.* New York: The Psychological Corporation.

Wechsler, D. (1949). *Wechsler Intelligence Scale for Children.* New York: The Psychological Corporation.

Wechsler, D. (1974). *Wechsler Preschool and Primary Scale of Intelligence.* New York: The Psychological Corporation.

Wechsler, D. (1991). *Wechsler Intelligence Scale for Children- Revised.* San Antonio, TX: The Psychological Corporation.

Wechsler, D. (1992). *Wechsler Intelligence Scale for Children- Third Edition UK.* London: Harcourt Assessment.

Wechsler, D. (1993). *Wechsler Objective Reading Dimensions.* London: Harcourt Assessment.

Wechsler, D. (1996). *Wechsler Objective Numerical Dimensions.* London: Harcourt Assessment.

Wechsler, D. (2003). *Wechsler Intelligence Scale for Children- Fourth Edition.* San Antonio, TX: The Psychological Corporation.

Wellesley, D. G., Hockey, K. A., Montgomery, P. D., & Stanley, F. J. (1992). Prevalence of intellectual handicap in Western Australia: a community study. *Medical Journal of Australia, 156,* 94-102.

Wilson, M. S., & Reschly, D. J. (1996). Assessment in school psychology training and practice. *School Psychology Review, 25,* 9-23.

World Health Organization (1993). Mental disorders: glossary and guide to their classification in accordance with the the tenth revision of the International Classification of Diseases. Geneva (Switzerland).

Zigler, E., & Hodapp, R. M. (1986). *Understanding mental retardation.* New York: Cambridge University Press.

In: Learning and Memory Developments...
Editors: L. C. Eklund, A. S. Nyman, pp. 173-187
ISBN: 978-1-60876-397-9

Chapter 7

FACILITATORY EFFECTS OF MUSIC ON MEMORY: A REVIEW OF THE POTENTIAL ROLE OF EMOTIONAL AROUSAL

Sherilene M. Carr and Nikki S. Rickard
School of Psychology, Psychiatry & Psychological Medicine, Monash University, Australia.

ABSTRACT

Research reveals background music played during learning can variously enhance or impair memory, although the conditions which determine its effect are not yet understood. Possible explanations for the differing effects of music on memory include characteristics of the music itself, such as tempo and lyrics, induced mood of the listener and personality differences. In this chapter, consideration of the type of music used to manipulate learning and memory will be reviewed, indicating that arousal may play an important moderating role, either as a means of reducing anxiety or increasing arousal to an optimum performance levels. As music is often reported to increase arousal via emotion induction or enjoyment, a well established theory of arousal-modulated memory will be argued to underly the facilitatory effects of music on memory. The methodology used within this research paradigm will be described, and adaptations will be proposed that make it amenable to investigating the effect of music induced arousal on memory. This approach provides a novel method for combining the knowledge gained from music and memory research with arousal and memory literature to further investigate the potential memory enhancing role of music.

INTRODUCTION

Memory consolidation is known to be sensitive to modulation by a range of exogenous sources, including emotional arousal, stress and exercise. The influence of music on various forms of memory has also been investigated, and in general, has also been found to be capable of modulating the strength of recall in a manner that is dependent on task, individual and music. The significance of this finding has, however, failed to yet be fully acknowledged. Music has become ubiquitous in most people's lives, chosen as a continuous accompaniment during travel, exercise and work via portable media players and omnipresent in public places, such as shops and dining establishments. The impact of this soundtrack on cognitive processes generally tends, however, to be assumed to be benign. The potential for music to be used to facilitate memory in study or therapeutic settings has been explored to some extent (see Rickard, Toukhsati, & Field, 2005 for a review). In this review, we re-examine this literature from a directed theoretical approach, that of the neuromodulatory arousal framework. The *arousal hypothesis* (Cahill & McGaugh, 1995; Cahill, Prins, Weber, & McGaugh, 1994), posits that emotionally arousing events elicit a neuro-endocrine response which culminates in strengthened consolidation of the event. As music can elicit powerful emotional responses in listeners (Gabrielsson, 2001), the majority of reported music effects on memory may be mediated by emotional arousal. We argue that this account of music-facilitated memory is therefore not only viable, but can be utilized to extend basic research into applied settings of everyday memory benefits.

The Effect of Music on Memory

Music has been used empirically as both the 'stimulus to be remembered' (musical memory, see review by Jancke, 2008) and as the 'facilitatory treatment'. The scope of the current review is confined to examination of the latter, with music being used as an experimental stimulus to manipulate learning and memory. The various mechanisms identified relate to attention (distracting stimuli, selective capture), arousal, memory network activation, and phonological working memory. This section will review studies that have used music as a stimulus to manipulate such mechanisms. The method in which music has been applied to test models of learning and memory will be described, and key findings outlined. Possible explanations for contradictory effects will be proposed in terms of the structural characteristics of the music used.

The literature indicates that a range of memory functions are amenable to music manipulation, including short-term memory, working memory, learning, retrieval, and storing knowledge. Short-term and working memory research has examined how speech sounds embedded in music can interfere with phonological memory storage. Music has been used as phonological properties (lyrics) can be changed whilst maintaining the integrity of the stimulus (same or similar music without lyrics). For example, Salame and Baddeley (1989, Exp 1) revealed more errors were made in a nine digit serial recall task when vocal music was played during digit encoding compared to instrumental music. They interpreted vocal music interference in terms of extra demands placed on the phonological store that was used to process the digits. A similar effect was revealed in a later study conducted by Crawford and Strapp (1994).

The effects of music on learning and storage of information into long-term memory have been investigated primarily in terms of context dependence (Balch, Bowman, & Mohler, 1992; Balch & Lewis, 1996; de l'Etoile, 2002; Thaut & de l'Etoile, 1993), schema consistency (Boltz, Schulkind, & Kantra, 1991; Boltz, 2001), and arousal (Hallam, Price, & Katsarou, 2002; Kiger, 1989; Morton, Kershner, & Siegel, 1990; Savan, 1999). Context (or state) dependence is the phenomenon of enhanced recall of information when an individual is placed in the same or similar context as learning. The context stimulus is posited to integrate learned material into associated memory networks. At retrieval, priming of the same memory network with the context stimulus acts to enhance retrieval of the associated learned information. Music has been successfully used to provide context by Balch et al. (1992; 1996; 1999). In a series of studies, they found memory could be manipulated with background music presented while information was learnt. Recall was superior when the same (rather than different) music was played at encoding and retrieval. Characteristics of the music were analyzed in these studies, revealing that tempo, but not genre or timbre, was the key moderator. That is, music that had a fast tempo at encoding and recall facilitated retrieval, whereas the same music played at a slow tempo at recall did not.

Schema consistency effects on memory can also be understood with an associated memory network model. Schemata are stored concepts that represent our knowledge of the world (Baddeley, 1999) and can be used to help interpret ambiguous situations. In doing so, attention will become selective to information that is consistent with that schema and subsequently influence encoding and memory. Boltz et al. (1991; 2001; 2004) tested this theory using ambiguous film clips accompanied by background positive or negative music. Their findings indicate that music provides a schematic framework for interpreting the ambiguous film and biasing attention to schema-consistent information. Attention in this context was operationalized by the successful long-term free recall of the film content. In addition, recall for the films was greater when background music was played compared to viewing the film in silence. Boltz (2001) interpreted this result within Marshal and Cohen's (1988) 'Congruence Associationist Model' in that congruent information from different sensory modalities combines to increase the potency of the information. Marshal and Cohen did not test memory, however it may be possible to interpret from their integration/potency theory that widespread (integrated) and strengthened (potency) activation at encoding increases the likelihood that the information will be retained. The studies conducted by Boltz et al. provide empirical support for the memory enhancing effects of background music within this theoretical framework.

The impact of distracting background sound on learning and memory has been intensively studied. Vocal music has often been chosen as the distracting stimulus as it is hypothesized to interfere with phonological working memory, thereby impairing performance (Crawford & Strapp, 1994; Salame & Baddeley, 1989). To optimize distraction, music selections have therefore typically included lyrics, have been arousing, complex, and played at a fast tempo. Performance on a range of memory tasks (digit span, short term word recall, delayed word recall, visual recall, serial word recall, language comprehension, word pair learning, lyrics recall) completed with distracting background music has then been compared to performance in silence or less distracting, usually instrumental, background music. Research in this context has yielded surprisingly contradictory findings. Vocal or distracting music has been found to both impair (Cassidy & MacDonald, 2007; Furnham & Allass, 1999; Nittono, 1997; Salame & Baddeley, 1989: Exp 1; Sousou, 1997) *and enhance* memory (Furnham & Allass, 1999; Morton, et al., 1990). In sum, while vocal background music does tend to impair performance, the variability of the results makes it difficult to conclude that these effects are clearly attributable to interference in phonological processing.

Instrumental background music has also been reported to variously enhance (de Groot, 2006; Hallam, et al., 2002; Kiger, 1989; Savan, 1999), impair (Alley & Greene, 2008; Cassidy & MacDonald, 2007; Crawford & Strapp, 1994; Kiger, 1989; Nittono, 1997; Salame & Baddeley, 1989, Exp 1; Sousou, 1997) or have no effect on memory (Boyle & Coltheart, 1996; Furnham & Allass, 1999; Salame & Baddeley, 1989: Exp 2; Woo Ee & Kanachi, 2005). De Groot (2006) played positively valenced music (part of the fourth Brandenburg Concerto, composed by J. S. Bach) in the background while participants learned foreign language word pairs. Participants who learnt in the presence of music recalled more word pairs than those who learnt in silence. Kiger (1989) played simple background music (Vangelis, repetitive synthesizer music with narrow tonal range) to a group of 15 year old participants while they read, and found comprehension scores were higher than when they read in silence or with high load music (Toccata, dissonant, arrhythmic and dynamic). In contrast, Hallam et al. (2002) played negatively valenced music (*Meditations* by John Coltrane, complex jazz) in the background whilst 11-12 year old participants read, and found recognition memory for words in the text was significantly worse than participants who learnt in silence, or heard calming background music (Albinoni's Adagio in G minor).

Consideration of the different types of music used in these experiments may provide some insight into the potential cause of performance variability. Music that was most detrimental to performance tended to be complex, percussive, have a fast tempo, and loud dynamic. Performance enhancing music, in contrast, had a slow tempo and soft flowing dynamic. These music characteristics coincide with the arousal inducing properties of music (Lundqvist, Carlsson, Hilmersson, & Juslin, 2009), with high-arousing music impairing, and low-arousing music enhancing performance. To add to the complexity, however, performance in the presence of arousing music can vary depending on whether it is presented before or during learning. For example, Morton et al. (1990) played arousing music (Pink Floyd's *The Wall*) to participants before they completed a dichotic listening task, and revealed increased memory capacity compared to a no-music control. In the presence of arousing background music, individual differences in sensitivity to distracting stimuli, usually measured in terms of the personality traits of extraversion/introversion, can significantly affect performance. Extraverts have been found to perform optimally with arousing background music compared to silence, and introverts perform worse (Crawford & Strapp, 1994; Furnham & Allass, 1999).

An alternative theoretical framework that offers a more consistent interpretation of these results is the arousal-performance framework. This well-established theory describes a relationship between arousal levels and performance, where performance is optimum with moderate levels of arousal but impaired with low or high arousal levels. The specific shape of the relationship can vary from an inverted U-shape (Yerkes & Dodson, 1908) to complex non-linear functions (Hardy, 1990). On the basis of this theory, the effects of music are interpreted with regard to the degree to which they modulate physiological arousal levels (see Meyer, 1956; Narmour, 1990, 1992). Empirical research has supported an inverted U shape relationship between the arousal response to music and preference (Berlyne, 1971; North &

Hargreaves, 1997), although a relationship between music and cognitive performance is yet to be demonstrated. If consistent with the broader arousal-performance literature, arousing music should (within limits) facilitate memory consolidation, while highly arousing (for instance, if perceived as highly complex) or unarousing (for instance, boring and repetitive) music will either have no effect on, or will impair, memory processing. This theory also explains potentially beneficial effects of music in stressful situations, in that simple, calming music may have an anxiolytic effect, thereby reducing arousal associated with stress to a more optimum level (Velik & Rickard, 2009). A separate body of research corroborates the music induced arousal effects on cognitive task performance. Rauscher, Shaw and Ky (1993) reported spatial abilities were enhanced after listening to ten minutes of a Mozart sonata (the *Mozart Effect*). Further research has indicated that the enhancing effect of music on spatial temporal performance may be due to positive and aroused mood induced by the music (Thompson, Schellenberg, & Husain, 2001). Arousal may be a likely means by which music can influence memory, yet at this point, no clear mechanism for the music-arousal-memory relationship has been proposed. One theory that may offer insight is the neurobiological 'arousal' hypothesis of memory consolidation. Emotional responses are associated with an adrenal *arousal* response, which is believed to trigger a chain of neuroendocrine events that culminate in enhanced consolidation of details surrounding the emotion elicitor (McGaugh, 2000). Given the breadth of empirical evidence that music is capable of affecting arousal levels (see reviews by Johnson-Laird & Oatley, 2008; Juslin & Vastfjall, 2008; North & Hargreaves, 1997), the arousal hypothesis offers a possible model for explaining the effect of music on memory.

The arousal hypothesis is predicated on the *arousal* (or sometimes termed *stress*) response to emotion elicitors. Increased physiological arousal is a primary component of an emotional response, and the neurobiological mechanism underlying this response has been posited to enhance memory for details of the event. Events that induce an emotional response, and are remembered, have survival value as they can inform future decision making. For example, remembering the close encounter with the bear in the woods (past fear experience), will inform the decision as to which route should be taken to get to the wild berry patch (past reward experience) without being hurt. There is widespread empirical support for neurobiological accounts of emotion-enhanced memory, initiated by seminal papers in the animal research literature published by Gold and McGaugh (1975) and Kety (1972), and in the human research literature published by Cahill, Prins, Weber and McGaugh (1994). Emotional arousal in human research is typically manipulated by exposing two groups of participants to a slideshow of 11 or 12 images presented for around 15 seconds each. The images are mostly neutral except for a highly aversive image towards the middle (a boy's severed and re-attached legs). The slideshow is accompanied by a simple narrative which is either neutral or negative in affective content. After a delay of one or two weeks, participants complete a surprise free recall and/or recognition memory test for details relating to the images and narrative in the slideshow. The two slideshows differ in content mostly in the narrative of the middle of three phases, where emotion is manipulated. The narrative of the first and third phase is near identical in content and meaning. The consistent finding from studies utilizing this paradigm is that memory is enhanced for the middle phase of the emotional slideshow compared to the neutral slideshow (Cahill, Gorski, Belcher, & Huynh, 2004; Hamann, Cahill, McGaugh, & Squire, 1997; O'Carroll, Drysdale, Cahill, Shajahan, & Ebmeier, 1999; van Stegeren, Everaerd, Cahill, McGaugh, & Gooren, 1998).

Importantly, Cahill et al. (1994) demonstrated that this effect was likely to be on consolidation of memory, as they controlled a number of additional factors known to influence the encoding of emotional information, such as attention and rehearsal. They also provided evidence that the effect on long-term memory was mediated by beta-adrenergic receptor activation. The consolidation hypothesis proposes that increased arousal in response to an emotional event activates the beta-adrenergic system peripherally and in the basolateral amygdala (BLA), which projects to important cortical memory structures (Sah, Faber, Lopez De Armentia, & Power, 2003), thereby enhancing consolidation of memory for the event (see review by McGaugh, 2004). There is considerable evidence to support the effect of beta-adrenergic modulation on the consolidation of long-term memory in both animals (e. g. Gibbs & Summers, 2002; McGaugh, 1983) and humans.

The arousal hypothesis of emotion-enhanced memory is a well validated model that is easily adapted to explore the effects of music on memory. Emotion within this paradigm is typically manipulated with a slideshow containing images and a narrative. Addition of various types of background music to the slideshow could enhance the emotional response (see review of effect of music soundtracks on interpretation of film by Cohen, 2001). The use of music as the source of emotional arousal may also make the slideshow methodology more amenable to controlling affective valence, both positive and negative. Additionally, emotion manipulation using related images and narrative means memory is enhanced for details related to that intrinsic information only. A potentially viable adaptation of the slideshow methodology would be to replace the intrinsic emotional information with arousing background music, thereby making the arousal source extraneous and applicable to any concomitantly presented but unrelated information. The arousal model of memory may be appliedto explain the effect of music on memory. The methodology used to test arousal effects of memory could easily be modified to include music, and in so doing also potentially lay the foundation for extending the arousal-memory effect to wider populations. The next section will review the music-emotion literature, identifying characteristics of music that make it ideal as a source of emotional arousal for applied memory enhancement.

Music and Emotional Arousal

There is debate as to whether music induces the evolutionarily adaptive 'basic' emotions, such as happiness, sadness, fear and anger, or whether the response is rather an appraisal or appreciation of the aesthetic qualities of the music (Konecni, 2008). Regardless of the cognitive label, there is considerable and growing behavioral, neuroimaging and physiological evidence that music does indeed result in experiential emotion responding and increases in physiological arousal (see reviews by Juslin & Vastfjall, 2008; Rickard, et al., 2005). The use of emotionally valent music could, therefore, be of great value as a method for understanding the relationship between emotion and memory.

Neuroimaging studies have demonstrated that similar brain regions are activated by non-music and music emotional stimuli. The amygdala (Hamann & Mao, 2002; Hamann, Ely, Hoffman, & Kilts, 2002; Kensinger & Schacter, 2006; Phan, Wager, Taylor, & Liberzon, 2002), basal ganglia and insula (Calder, Lawrence, & Young, 2001), and medial pre-frontal cortex, anterior cingulate cortex and sub callosal cingulate (Phan, et al., 2002; Wager, Phan,

Liberzon, & Taylor, 2003) are all implicated in processing of basic emotions. Activation of brain regions in response to music is similar. Brown, Martinez and Parsons (2004) reported widespread activation, measured by positron emission tomography (PET), of the sub callosal cingulate gyrus, prefrontal anterior cingulate, retrosplenial cortex, hippocampus, anterior insula and nucleus accumbens in response to liked but unfamiliar emotional music. In addition to amygdala activation, Blood and Zatorre (2001) reported cerebral blood flow increases to ventral striatum, midbrain, orbitofrontal cortex, and ventral medial prefrontal cortex in response to participant selected arousing music compared to control pieces matched on musical features.

The autonomic nervous system (ANS) is a central component of the bodily response to an emotion elicitor. High-arousal emotions, such as anger and joy, activate the sympathetic arm of the ANS, which prepares the body for action (e.g., by stimulating heart rate). Whereas low-arousal emotions, such as sadness or peace, activate the parasympathetic arm of the ANS, which de-activates the body (Larsen, Berntson, Poehlmann, Ito, & Cacioppo, 2008). ANS mediated changes in heart rate, diastolic blood pressure and skin conductance in response to the basic emotions of fear, anger, sadness and happiness have been consistently found (reviewed by Cacioppo, Berntson, Larsen, Poehlmann, & Ito, 2000). Similarly, emotionally arousing music significantly increases skin conductance (Baumgartner, Esslen, & Jancke, 2006; Ellis & Simons, 2005; Khalfa, Isabelle, Jean-Pierre, & Manon, 2002; Krumhansl, 1997; Lundqvist, et al., 2009; Rickard, 2004; Taylor, 1973; Vanderark & Ely, 1993), and heart rate (Baumgartner, Esslen, et al., 2006; Iwanaga & Moroki, 1999; Mockel, et al., 1994; Taylor, 1973), but not always (Lundqvist, et al., 2009). Respiratory rate increases have also been reported as a reliable measure of musically elicited emotional arousal (Nyklicek, Thayer, & Van Doornen, 1997), but this result could be confounded by potential entrainment effects induced by the tempo of the music (high arousal music typically has a fast tempo), that are independent of emotional arousal. Low-arousal music generally decreases heart rate, skin conductance, and skin temperature (Bartlett, 1996).

The Problem of Variability

It has been argued that music may be a viable source of emotional arousal when considering methods of extending the well established *arousal hypothesis* of memory enhancement. However, the use of music for this purpose is offset by many variables that potentially moderate or confound the response. Variability in response to music may have contributed to the inconsistent music-memory research results reviewed earlier. Emotional response by nature is highly variable, both inter-individually and intra-individually (Hamann & Canli, 2004). Emotional response to music is further complicated by the highly personal and often idiosyncratic interpretations of music that are not easily reproduced in an experimental environment. An individual's response to free form jazz music for example, may be quite different to that of 1970's British punk. To add to this complexity, the response to the same music by the same individual may also vary depending on extra-musical variables, such as one's current mood state, and frequency of listening (music that was once loved can quickly become irritating with over-exposure). The literature reveals other variables that may also moderate this response, such as level of musical training, musical engagement, personality, familiarity and liking of the music.

Music Experience

Differences in emotional and physiological arousal responses between musicians and non-musicians may have a moderating effect on emotion enhanced memory. Bigand et al. (2005) reported that musicians and non-musicians were no different in their ability to categorize the emotional valence and arousal of musical excerpts. However, VanderArk and Ely (1992, 1993) reported significantly greater skin conductance responses to arousing music for music majors compared to non-music majors. A possible explanation for the difference in physiological response in musicians may be the activation of sympathetic motor movement in response to hearing familiar music. This hypothesis has been explored by D'Ausilio, Altenmuller, Belardinelli and Lotze (2006), who found increased motor neuron excitability by transcranial magnetic stimulation when pianists heard excerpts they had been rehearsing. It is therefore unknown whether the physiological differences between musicians and non-musicians are solely due to the emotion inducing properties of the music, or to some other response related to the perceptual elements of the music. The results of this research imply that musicians and non-musicians may not differ on their emotional *categorization*, but rather differ on their emotional *arousal* response. These differences are highly relevant in research on music and memory where physiological arousal has been identified as a central requirement for the memory enhancing effect of emotion.

An alternative concept that may be a less confounded method of gauging an individual's propensity to be emotionally aroused by music is their level of active interest, participation or engagement in music activities. There are a number of studies investigating people's everyday use of music which show individuals engage with and use music often for a wide variety of functions (Juslin & Vastfjall, 2008; North, Hargreaves, & Hargreaves, 2004; Sloboda & O'Neill, 2001). For example, music is used as a mood regulator, for catharsis, to aid sleep, or simply as something to listen to in the background whilst undertaking other activities. It may therefore also be important to assess the importance and use of music in an individual's life, or how much they *engage* with music, in addition to their musical expertise. Werner, Swope and Heide (2006) have devised a music experience questionnaire with the factors of commitment to music, positive psychotropic effect, affective reactions, reactive behavior, innovative aptitude, and social uplift; which may assist with the identification and control of variables that influence emotional response to music.

Liking, Enjoyment, Preference and Familiarity

Thus far, emotional arousal in response to music has been argued to be a modulator of memory worthy of theoretical consideration. Another important factor not yet fully discussed in this review, and which has implications for the music induced elicitation of arousal, is music induced 'enjoyment-arousal' (reviewed by Husain, Forde Thompson, & Schellenberg, 2002). Enjoyment-arousal is a response to music that is variously described as liked, enjoyed or preferred, thereby inducing increased arousal and a positive mood. It is the arousal and mood effects of the music that are argued to enhance cognitive performance (often tasks of spatial ability). For example, experiments conducted by Nantais and Schellenberg (1999) reveal enhanced cognitive abilities after participants listened to three sound conditions (Mozart, Schubert, or a narrated story) depended on whether the sound condition was preferred. They concluded enhanced ability was a consequence of preference, which induced arousal levels and mood states that facilitated performance. Additionally, evidence of an enjoyment dependent effect was revealed by Thompson et al. (2001), in that improved spatial task performance after listening to a fast, upbeat Mozart sonata compared to slow, sad music (Albinoni's adagio) depended on whether the music was enjoyed and considered arousing. Theoretical models that may explain differences in cognitive performance based on enjoyment are posited in terms of differing effects of mood on information processing (Levine & Pizarro, 2004). Positive moods induce a 'paint with broad strokes' style of heuristic information processing, a style that is quick and relies on top-down representations to process information. Negative moods induce a slower systematic processing approach that is more analytical, and relies on data to process information. Music enjoyment-arousal has been found to have a significant effect on spatial task performance, but as yet is not tested on memory performance.

Based on Levine and Pizarro's (2004) theory of mood valence effects on information processing speed, hypotheses could be derived to test whether enjoyed music could increase information processing at the registration stage of memory. However, a further potential moderator of music induced arousal-enjoyment, music familiarity, will need to be considered. Music that is familiar is often rated as more positive (e.g., Iwanaga & Moroki, 1999; Ritossa & Rickard, 2004). Familiar music is also more likely to prime autobiographical memories which could influence performance. Known as the 'they're playing our song' phenomenon, familiar music can act as a reminder of past experiences, and thus potentially modulate mood independently of that intended by the experimental manipulation, confounding interpretation of task performance. An effective way of minimizing the effects of familiarity is to use unfamiliar music; with younger samples, this is usually from the western classical genre.

Concluding Comments

There are a number of powerful advantages of music over other forms of emotion-inducing stimuli as a means of enhancing memory. Increasing research indicates music can activate emotion centers in the brain and induce physiological responses consistent with those induced with non-music emotional stimuli. The advantage of using emotionally salient music, however, is that these responses are rapid and require little effort (Johnson-Laird & Oatley, 2008), and can bias our interpretation of otherwise neutral information. For example, Grady (2007) revealed that musical mood induction changed participants' valence judgments of neutral faces; Tan, Spackman and Bezdek (2007) revealed that emotionally valent music played before or after presentation of a film affected interpretation of the neutral character's emotion in a valence congruent way; and Logeswaran and Bhattacharya (2009) revealed that emotionally valent music played before presentation of neutral faces influenced judgment of emotion facial expression.

Music can also strengthen the emotional impact of concomitant events or stimuli, as revealed by Marshal and Cohen (1988) reviewed earlier. The 'Congruence Associationist Model' was used by Boltz (2001) to explain how memory for details was enhanced most by a combination of film and music. Corroborating Boltz's finding, Baumgartner et al. (2006; 2006; 2007) found electrophysiological and functional neural activation to be strongest when emotionally arousing music was combined with emotional images. The pattern of activation for the music and image combinations correlated with areas known to be involved in emotion, however this pattern of activation was absent when the images were presented on their own. These results indicate that music may be used as an implicit method of influencing the emotional content of a neutral situation, with minimal information processing interference, by enhancing the emotional significance of visual stimuli. That is, music can become intrinsically associated with neutral stimuli at minimal information processing cost. Emotionally arousing background music may therefore be a simple and effective means of increasing the emotional impact of visual stimuli, thereby enhancing memory via the neurobiological mechanism of memory consolidation. There are few alternative emotion inducing stimuli that can be so easily 'added on' to an event to significantly increase its emotional meaning, and hence memorability.

REFERENCES

Alley, T. R. & Greene, M. E. (2008). The relative and perceived impact of irrelevant speech, vocal music and non-vocal music on working memory. *Current Psychology, 27(4)*, 277-289.

Baddeley, A. D. (1999). *Essentials of human memory*. Hove, England: Psychology Press/Taylor & Francis (UK).

Balch, W. R., Bowman, K. & Mohler, L. A. (1992). Music-dependent memory in immediate and delayed word recall. *Memory & Cognition, 20(1)*, 21-28.

Balch, W. R. & Lewis, B. S. (1996). Music-dependent memory: The roles of tempo change and mood mediation. *Journal of Experimental Psychology: Learning, Memory, and Cognition, 22(6)*, 1354-1363.

Balch, W. R., Myers, D. M. & Papotto, C. (1999). Dimensions of mood in mood-dependent memory. *Journal of Experimental Psychology: Learning, Memory & Cognition, 25(1)*, 70-83.

Bartlett, D. L. (1996). Physiological responses to music and sound stimuli. In: D. A., Hodges, (Eds.), *Handbook of music psychology* (2nd ed., 343-385). San Antonio IMR Press.

Baumgartner, T., Esslen, M. & Jancke, L. (2006). From emotion perception to emotion experience: Emotions evoked by pictures and classical music. [peer reviewed]. *International Journal of Psychophysiology, 60*, 34-43.

Baumgartner, T., Lutz, K., Schmidt, C. F. & Jancke, L. (2006). The emotional power of music: How music enhances the feeling of affective pictures. *Brain Research 1075*, 151-164.

Baumgartner, T., Willi, M. & Jancke, L. (2007). Modulation of corticospinal activity by strong emotions evoked by pictures and classical music: a transcranial magnetic stimulation study. *Neuroreport, 18(3)*, 261-265.

Berlyne, D. E. (1971). *Aesthetics and psychobiology*. East Norwalk, CT: Appleton-Century-Crofts.

Bigand, E., Vieillard, S., Madurell, F., Marozeau, J. & Dacquet, A. (2005). Multidimensional scaling of emotional responses to music: The effect of musical expertise and of the duration of the excerpts. *Cognition & Emotion, 19(8)*, 1113-1139.

Blood, A. J. & Zatorre, R. J. (2001). Intensely pleasurable responses to music correlate with activity in brain regions implicated in reward and emotion. *Proc Natl Acad Sci,* U S A, *98(20)*, 11818-11823.

Boltz, M., Schulkind, M. & Kantra, S. (1991). Effects of background music on the remembering of filmed events. *Memory & Cognition, 19(6)*, 593-606.

Boltz, M. G. (2001). Musical soundtracks as a schematic influence on the cognitive processing of filmed events. *Music Perception, 18(4),* 427-454.

Boltz, M. G. (2004). The cognitive processing of film and musical soundtracks. *Memory & Cognition, 32(7)*, 1194-1205.

Boyle, R. & Coltheart, V. (1996). Effects of irrelevant sounds on phonological coding in reading comprehension and short-term memory. *The Quarterly Journal of Experimental Psychology A: Human Experimental Psychology, 49A(2)*, 398-416.

Brown, S., Martinez, M. J. & Parsons, L. M. (2004). Passive music listening spontaneously engages limbic and paralimbic systems. *Neuroreport: For Rapid Communication of Neuroscience Research, 15(13)*, 2033-2037.

Cacioppo, J. T., Berntson, G. G., Larsen, J. T., Poehlmann, K. M. & Ito, T. A. (2000). The Psychophysiology of Emotion. In M. Lewis & J. M. Haviland-Jones (Eds.), *Handbook of Emotions* (2nd ed., 173-191). NY, London: Guilford Press.

Cahill, L., Gorski, L., Belcher, A. & Huynh, Q. (2004). The influence of sex versus sex-related traits on long-term memory for gist and detail from an emotional story. *Consciousness & Cognition, 13(2)*, 391-400.

Cahill, L. & McGaugh, J. L. (1995). A novel demonstration of enhanced memory associated with emotional arousal. *Consciousness and Cognition: An International Journal, 4(4)*, 410-421.

Cahill, L., Prins, B., Weber, M. & McGaugh, J. L. (1994). β-Adrenergic activation and memory for emotional events. *Nature, 371(6499)*, 701-704.

Calder, A. J., Lawrence, A. D. & Young, A. W. (2001). Neuropsychology of fear and loathing. *Nat Rev Neurosci, 2(5)*, 352-363.

Cassidy, G. & MacDonald, R. A. (2007). The effect of background music and background noise on the task performance of introverts and extraverts. *Psychology of Music, 35(3)*, 517-537.

Cohen, A. J. (2001). *Music as a source of emotion in film*. Juslin, Patrik N (Ed); Sloboda, John A (Ed). (2001). Music and emotion: Theory and research.

Crawford, H. J. & Strapp, C. M. (1994). Effects of vocal and instrumental music on visuospatial and verbal performance as moderated by studying preference and personality. *Personality and Individual Differences, 16(2)*, 237-245.

D'Ausilio, A., Altenmuller, E., Olivetti Belardinelli, M. & Lotze, M. (2006). Cross-modal plasticity of the motor cortex while listening to a rehearsed musical piece. *Eur J Neurosci, 24(3)*, 955-958.

de Groot, A. M. B. (2006). Effects of Stimulus Characteristics and Background Music on Foreign Language Vocabulary Learning and Forgetting. *Language Learning. Vol, 56(3)*, 463-506.

de l'Etoile, S. K. (2002). The effect of musical mood induction procedure on mood state-dependent word retrieval. *Journal of Music Therapy, 39(2)*, 145-160.

Ellis, R. J. & Simons, R. F. (2005). The Impact of Music on Subjective and Physiological Indices of Emotion While Viewing Films. *Psychomusicology, 19(1)*, 15-40.

Furnham, A. & Allass, K. (1999). The influence of musical distraction of varying complexity on the cognitive performance of extroverts and introverts. *European Journal of Personality, 13(1)*, 27-38.

Gabrielsson, A. (2001). *Emotions in strong experiences with music*. Juslin, Patrik N (Ed); Sloboda, John A (Eds.), (2001). Music and emotion: Theory and research.

Gibbs, M. E. & Summers, R. J. (2002). Role of adrenoceptor subtypes in memory consolidation. *Progress in Neurobiology, 67(5)*, 345-391.

Gold, P. E. & McGaugh, J. L. (1975). A single-trace, two-process view of memory storage processes. In: D., Deutsch, & J. A. Deutsch (Eds.), *Short-term Memory* (355-378). New York: Academic Press.

Grady, M. K. M. K. (2007). The Effect of Age on Memory for Emotional Faces. *Neuropsychology, 21(3)*, 371-380.

Hallam, S., Price, J. & Katsarou, G. (2002). The effects of background music on primary school pupils' task performance. *Educational Studies. Vol, 28(2)*, 111-122.

Hamann, S. & Canli, T. (2004). Individual differences in emotion processing. *Curr Opin Neurobiol, 14(2)*, 233-238.

Hamann, S. & Mao, H. (2002). Positive and negative emotional verbal stimuli elicit activity in the left amygdala. *Neuroreport, 13(1)*, 15-19.

Hamann, S. B., Cahill, L., McGaugh, J. L. & Squire, L. R. (1997). Intact enhancement of declarative memory for emotional material in amnesia. *Learning and Memory, 4(3)*, 301-309.

Hamann, S. B., Ely, T. D., Hoffman, J. M. & Kilts, C. D. (2002). Ecstasy and agony: activation of the human amygdala in positive and negative emotion. *Psychol Sci, 13(2)*, 135-141.

Hardy, L. (1990). *A catastrophe model of performance in sport*. Oxford, England: John Wiley & Sons.

Husain, G., Forde Thompson, W. & Schellenberg, E. G. (2002). Effects of Musical Tempo and Mode on Arousal, Mood, and Spatial Abilities. *Music Perception, 20(2)*, 151.

Iwanaga, M. & Moroki, Y. (1999). Subjective and physiological responses to music stimuli controlled over activity and preference. *Journal of Music Therapy, 36(1)*, 26-38.

Jancke, L. (2008). Music, memory and emotion. *J Biol, 7(6)*, 21.

Johnson-Laird, R. N. & Oatley, K. (2008). *Emotions, music, and literature*. New York, NY: Guilford Press.

Juslin, P. N. & Vastfjall, D. (2008). Emotional responses to music: the need to consider underlying mechanisms. *Behav Brain Sci, 31(5)*, 559-575, discussion 575-621.

Kensinger, E. A. & Schacter, D. L. (2006). Processing emotional pictures and words: Effects of valence and arousal. *Cognitive Affective & Behavioral Neuroscience, 6(2),* 110-126.

Kety, S. (1972). *Brain catecholamines, affective states and memory.* Oxford, England: Plenum.

Khalfa, S., Isabelle, P., Jean-Pierre, B. & Manon, R. (2002). Event-related skin conductance responses to musical emotions in humans. *Neuroscience Letters, 328(2),* 145-149.

Kiger, D. M. (1989). Effects of music information load on a reading comprehension task. *Perceptual & Motor Skills, 69,* 531-534.

Konecni, V. J. (2008). Does music induce emotion? A theoretical and methodological analysis. *Psychology of Aesthetics, Creativity, and the Arts, in press.*

Krumhansl, C. L. (1997). An exploratory study of musical emotions and psychophysiology. *Canadian Journal of Experimental Psychology Vol 51(4) Dec 1997, 336-352.*

Larsen, J. T., Berntson, G. G., Poehlmann, K. M., Ito, T. A. & Cacioppo, J. T. (2008). *The psychophysiology of emotion.* New York, NY: Guilford Press.

Levine, L. J. & Pizarro, D. A. (2004). Emotion and memory research: A grumpy overview. *Social Cognition, 22(5),* 530-554.

Logeswaran, N. & Bhattacharya, J. (2009). Crossmodal transfer of emotion by music. *Neurosci Lett, 455(2),* 129-133.

Lundqvist, L. O., Carlsson, F., Hilmersson, P. & Juslin, P. N. (2009). Emotional responses to music: Experience, expression, and physiology. *Psychology of Music, 37(1),* 61-90.

Marshall, S. K. & Cohen, A. J. (1988). Effects of musical soundtracks on attitudes toward animated geometric figures. *Music Perception, 6(1),* 95-112.

McGaugh, J. L. (1983). Hormonal influences on memory. *Annual Review of Psychology, 34,* 297-323.

McGaugh, J. L. (2000). Memory: A century of consolidation. *Science Vol 287(5451) Jan 2000, 248-251.*

McGaugh, J. L. (2004). The amygdala modulates the consolidation of memories of emotionally arousing experiences. *Annual Review of Neuroscience, 27,* 1-28.

Meyer, L. B. (1956). *Emotion and meaning in music*: (1956) Emotion and meaning in music University of Chicago Press: Chicago.

Mockel, M., Rocker, L., Stork, T., Vollert, J., Danne, O., Eichstadt, H., et al. (1994). Immediate physiological responses of healthy volunteers to different types of music: cardiovascular, hormonal and mental changes. *Eur J Appl Physiol Occup Physiol, 68(6),* 451-459.

Morton, L. L., Kershner, J. R. & Siegel, L. S. (1990). The potential for therapeutic applications of music on problems related to memory and attention. *Journal of Music Therapy. Vol, 27(4),* 195-208.

Nantais, K. M. & Schellenberg, E. (1999). The Mozart effect: An artifact of preference. *Psychological Science, 10(4),* 370-373.

Narmour, E. (1990). *The analysis and cognition of basic melodic structures: The implication-realization model.* Chicago, IL: University of Chicago Press.

Narmour, E. (1992). *The influence of embodied registral motion on the perception of higher-level melodic implication.* Washington, DC: American Psychological Association.

Nittono, H. (1997). Background instrumental music and serial recall. *Perceptual & Motor Skills, 84,* 1307-1313.

North, A. C. & Hargreaves, D. J. (1997). Liking, arousal potential, and the emotions expressed by music. *Scandinavian Journal of Psychology, 38(1)*, 45-53.

North, A. C., Hargreaves, D. J. & Hargreaves, J. J. (2004). Uses of music in everyday life. *Music Perception Vol 22(1) Fal 2004, 41-77.*

Nyklicek, I., Thayer, J. F. & Van Doornen, L. J. (1997). Cardiorespiratory differentiation of musically-induced emotions. *Journal of Psychophysiology, 11(4)*, 304-321.

O'Carroll, R., Drysdale, E., Cahill, L., Shajahan, P. & Ebmeier, K. (1999). Memory for emotional material: A comparison of central versus peripheral beta blockade. *Journal of Psychopharmacology, 13(1)*, 32-39.

Phan, K. L., Wager, T., Taylor, S. F. & Liberzon, I. (2002). Functional neuroanatomy of emotion: a meta-analysis of emotion activation studies in PET and fMRI. *Neuroimage, 16(2)*, 331-348.

Rauscher, F. H., Shaw, G. L. & Ky, K. N. (1993). Music and spatial task performance. *Nature, 365*(6447), 611.

Reisberg, D. (2006). *Memory for emotional episodes: The strengths and limits of arousal-based accounts*. Uttl, Bob (Ed); Ohta, Nobuo (Ed); Siegenthaler, Amy L (Ed). (2006). Memory and emotion: Interdisciplinary perspectives.

Rickard, N. S. (2004). Intense emotional responses to music: A test of the physiological arousal hypothesis. *Psychology of Music Vol 32(4) Oct 2004, 371-388.*

Rickard, N. S., Toukhsati, S. R. & Field, S. E. (2005). The Effect of Music on Cognitive Performance: Insight From Neurobiological and Animal Studies. *Behavioral and Cognitive Neuroscience Reviews 4(4)*, 235-261.

Ritossa, D. A. & Rickard, N. S. (2004). The relative utility of 'pleasantness and liking' dimensions in predicting the emotions expressed by music. *Psychology of Music, 32(1)*, 5-22.

Sah, P., Faber, E. S. L., Lopez De Armentia, M. & Power, J. (2003). The amygdaloid complex: anatomy and physiology. *Physiological Reviews, 83(3)*, 803-834.

Salame, P. & Baddeley, A. D. (1989). Effects of background music on phonological short-term memory. *The Quarterly Journal of Experimental Psychology A: Human Experimental Psychology. Vol, 41*(1-A), 107-122.

Savan, A. (1999). The effect of background music on learning. *Psychology of Music, 27(2)*, 138-146.

Sloboda, J. A. & O'Neill, S. A. (2001). Emotions in everyday listening to music. *Juslin, Patrik N (Ed); Sloboda, John A (Ed), (2001). Music and emotion: Theory and research. (415-429). viii*, NY, US: Oxford University Press.

Sousou, S. D. (1997). Effects of melody and lyrics on mood and memory. *Perceptual & Motor Skills, 85*, 31-40.

Tan, S. L., Spackman, M. P. & Bezdek, M. A. (2007). Viewers' interpretations of film characters' emotions: Effects of presenting film music before or after a character is shown. *Music Perception Vol 25(2) Win 2007, 135-152.*

Taylor, D. B. (1973). Subject resonses to precategorized stimulative and sedative music. *Journal of Music Therapy, 10*, 86-94.

Thaut, M. H. & de l'Etoile, S. K. (1993). The effects of music on mood state-dependent recall. *Journal of Music Therapy, 30(2)*, 70-80.

Thompson, W. F., Schellenberg, E. G. & Husain, G. (2001). Arousal, mood, and the Mozart effect. *Psychol Sci, 12(3)*, 248-251.

van Stegeren, A. H., Everaerd, W., Cahill, L., McGaugh, J. L. & Gooren, L. J. (1998). Memory for emotional events: Differential effects of centrally versus peripherally acting beta -blocking agents. *Psychopharmacology, 138*(3-4), 305-310.

Vanderark, S. D. & Ely, D. (1992). Biochemical and galvanic skin responses to music stimuli by college students in biology and music. *Perceptual & Motor Skills, 74*, 1079-1090.

Vanderark, S. D. & Ely, D. (1993). Cortisol, biochemical, and galvanic skin responses to music stimuli of different preference values by college students in biology and music. *Perceptual & Motor Skills, 77(1)*, 227-234.

Velik, L. & Rickard, N. S. (2009). A Novel Approach to Memory Neuromodulation Using Music: A Literature Review In B. Figueredo & F. Meléndez (Eds.), *Neuroscience Research Advances*: Nova.

Wager, T. D., Phan, K. L., Liberzon, I. & Taylor, S. F. (2003). Valence, gender, and lateralization of functional brain anatomy in emotion: a meta-analysis of findings from neuroimaging. *Neuroimage, 19(3)*, 513-531.

Werner, P. D., Swope, A. J. & Heide, F. J. (2006). The Music Experience Questionnaire: development and correlates. *Journal of Psychology, 140(4)*, 329-345.

Woo Ee, W. & Kanachi, M. (2005). The Effects of Music Type and Volume on Short-Term Memory. *Tohoku Psychologica Folia. Vol, 64*, 68-76.

Yerkes, R. M. & Dodson, J. D. (1908). The relation of strength of stimulus to rapidity of habit-formation. *Journal of Comparative Neurology and Psychology, 18*, 459-482.

In: Learning and Memory Developments...
Editors: L. C. Eklund, A. S. Nyman, pp. 189-207
ISBN: 978-1-60876-397-9

Chapter 8

SPATIAL MEMORY AND LARGE-SCALE ECOLOGICAL ENVIRONMENTS

Tina Iachini, Gennaro Ruggiero and Francesco Ruotolo
Department of Psychology, Second University of Naples
Via Vivaldi 43, 81100, Caserta, Italy.

ABSTRACT

Spatial memory is a necessary prerequisite of most everyday activities. We usually define "spatial" that information useful to locate objects and to interact with them. Therefore, it is "spatial" information about relational and metric properties, such as relative positions (e.g., left/right), distance, size, orientation, as well as dynamic properties, such as velocity and strength. Clearly, the ability to navigate in the environment requires an understanding of all these properties and a representation in memory of structured information. To organize spatial memory, egocentric (i.e. based on body's position) or allocentric (i.e. based on external positions) frames of reference are used. Although research on spatial memory has a long history, in the majority of the cases experimental settings and procedures are restricted to laboratory situations, and the results are typically generalized to real world contexts. Consequently, little is known on the characteristics of spatial memory based on bodily interactions with large-scale everyday environments. In this paper we review evidence about laboratory-based and environment-based research on spatial memory. Further, a research is presented that investigated whether familiarity with a large-scale regular environment affects the spatial frames of reference necessary to represent it in memory. It was tested the hypothesis that familiarity facilitates an allocentric representation of the environment. Familiar and unfamiliar participants had to study 5 triads of buildings by walking along a path surrounding each triad. Afterwards, they had to provide relative distance judgments in relation either to their body (egocentric) or external buildings (allocentric). Results showed that familiar participants were more accurate than unfamiliar participants in the allocentric judgments and faster on the whole. Unfamiliar participants performed similarly in both judgments and were better than familiar participants in the egocentric

· Corresponding author: Tel: +39-0823-274789 Fax: +39-0823-323000 E-mail: santa.iachini@unina2.it judgments. These findings suggest that when the environment is familiar and regular it is represented on the basis of allocentric frames of reference. The results are discussed in relation to models of spatial memory that emphasize the importance of experience and of the geometric structure.

Keywords: Spatial memory, environmental memory, frames of reference.

INTRODUCTION

Spatial Memory of Environments and Objects

Spatial memory is implied in most everyday activities, such as grasping objects or reaching places. However, the term "spatial" is somewhat ambiguous as it has been used with different meanings. For example, it is spatial the processing of static geometric and metric properties, such as configuration, distance and size, as well as dynamic properties, such as velocity and strength. Clearly, the ability to navigate in the environment requires an understanding of all these properties, thus linking the idea of spatial competence with that of an intuitive physics (Eilan, 1993). This ability is so fundamental to our survival that spatial abilities are often synonymous of navigational abilities, including sense of direction and capacity to represent the environment. This research domain has often been indicated as topographical memory (e.g., Ball, Smith, Ellison & Schenk, 2009).

Besides spatial competence in environmental settings, also characteristics of objects such as size, orientation and location are defined "spatial" (Pinker, 1984). Ungerleider and Mishkin (1982) proposed a distinction between spatial information and object information in terms of "where" and "what" systems. According to the authors, the visual system comprises two different streams: the dorsal stream processes spatial or "where" information useful for object localization, whereas the ventral stream processes visual or "what" features (such as, shape, color, luminance) useful for object recognition. We can use diverse spatial strategies to find out our way in the environment and to act with objects. The fundamental role of spatial processes in action and cognition is highlighted by Milner and Goodale (1995) in their re-interpretation of Ungerleider and Mishkin's model. They proposed that the ventral stream generates object-centered, allocentric representations to the purpose of building up long-term representations of objects, whereas the dorsal stream generates egocentric representations necessary to plan and execute reaching movements under the guidance of vision.

The concept of frames of reference encompasses the distinction in spatial competence for environments and objects. To encode the position of an object or a building a second object is needed that acts as a frame of reference. Humans can use two fundamental classes of frames of reference to encode and organize in memory spatial information: egocentric and allocentric (e.g., Levinson, 1996; Paillard, 1991; Pani & Dupree, 1994).

Egocentric frames of reference use the organism as the centre of the organization of surrounding space; the whole body, the head, the trunk, the eyes may serve like anchor-points (e.g., Kosslyn, 1994). Egocentric spatial representations maintain the perspective under which spatial information was experienced. Consequently, access to spatial locations is not equally easy but depends on the relation between the required location and the organism. Egocentric frames of reference are often defined as viewer-based (e.g., Kosslyn, 1994) or orientation-dependent (e.g., Presson, DeLange & Hazelrigg, 1989). Allocentric frames of reference specify spatial information independently of the organism's position. According to some authors, this would imply that spatial positions in the environment are equally accessible and hence derived spatial representations are called "orientation-free" (Rieser, 1989; Roskos-Ewoldsen, McNamara, Shelton & Carr, 1998; Waller, Montello, Richardson & Hegarthy, 2002). Other authors highlight that external positions may constitute privileged anchor-points, such as salient landmarks, local features like walls and global features like mountains (see Mou & McNamara, 2002), salient geometric axes (McNamara, Rump & Werner, 2003), the azymuth of the sun, and even the direction of gravity (Paillard, 1991). For these reasons, allocentric frames of reference are also called "environmental" or "geocentric" (McNamara et al., 2003; Paillard, 1991).

Spatial Memory and Familiarity with the Environment

Although research on spatial memory has a long history, in the majority of the cases experimental settings and procedures are restricted to laboratory situations, and the results are typically generalized to real world contexts. Consequently, little is known on the characteristics of spatial memory based on bodily interactions with large-scale everyday environments. The focus of this paper is on memory for actual environments that, obviously, may be familiar or unfamiliar. Our common experience tells us that the more we travel through a specific area the better we remember its spatial structure, that is its locations, directions and distances. Spatial representations of heavily travelled areas are more integrated than those of less travelled areas, suggesting a transition to a map-like representation (Hart & Moore, 1973; Golledge & Spector, 1978; Bryant, 1982). Does this mean that with increasing familiarity there is a transition to more allocentric spatial representations? In this research we seek to investigate whether familiarity with a large-scale outdoor environment affects the spatial frames of reference necessary to represent it in memory.

The literature about spatial memory has assessed the influence of several factors on the selection of the frames of reference, for example: way of learning (Presson & Hazelrigg, 1984), size (Presson & Montello, 1994; Roskos-Ewoldsen et al., 1998), number of experienced orientations (Presson et al., 1989), geometric structure of the environment (McNamara et al., 2003; Mou & McNamara, 2002), processes of spatial updating (Presson & Montello, 1994; Farrell & Robertson, 2000; Waller et al., 2002). It has not been sufficiently investigated the effect of familiarity on spatial representations.

Spatial representations should include knowledge of locations, distances and directions of the places people experience. The acquisition of this knowledge begins as soon as one arrives in a place, but presumably continues over long time periods, for months and years. The developmental process of acquiring knowledge about the spatial layout of places over time is termed. In several disciplines, such as psychology, geography, architecture and computer science, models of development of spatial knowledge have been proposed. Perhaps the most influential framework is by Hart and Moore (1973) and Siegel and White (1975). Hart and Moore (1973) discussed the evolution from egocentric to allocentric frames of reference, on whose basis Siegel and White (1975) proposed a model of acquisition of spatial knowledge which develops along three stages: landmark, route and survey. A landmark representation is based on the visual salience of landmarks, without knowledge of their relative spatial relations. A route representation is based on knowledge of the routes connecting landmarks as seen from a first-person perspective, and therefore implies an egocentric representation. A survey representation is a global, integrated and map-like representation of the environment which is independent of the person's position and emphasizes the allocentric relationships between objects. This model has been extended to the development by adults of familiarity with the environment. As experience with an environment increases, the adult would progress through these stages whose final output, then, is the allocentric representation of the environment (Golledge, Smith, Pellegrino, Doherty & Marshall, 1985).

Several studies with adults are consistent with the developmental model but others are not. It has been suggested that the physical structure of natural settings may afford different kinds of representation and that the final survey stage based on allocentric frames of reference may not be reached (McDonald & Pellegrino, 1993; see also Lindberg & Gärling, 1982). For example, Moeser (1988) studied memory for a complex and irregularly shaped building, the Health Sciences Centre (CDN). After inspecting several measures, it was shown that the student nurses could not form survey allocentric maps of the building even after traversing it for two years. Instead, Gärling and colleagues (Gärling, Lindberg, Carreiras & Böök, 1986) reported that the presence of a regular street greed favored the acquisition of allocentric spatial relations between places in the city of Umeå, Sweden. The features of the environment, then, can make a difference. However, we cannot forget that even within the same environment large individual differences in spatial knowledge may emerge (e.g., Hirtle & Hudson, 1991; Kozlowski & Bryant, 1977; Montello & Pick, 1993; Lawton, 1996; Schmitz, 1999; Montello, Lovelace, Golledge & Self, 1999). These considerations imply that both the characteristics of the environment, such as the degree of regularity, and the characteristics of individuals, such as familiarity and gender, should be taken into account (see Iachini, Ruotolo & Ruggiero, 2009; Montello et al., 1999). In the next paragraph we review research on spatial memory in laboratory-based and environment-based settings by focusing on the possible influence of familiarity on the frames of reference used to organize spatial information in memory.

Pioneering Studies on Spatial Memory

In their seminal work, Evans and Pezdek (1980) studied the effect of familiarity on spatial representations by comparing participants who were familiar or unfamiliar with the same real-world setting: the University campus of San Bernardino (USA). Participants had to assess whether maps reproducing triads of locations and presented in various orientations, reproduced correctly the reciprocal relations between the locations. The results showed orientation effects only with unfamiliar participants, but not with familiar participants. Unfamiliar participants learned the environment through a map, whereas familiar participants relied on their long-term experience with the environment. Therefore, the results were interpreted as evidence that learning spatial relationships from maps produces orientation-specific, i.e. egocentric, representations, whereas learning spatial information from direct bodily exploration results in orientation-free, i.e. allocentric, representations. However, the authors recognized that it was difficult to disentangle whether the results were due to the way of learning spatial information (map vs direct exploration) or to the amount of experience.

Thorndyke and Hayes-Roth (1982) tested the knowledge of one floor of a building of participants with different degrees of familiarity. They compared familiar participants who had learned the layout of the building from direct exploration (familiarity defined as amount of exposure ranging from 1 to 24 months) and unfamiliar participants who had learned the same layout from a map. The unfamiliar group was worse in pointing to locations within the building from different positions than the familiar group and was equally accurate in estimating straight-line and route distances, whereas the navigation group was better at estimating route than straight-line distances. The results suggested that spatial knowledge derived from direct experience is allocentric, whereas spatial knowledge derived from maps is egocentric.

Studies of Spatial Memory in Laboratory

Following Evans and Pezdek (1980), several laboratory studies have examined more closely some factors supposed to make a difference between navigable large-scale environments and small spatial layouts, such as maps. According to Roskos-Ewoldsen and colleagues (1998), these factors can be summarized as follows: number of experienced orientations, size and way of learning spatial information. Presson and Hazelrigg (1984) focused on the effect of primary learning, that is visual and/or kinaesthetic exploration of the environment, and of secondary learning, that is the indirect achievement of spatial information by symbolic means, such as maps. They found orientation effects after learning a map but not after learning a path by looking at it from a single viewpoint and by walking along the path while blindfolded. This confirmed that primary learning of spatial information leads to orientation-free representations. Subsequently, Presson, DeLange and Hazelrigg (1987) manipulated the number of experienced orientations. They found that when participants experienced only one orientation while walking blindfolded, the derived spatial representation was orientation-specific; on the contrary, when they experienced multiple orientations, the derived spatial representation was orientation-free. The same authors (Presson et al., 1989) also examined the effect of the size of the spatial layout; they found orientation effects only after learning small maps and short paths, but not large maps and long paths.

Overall, these early findings would indicate that mental representations of small spatial layouts are based on egocentric systems of reference, whereas large-scale spaces are represented according to allocentric systems of reference. However, recent evidence has shown that room-sized spatial layouts are represented in an orientation-dependent way (Christou & Bülthoff, 1999; Diwadkar & McNamara, 1997; Easton & Sholl, 1995; Presson & Montello, 1994; Richardson, Montello & Hegarty, 1999, map & virtual-walk conditions; Rieser, 1989; Roskos-Ewoldsen et al., 1998; Shelton & McNamara, 1997, 2001; Sholl & Nolin, 1997, Exps. 1, 2 & 5; Waller et al., 2002). Of special interest is that some studies failed to replicate Presson's results, although they used a similar experimental setting and procedure. Indeed, it has been shown that sensorimotor awareness of the relationship between one's body and the surrounding environment (Waller et al., 2002; see also Roskos-Ewoldsen et al., 1998) and the regularity of the spatial array (Easton & Sholl, 1995) would facilitate the allocentric processing of spatial information.

In a series of studies, McNamara and collaborators (Shelton & McNamara, 2001; Mou & McNamara, 2002; for a review see McNamara, 2003) examined the relative importance of egocentric and allocentric (that is geocentric) reference systems in memory of room-sized spatial layouts. Shelton and McNamara (2001) studied the influence of the surrounding environment on how inter-objects spatial relations are represented in memory. Their participants had to learn the location of seven objects in a room and subsequently they had to give direction judgments from memory. There were two main manipulations: the number of views from which the layout was studied, and the presence or absence of local and global frames of reference (that is a rectangular mat on which objects were placed and the walls of the room). Results showed that judgments of direction were more accurate for imagined headings parallel to egocentric reference points (i.e. study views) which were aligned with salient environmental axes. Subsequent research (Mou & McNamara, 2002) confirmed that spatial memories are defined in relation to intrinsic (i.e. allocentric) frames of reference, which are selected on the basis of egocentric experience and environmental cues.

In sum, it is still unclear whether spatial memories of navigable spaces learned by direct exploration are represented on the basis of egocentric or allocentric frames of reference. Furthermore, these laboratory-based studies have weak ecological validity. Even if they are intended to study navigable spaces, they reduce the environmental setting to the size of a room where simple four-point paths (maximum extent 4 x 4m, see for example Presson et al., 1989; Roskos-Ewoldsen et al., 1998) or six objects (Rieser, 1989) are displayed. The exploration of these settings is often based exclusively on vision or on a restricted range of movements. As a consequence, the generalization of results obtained in room-sized settings to real and complex environments should be taken with caution (Siegel, Kirasic & Kail, 1979). As anticipated, in natural settings different types of spatial knowledge may be acquired (McDonald & Pellegrino, 1993; see also Lindberg & Gärling, 1982). For example, if the environment is irregularly shaped it may prevent from the acquisition of allocentric knowledge (Moeser, 1988), whereas if it is regular it may facilitate the knowledge of allocentric spatial relationships between locations (Gärling et al., 1986). Therefore, the complexity of real environments might undermine the experimental control of the variables under investigation or lead to designs that can be insensitive to the phenomena of interest (see Davies & Logie, 1993).

Studies of Spatial Memory in Large-Scale Ecological Environments

Despite its ecological impact, then, it is not surprising that few studies about spatial frames of reference are settled in large-scale everyday environments and take into account the different degrees of familiarity with which they may be known. Below we describe a sample representative of these studies. Some studies considered separately either familiar or unfamiliar real-world environments. Sholl (1987) asked students at Boston college to point to landmarks within the campus in order to compare mental representations acquired through navigation and map presentation. Results indicate that, other things being equal, the accessibility of a landmark's location was a function of where it was located within body-centred coordinates.

Werner and Schmidt (1999) studied the frames of reference used to represent in memory a familiar environment, that is the city of Göttingen, Germany. They asked students living in the city to imagine themselves at the intersection of two main streets in town, facing down either the streets or the corners, and to point to landmarks placed at different angular distances. The results showed that spatial performance was faster and more accurate when participants imagined themselves aligned with the streets than when they did not. Further, landmarks in front of the participants' imagined position were identified faster and more accurately than landmarks behind. These findings suggest that both allocentric reference systems, based on environmental characteristics, and egocentric reference systems may be used to represent the spatial structure of a large-scale familiar environment.

McNamara, Rump and Werner (2003) obtained similar results in a study settled in an unfamiliar city park. Participants had to learn the locations of eight objects in the park by walking along one of two paths, one aligned with a salient regular building, a reproduction of the Parthenon, and one misaligned with the Parthenon. After learning, participants were led to the laboratory where were asked to point to target objects from imagined headings. Results showed that pointing accuracy was better for aligned than misaligned paths, and in particular accuracy was higher when the imagined heading was parallel to the legs of the path or was oriented towards a salient landmark, that is a nearby lake. In the misaligned condition, accuracy decreased with angular disparity but increased when the imagined heading was oriented towards the lake. The authors interpreted the results as evidence that the spatial structure of the environment was represented according to frames of reference anchored on the environment but selected on the basis of egocentric experience.

Iachini and Logie (2003) studied how an unfamiliar environment, the University campus of Aberdeen (Scotland), was represented in memory. Participants had to observe real buildings from a starting position, then were led to a testing position that differed from the initial orientation by various degrees (from 0° to 180°, with 45° in step) and finally had to mark their positions on a map. The results showed that the latency of self-localization increased as the angular distance between initial and final perspectives increased. This finding suggests that spatial information acquired from an unfamiliar real-world environment is egocentrically represented.

Few studies compared directly participants familiar or unfamiliar with the same setting, apart from Evans and Pezdek (1980) and Thorndyke and Hayes-Roth (1982). Two experiments compared participants with different degrees of familiarity with the same University campus on distance (Foley & Cohen, 1984) and distance and direction (Kirasic, Allen & Siegel, 1984) estimation tasks. Kirasic and colleagues (1984) found that students who had at least one year of experience with their University campus revealed a more abstract and flexible spatial map than students who were less familiar (less than six months of experience). Foley and Cohen (1984) showed that first year students used a perspective-dependent strategy and were less accurate in distance estimates with respect to fourth year students who instead used a more abstract map-like representation.

Iachini, Ruotolo and Ruggiero (2009) compared participants familiar or unfamiliar with a pool of buildings in the city of Naples, Italy. Participants learned the locations of three triads of buildings by walking on a path that encircled each triad. Then they were shown with maps reproducing these triads at five different orientations (from 0° to 180°) and had to judge whether each triad represented correctly the relative positions between the buildings. Results suggested that locations of unfamiliar buildings were mentally represented in terms of egocentric frames of reference; instead, allocentric frames of reference defined by salient and regular environmental axes were used when the environment was familiar.

Overall, these environment-based studies show that spatial information acquired from unfamiliar environments is represented in an egocentric way (Kirasic et al., 1984; Foley & Cohen, 1984; Sholl, 1987; Iachini & Logie, 2003; Iachini et al., 2009; see also Evans & Pezdek, 1980; Thorndyke & Hayes-Roth, 1982), although geometrical salience and regularity may facilitate an allocentric processing (McNamara et al., 2003). Less conclusive are the results about familiar environments as data in support of an allocentric representation (Evans & Pezdek, 1980; Thorndyke & Hayes-Roth, 1982; Kirasic et al., 1984; Foley & Cohen, 1984; Iachini et al., 2009), or of an egocentric representation (Easton & Sholl, 1995) or of both kinds of representations (Werner & Schmidt, 1999) have been reported. Of particular interest is the fact that these studies typically use pointing tasks where participants are required to point to target-objects from a real or imagined orientation (e.g., McNamara et al., 2003) or tasks such as relative position judgments (Evans & Pezdek, 1980; Iachini et al., 2009). Consequently, the type of frame of reference used to perform the task is never manipulated directly but inferred from the pattern of results. Even when distance judgment tasks are used, only the spatial relationships between landmarks, i.e. allocentric relationships, are assessed (Kirasic et al., 1984; Foley & Cohen, 1984).

Aims and Hypotheses

Our primary intention is to study the effect of familiarity on the frames of reference used to represent a large-scale outdoor environment by comparing directly egocentric and allocentric spatial judgments. As with our previous research (Iachini et al., 2009), the experiment reported here took place in a wide pedestrian area comprising several buildings within the administrative district of the city of Naples (Italy) and involved participants who had an extensive experience with this area and participants who had never been there before. As shown in Figure 1, the setting was characterized by a global rectangular shape and two main streets forming a T-junction. The choice of a regular environment was due to the consideration that too complex natural settings may undermine the experimental design and prevent from the acquisition of allocentric spatial information (e.g., Moeser, 1988; McDonald & Pellegrino, 1993). By manipulating the required spatial frame of reference during a task of relative distance estimation, it was possible to compare directly egocentric and allocentric processing of environmental information. In order to avoid the confounding between the way of learning spatial information and the degree of familiarity (see Evans & Pezdek, 1980), unfamiliar participants had to experience the environment by visual locomotion. Familiar participants were also submitted to the same learning phase to rule out the possibility of spurious factors due to differences in the procedure. Therefore, all participants had to learn triads of buildings and then provide spatial judgments of relative distance either in relation to the viewer ("Which building was closest to you?") or to another building ("Which building was closest to the building F3?"). If increasing experience with the environment leads to a transition from egocentric to allocentric representations, then familiar participants should perform better and be faster than unfamiliar participants in the allocentric distance judgments.

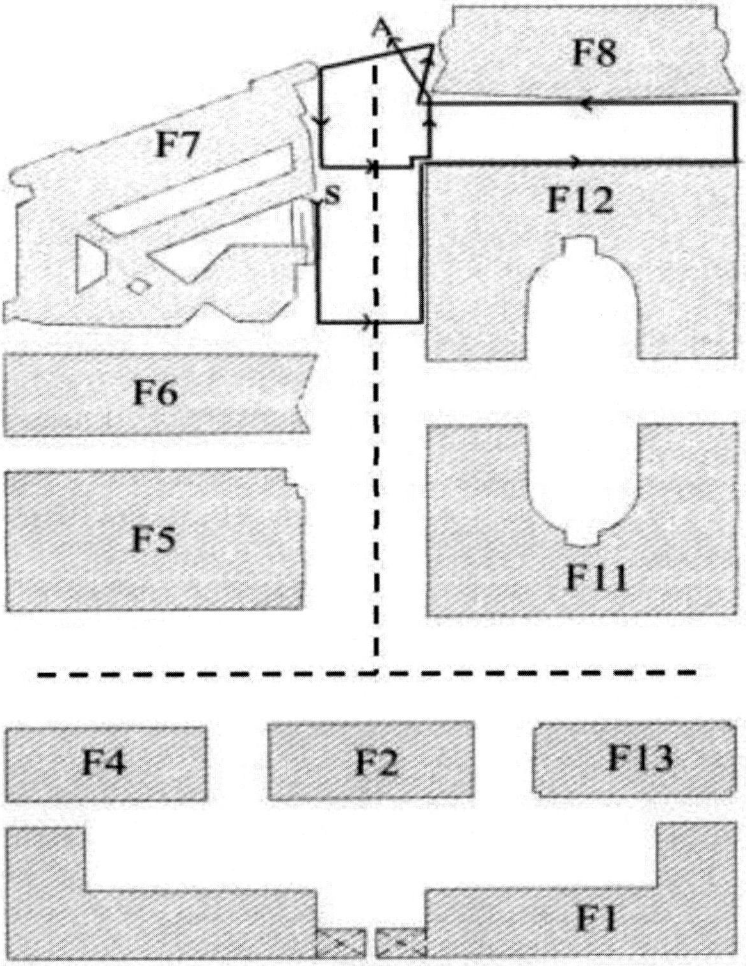

Fig. 1. The two-dimensional map of area F of the administrative district of the city of Naples is shown. All labelled buildings were used in the experiment. The black line circumscribing three buildings (F7, F8, F12) gives an example of the path taken during the learning phase. S = starting position; A = arrival position, also used as Testing position. The dashed lines show the two main

METHOD

Participants. Forty participants took part in the experiment, 20 were unfamiliar (9 men; 11 women; mean age= 25.7, SD= 3.6, range= 20-32) and 20 familiar (10 men, 10 women; mean age= 25.7, SD= 3.4, range= 21-31). Familiar participants were employed in several buildings of area F and were recruited through the intervention of the office of Public Relations of the Council of Naples. They all volunteered to take part in the experiment. Fourteen participants worked for a call centre placed at the 17th floor of building F2, from five- to seven day a week. From their workplace they could see all the other buildings of the area and the two main streets. The layout of the area F is shown in Figure 1. Four participants worked as secretaries at building F6, 5th floor, a five-day week. Two participants attended a 2-year master course at building F12, 5th floor, a three-day week. All familiar participants had worked in the selected area from 1 to 5 years before testing, mean= 3, SD= 1.68. Further, they all traversed the two main streets day by day to reach their workplace and to go out for lunch. Unfamiliar participants had never been in area F before the experiment. They were undergraduate students recruited from the Second University of Naples and members of the general public who volunteered to participate in the experiment. All participants gave informed consent to take part in the experiment and had normal or corrected to normal sight.

Experimental setting. An area of the administrative district of Naples, called area F, was chosen as setting for the Experiment. The administrative district comprises buildings of different height (from 5 to 28 floors) grouped in 7 areas, labelled with letters from A to G. Each area is separated from the others by streets or gardens and includes several buildings identified by a letter and a number. On the basis of a two-dimensional, black and white map of the district (ratio 1: 1000), area F was chosen as setting for the Experiment. This area has a surface of 26.578m^2 and comprises 11 buildings. It has a rectangular shape and is characterized by two salient main streets forming a T-junction (see Figure 1). Finally, it is situated in a flat land, is far from traffic noise and accessible only by pedestrians. Within this area, 10 buildings were selected as stimuli on the basis of the following criteria: they could be circumnavigated with no problems, could form triads of buildings that were all visible from the same vantage point and allowed for paths around each triad of homogeneous length (about 250m). The relative distances among the buildings varied from 6 to 26meters (mean=16.45m; SD=6.94m). The 10 buildings (called F1, F2, F4, F5, F6, F7, F8, F11, F12, F13) were combined in such a way as to produce 5 triads. These triads were: a) F4-F5-F2; b) F6-F7- F8; c) F7-F12-F8; d) F1-F2-F13; e) F4-F5-F11. Figure 1 shows the setting of the experiment. Two different positions (one starting position and one arrival position) for each triad were first marked on the map and then reproduced in the real environment by marking a black dot on the ground. The arrival position allowed participants to see the three buildings at the same time. A route connecting the two positions and circumnavigating each triad was first highlighted on the map and then reproduced in the environment. For each triad a building was chosen as target for the allocentric judgment (see Figure 1 again). The arrival position was also used as testing position (i.e. where distance judgments were provided). This position was defined in such a way that the difficulty to compare the egocentric distances (i.e. the distances between the 2 buildings closest to the participant's body) was the same as the allocentric distances (i.e. the distances between the 2 buildings and the target-building). On the basis of previous research (Iachini et al., 2009), the duration of the learning time was established in two turns around triads. Three buildings (G6, G7 and G8) of an area far from area F, called area G, were selected for a practice trial.

Procedure. Participants were led to area G of the Administration Centre. Here they read written instructions about the task, which were then revised orally by the experimenter. Afterwards, there was the training session. Participants had to learn the names and the positions of three buildings (G6, G7 and G8) located along a route and subsequently to give egocentric and allocentric distance judgments. If the entire procedure was clear, participants were blindfolded and conducted to area F where the experimental session started.

Learning phase. Participants were instructed to memorize as accurately as possible the names and the locations of buildings that they encountered as they were guided along the route by the experimenter. Moreover, the experimenter emphasized that participants had to focus on these buildings and their locations as they were encountered and not on additional contextual information. In order to avoid the acquisition of additional information, participants were blindfolded at entering area F and when led from one triad to another. Once arrived at the starting position of each triad, the experimenter removed the participant's blindfold and named the first building. Participants were given 6 sec to observe the building and then were conducted to the next building that was named and observed for 6 sec. The procedure was repeated for the third building. After walking twice the path, participants were led to the arrival position where they had to observe the three buildings together for 20 sec. Afterwards, participants were blindfolded and there was a memory check: they had to name the buildings in their order of occurrence (for a similar procedure see McNamara, Rump & Werner, 2003). The learning procedure lasted about 6 minutes per triad. If the memorization was accurate, the testing phase started; if not, the learning procedure was repeated once more. Once the testing phase for the first triad had finished, participants were led to the next triad. The order of presentation of triads was counterbalanced among participants.

Testing phase. In the testing position (corresponding to the arrival position), the experimenter asked blindfolded participants to provide 4 judgments for each triad of buildings. There was one egocentric question: "Which building was closest to you?"; and one allocentric question: "Which building was closest to building X (i.e. Target-building, as shown in Figure 1)?". In addition, there were 2 distractors: "Which building was tallest?" and "Which building was largest?". For each judgment, accuracy and latency were recorded. Correct judgments were scored 1, incorrect 0. Latency was recorded by means of a hand-held stopwatch, starting from when the experimenter named the required frame until the participant gave the response. The order of presentation of questions was counterbalanced across participants. At the ending of the testing phase, participants were interviewed to be sure that they had followed the instructions accurately. Participants were also asked to describe the way in which they performed the task and if there were triads more difficult than others. As soon as the testing phase ended the participant, still blindfolded, was led to the next triad, and the procedure was repeated. The entire session took about one hour.

The experimental design was based on two independent variables: a 2-level "between" variable Familiarity (Familiar vs. Unfamiliar) and a 2-level "within" variable Spatial judgments (Egocentric/Allocentric). As dependent variables there were accuracy (mean of correct judgments based on the range 0-5) and mean latency for correct responses (sec).

RESULTS

Analyses were based on 2-way Anovas for mixed designs with terms for Familiarity (between) and Spatial Judgments (within). The Bonferroni correction was used to analyze post-hoc effects.

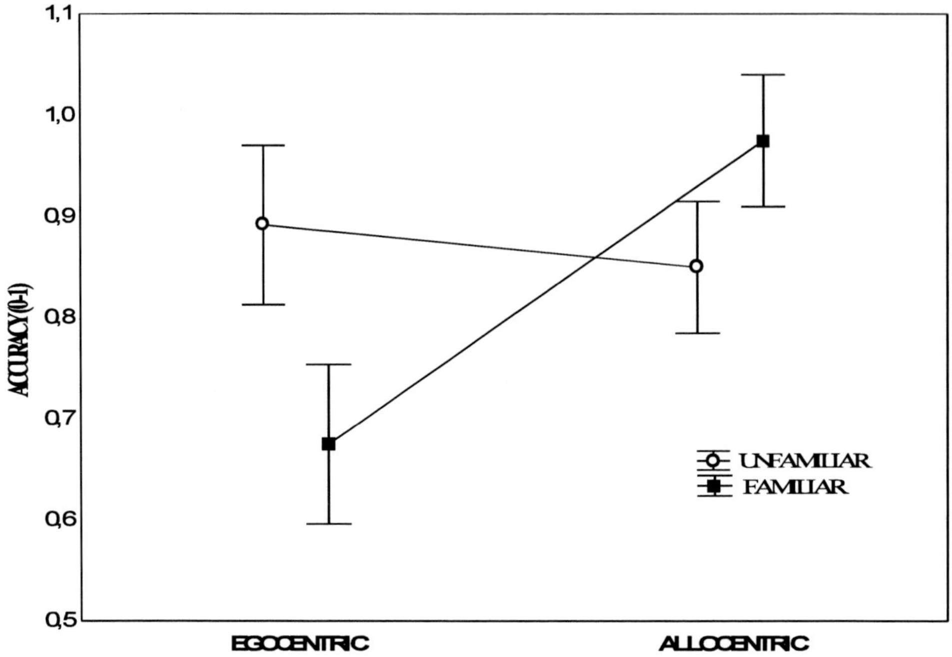

Figure 2. Mean accuracy of Familiar and Unfamiliar participants as a function of egocentric and allocentric spatial judgments.

Table 1. Mean of accuracy and latency of spatial judgments as a function of familiar and unfamiliar participants.

Spatial judgments	*Familiar*		*Unfamiliar*	
Accuracy (0-1)	*Mean*	*SD*	*Mean*	*SD*
Egocentric	.67	.16	.89	.18
Allocentric	.97	.06	.85	.19
Latency (sec)				
Egocentric	2.01	.64	2.54	.95
Allocentric	2.35	.87	3.25	.85

As regards accuracy, no main effect of Familiarity emerged ($F(1, 38)= 1.50$, $\eta^2= .03$, $p> .05$). A main effect of Spatial Judgments was found ($F(1, 38)= 14.503$, $\eta^2= .27$, $p< .001$), due to allocentric judgments (mean= .912, SD= .128) being more accurate than egocentric ones (mean= .783, SD= .174). A significant interaction between the two factors was found ($F(1, 38)= 25.368$, $\eta^2= .40$, $p< .001$) (see Figure 2). The Post-hoc analyses (with $\alpha= .0125$) showed that Familiar participants were more accurate than Unfamiliar participants in allocentric judgments ($F(1, 38)= 7.546$, $\eta^2= .17$, $p< .01$). Conversely, Unfamiliar participants were more accurate than Familiar participants in egocentric judgments ($F(1, 38)= 15.474$, $\eta^2= .29$, $p< .001$) (see Table 1). Familiar participants performed better in allocentric than egocentric judgments ($F(1, 38)= 71.581$, $\eta^2= .65$, $p< .001$), whereas Unfamiliar participants performed similarly in both judgments ($F < 1$).

As concerns latency, the Anova revealed a main effect of Familiarity ($F(1, 38)= 9.123$, $\eta^2= .19$, $p< .001$) and of Spatial judgments ($F(1, 38)= 19.177$, $\eta^2= .33$, $p< .05$). Familiar participants (mean= 2.185, SD= .753) were faster than Unfamiliar participants (mean= 2.894, SD= .901). Egocentric judgments (mean= 2.275, SD= .794) were faster than allocentric judgments (mean= 2.804, SD= .860). No significant interaction between the two factors appeared: $F(1, 38)= 2.390$, $\eta^2= .06$, $p> .05$ (see Table 1 again).

CONCLUSION

In this research we aimed at investigating whether spatial memories of navigable spaces learned by direct exploration are represented on the basis of egocentric or allocentric frames of reference. The purpose was to assess whether with increasing familiarity there is a progression from egocentric to allocentric spatial representations, as suggested by Golledge and colleagues (1985) on the basis of the developmental model proposed by Siegel and White (1975). We are aware that the rigid version of the developmental model is no longer tenable both for architectural characteristics of the environment (Lindberg & Gärling, 1982; McDonald & Pellegrino, 1993; Moeser, 1988) and individual differences (e.g., Hirtle & Hudson, 1991; Kozlowski & Bryant, 1977; Montello & Pick, 1993; Lawton, 1996; Schmitz, 1999; Montello et al., 1999). Different kinds of spatial representations of an environment may be construed even at first encounters (see Montello, 1998). This led some theoreticians to support that with increasing experience changes are more quantitative than qualitative (Montello, 1998). Nevertheless, it is also true that with increasing familiarity our mental spatial representation of an environment becomes more integrated and detached by egocentric perspective, as suggested by our subjective experience and by several data in the literature. The research reported here represents a first endeavour to compare directly egocentric and allocentric representations of the environment on the basis of the explicit manipulation of the required spatial frames of reference (see Iachini & Ruggiero, 2006; Iachini, Ruggiero, Conson & Trojano, 2009). The idea behind is that familiarity pushes towards a more allocentric representation, but other factors beside this may determine the final output. In short, a flexible model of the development of spatial memory is proposed that takes into account the simultaneous interaction of multiple factors (see Iachini et al., 2009). Below, the results are analyzed to see whether or not they are compatible with this model.

Familiarity and Frames of Reference

Bearing in mind the ecological limitations of laboratory-based studies of spatial memory (e.g. Siegel et al., 1979), the present experiment was set within a large-scale regular environment combined, as far as possible, with the apparatus and experimental procedures typical of laboratory studies. With all the cautions due to an ecological study, the pattern of results suggests that the experimental manipulations have been sensitive to the phenomena of interest. Indeed, familiar participants performed better than unfamiliar participants in judging the allocentric distances between landmarks and were also better in using allocentric than egocentric frames of reference. On the contrary, unfamiliar participants performed equally well in both kinds of judgments and better than familiar participants in judging the egocentric distances. These findings can be attributed with no ambiguity to the amount of previous experience per se and not to the way of learning spatial information, as instead happened with Evans and Pezdek (1980) and Thorndyke and Hayes-Roth (1982). The confounding between the two factors was controlled in the present learning procedure by having both familiar and unfamiliar participants experiencing the environment by direct bodily exploration.

From one side, the pattern of results suggests that familiarity with the real-world environment facilitates the selection of allocentric frames of reference, as predicted by the developmental model (Siegel & White, 1975; Golledge et al., 1985). The crucial finding that familiar participants are more accurate than unfamiliar participants in the allocentric judgments clearly verifies the experimental hypothesis. The final output of long-term experience with the environment, then, should be an integrated, complete configurational map that is based on allocentric frames of reference. Since allocentric spatial information is not biased by the body's egocentric position, it can be easily reorganized to the service of the task at hand (see also Ruggiero, Sergi & Iachini, 2008). This kind of spatial representation, then, should be useful for multiple purposes and allow for flexible behaviours such as taking shortcuts and detours that are apparently more difficult in unfamiliar environments. Previous studies comparing unfamiliar and familiar participants (Evans & Pezdek, 1980; Thorndyke & Hayes-Roth, 1982; Iachini et al., 2009) and different levels of familiarity (Foley & Cohen, 1984; Kirasic et al., 1984) can be considered as consistent with this model predicting a transition to an allocentric spatial representation as familiarity with the environment increases.

From the other side, two findings conflict with the rigid version of the developmental model. First, the unexpected drop of familiar participants in the egocentric performance. The Siegel and White's model is cumulative and predicts that the final survey and allocentric stage of spatial representation incorporates the previous stages. Therefore, familiar participants should have performed at least as accurately as unfamiliar participants in the egocentric judgments. Although it is difficult to find out a convincing explanation for this drop, we might argue that it is due to an artifactual factor. Familiar participants were forced to learn new spatial relationships that differed from the ones experienced during their usual path to reach the workplace: pre-experimental knowledge might have interfered with the task, and this was informally suggested by several participants in the post-experimental interviews.

Second, unfamiliar participants showed almost the same level of accuracy in egocentric and allocentric spatial judgments. Instead, the lack of familiarity with the environment should have resulted in a worse performance in allocentric than egocentric judgments. Although we cannot discard the possibility that the extensive learning procedure made it equally easy to retrieve egocentric and allocentric distances, we can also speculate that the regularity of the environment facilitated the processing of allocentric information (Easton & Sholl, 1995). For example, Gärling and colleagues (1986) compared participants who had lived one or two months or one year in the city of Umeå, Sweden. They found that the presence of a regular street grid facilitated the acquisition of the allocentric spatial relationships between locations in less familiar participants. The theoretical model proposed by McNamara and collaborators (e.g., Shelton & McNamara, 2001; Mou & McNamara, 2002; McNamara et al., 2003), emphasizes the importance of the geometric structure of the environment. According to this model, learning an unfamiliar environment implies interpreting its spatial structure in terms of frames of reference.

The frames of reference can be selected on the basis of egocentric experience and properties of the environment. If the environment, though unfamiliar, is characterized by a regular structure and incorporates salient features, it affords the selection of allocentric frames of reference. If the environment is too complex and irregular, egocentric cues are dominant. These predictions were consistent with the pattern of results obtained when assessing spatial knowledge of participants unfamiliar with a regular and geometrically salient environment (McNamara et al., 2003). More specifically, a facilitation was found for pointing to positions aligned or orthogonal with the main environmental axes (the legs of the Parthenon, see above). This effect emerged only in the condition (aligned path) where participants could appreciate the salience of the environment. The authors concluded that spatial locations were mentally represented in terms of frames of reference defined by the environment but selected on the basis of egocentric experience.

Coming back to our results, we could say that egocentric judgments were facilitated because the environment was unfamiliar, but the geometric salience of that environment made it equally easy to work out allocentric judgments. However, we should notice that the level of allocentric accuracy was not as high as with familiar participants, and this suggests that familiarity per se plays an important role. From a theoretical point of view, then, the three-stage model predicting a linear progression from egocentric to allocentric representations does not appear to apply rigidly to real contexts (see McDonald & Pellegrino, 1993; Iachini et al., 2009). Although individuals who are familiar with an environment tend to represent it in an allocentric way, the regularity of the environment may facilitate the allocentric processing of the environment even when it is unfamiliar (as predicted by the McNamara's model).

Ecological Validity and Experimental Caveats

The pattern of results we obtained might partially reflect a lack of sensitivity that almost necessarily accompanies studies settled in ecological contexts (Davies & Logie, 1993; Logie, Baddeley & Woodhead, 1987). Given this possibility, it is notable that the better allocentric performance in familiar than unfamiliar participants is sufficiently robust to be observed in a real environment. Further, we should consider that in the literature about spatial memory spatial performance is typically measured by pointing tasks (e.g., McNamara et al., 2003; Easton & Sholl, 1995) and, to a lesser extent, by spatial judgments about positions (Evans & Pezdek, 1980; Iachini et al., 2009), directions and distances (Thorndyke & Hayes-Roth, 1982; Foley & Cohen, 1984; Kirasic et al., 1984; Gärling et al., 1986). The pattern of results is interpreted as consistent with an egocentric or an allocentric spatial representation depending on how the frames of reference are theoretically defined (see as an example Rieser, 1989; and McNamara et al., 2003). To the best of our knowledge, this is the first study that directly compared egocentric and allocentric processing of environmental information. The task adopted here was simple as required learning and then retrieving spatial relations between the buildings and the participant (egocentric judgments) or between the buildings (allocentric judgments). The underlying logic was similar to the distance estimation task devised by Committeri and colleagues to assess egocentric and allocentric processing of spatial information in a fMRI study (Committeri, Galati, Paradis, Pizzamiglio, Berthoz & LeBihan, 2004; see also Ruggiero & Iachini, 2006; Iachini et al., 2009).

One last comment deserves the high global accuracy (84%) of the spatial task. This suggests that the real world setting and the realistic procedure have provided participants with information that facilitated the task. Two factors might have played a crucial role: presence of a fully three-dimensional real environment versus reproduction of the environment by means of maps or simple linear paths, actual movement around buildings versus static observation of spatial layouts (for a similar analysis see Iachini & Logie, 2003). Two-dimensional visual stimuli can provide only simplified information about the environment. In a real environment, the participants can study the buildings but can also pick up more general information about the metric structure of the environment. Indeed, actual movement around three-dimensional buildings might provide kinaesthetic information about the approximate direction and distance travelled. A bulk of evidence suggests that locomotor experience with the environment provides proprioceptive feedbacks that contribute to process spatial information (e.g. Rieser, 1989; Presson & Montello, 1994; Waller et al., 2002).

In conclusion, the results are in agreement with a flexible model of development of spatial memory that is based on the reciprocal interaction of multiple factors. Increasing familiarity with the spatial surroundings pushes towards the progression from egocentric to allocentric types of representation. The geometric characteristics of the environment determine the possibility to reach or not this final output. If the environment is too irregular, it may contrast the acquisition of allocentric information; if the environment is regular, it may facilitate the encoding of this kind of information even at first encounters. Individual differences also play an important role. Therefore, the representation of environmental information is influenced by multiple factors and future research should allow further insights into this complex issue. Studies set in real environments could be particularly informative as they reflect the conditions in which spatial information is processed in everyday life. The challenge would be to match as much as possible ecological validity and experimental paradigms.

REFERENCES

Ball, K., Smith, D., Ellison, A., & Schenk, T. (2009). Both egocentric and allocentric cues support spatial priming in visual search. *Neuropsychologia, 47,* 1585-1591.

Bryant, K. J. (1982). Personality correlates of sense of direction and geographic orientation. *Journal of Personality and Social Psychology, 43,* 1318–1324.

Christou, C. G. & Bülthoff, H. H. (1999). View dependence in scene recognition after active learning. *Memory & Cognition, 27,* 996–1007.

Committeri, G., Galati, G., Paradis, A., Pizzamiglio, L., Berthoz, A., & LeBihan, D. (2004). Reference frame for spatial cognition: different brain areas are involved in viewer-, object-, and landmark-centered judgments about object location. *Journal of Cognitive Neuroscience, 16,* 1517-1535.

Davies, G. M. & Logie, R. H. (1993). *Memory in everyday life.* Amsterdam: Elsevier Publishers BV.

Diwadkar, V. A. & McNamara, T. P. (1997). Viewpoint dependence in scene recognition. *Psychological Science, 8,* 302–307.

Easton, R. D. & Sholl, M. J. (1995). Object-array structure, frames of reference, and retrieval of spatial knowledge. *Journal of Experimental Psychology: Learning, Memory, & Cognition, 21*, 483-500.

Eilan, N. (1993). Molyneux's question and the idea of an external world. In: N. Eilan, R.A. McCarthy, & B. Brewer (Eds.) *Spatial representation: Problems in philosophy and psychology* (236-255). Malden, MA, US: Blackwell Publishing.

Evans, G. W. & Pezdek, K. (1980). Cognitive mapping: knowledge of a real world distance and location information. *Journal of Experimental Psychology: Human Learning and Memory, 6*, 13-24.

Farrell, M. J. & Robertson, I. H. (2000). The automatic updating of egocentric spatial relationships and its impairment due to right posterior cortical lesions. *Neuropsychologia, 38*, 585-595.

Foley, J. E. & Cohen, A. J. (1984). Working mental representations of the environment. *Environment and Behavior, 16,* 713–729.

Gärling, T., Lindberg, E., Carreiras, M., & Böök, A. (1986). Reference systems in cognitive maps. *Journal of Environmental Psychology, 6,* 1–18.

Golledge, R. G, Smith, T. R., Pellegrino, J. W., Doherty, S., & Marshall, S. P. (1985). A conceptual model and empirical analysis of children's acquisition of spatial knowledge. *Journal of Environmental Psychology, 5*, 125–152.

Golledge, R. G. & Spector, N. A. (1978). Comprehending the urban environment: theory and practice. *Geographical Analysis, 14*, 305-325.

Hart, R. A. & Moore, G. T. (1973). The development of spatial cognition: A review. In R. Downs & D. Stea (Eds.), *Image and environments* (246–288). Chicago: Aldine.

Hirtle, S. C. & Hudson, J. (1991). Acquisition of spatial knowledge for routes. *Journal of Environmental Psychology, 11,* 335–345

Iachini, T. & Logie, R. H. (2003). The role of perspective in locating position in a real-world, unfamiliar environment. *Applied Cognitive Psychology, 17*, 1-18.

Iachini, T. & Ruggiero, G. (2006). Egocentric and allocentric spatial frames of reference: a direct measure. *Cognitive Processing, 7, supplement 5*, 126-127.

Iachini, T., Ruggiero, G., Conson, M., & Trojano, L. (2009). Lateralization of egocentric and allocentric spatial processing after parietal brain lesions. *Brain and cognition, 69,* 514-520.

Iachini, T., Ruotolo, F., & Ruggiero, G. (2009). The effects of familiarity and gender on spatial representation of a real environment. *Journal of Environmental Psychology, 29*, 227-234.

Kirasic, K. C., Allen, G. L., & Siegel, A. W. (1984). Expression of configurational knowledge of large scale environments. *Environment and Behavior, 16,* 687–712.

Kosslyn, S. M. (1994). *Image and brain: the resolution of the imagery debate.* Cambridge, MA: MIT Press.

Kozlowski, L. T. & Bryant, K. J. (1977). Sense of direction, spatial orientation, and cognitive maps. *Journal of Environmental Psychology: Human Perception and Performance, 3,* 590–598.

Lawton, C. A. (1996). Strategies for indoor wayfinding: the role of orientation. *Journal of Environmental Psychology, 16,* 137–145.

Levinson, S. C. (1996). Frames of reference and Molyneux's question. In P. Bloom, M.A. Peterson, L. Nadel & M. F. Garrett (Eds.), *Language and space* (109-169). Cambridge, MA: MIT Press.

Lindberg, E. & Gärling, T. (1982). Acquisition of locational information about reference points during locomotion: the role of central information processing. *Scandinavian Journal of Psychology, 23,* 207–218.

Logie, R., Baddeley, A. D., & Woodhead, M. M. (1987). Face recognition, pose and ecological validity. *Applied Cognitive Psychology, 1,* 53-69.

McDonald, T. P. & Pellegrino, J. W. (1993). Psychological perspectives on spatial cognition. In T. Gärling & R. G. Golledge (Eds.) *Behavior and Environment: Psychological and Geographic Perspectives.* N. Holland: Elsevier.

McNamara, T. P. (2003). How are the locations of objects in the environment represented in memory? In C. Freksa, W. Brauer, C. Habel, & K. Wender (Eds.) *Spatial cognition III: Routes and navigation, human memory and learning, spatial representation and spatial reasoning* (174-191). Berlin: Springer-Verlag.

McNamara, T. P., Rump, B., & Werner, S. (2003). Egocentric and geocentric frames of reference in memory of large-scale space. *Psychonomic Bulletin and Review, 10*, 589-595.

Milner, A. D. & Goodale, M. A. (Eds.) (1995). *The visual brain in action.* Oxford, England: Oxford University Press.

Moeser, S. D. (1988). Cognitive mapping in a complex building. *Environment and Behavior, 20,* 21–49.

Montello, D. R. (1998). A new framework for understanding the acquisition of spatial knowledge in large-scale environments. In M. J. Egenhofer & R. G. Golledge (Eds.) *Spatial and temporal reasoning in geographic information systems* (143-154). New York: Oxford University Press.

Montello, D. R., Lovelace, K. L., Golledge, R. G., & Self, C. M. (1999). Sex-related differences and similarities in geographic and environmental spatial abilities. *Annals of the Association of American Geographers, 89,* 515–534.

Montello, D. R. & Pick, H. L. (1993). Integrating knowledge of vertically aligned large-scale spaces. *Environment and Behavior, 25,* 457–484.

Mou, W. & McNamara, T. P. (2002). Intrinsic frames of reference in spatial memory. *Journal of Experimental Psychology: Learning, Memory, and Cognition, 28*, 162-170.

Paillard, J. (1991). *Brain and space.* Oxford : Oxford University Press.

Pani, J. R. & Dupree, D. (1994). Spatial reference systems in the comprehension of rotational motion. *Perception, 23*, 929–946.

Pinker, S. (1984). Visual cognition: an introduction. *Cognition, 18,* 1-63.

Presson, C. C., DeLange, N., & Hazelrigg, M. D. (1987). Orientation specificity in kinesthetic spatial learning: The role of multiple orientations. *Memory & Cognition, 15*, 225-229.

Presson, C. C., DeLange, N., & Hazelrigg, M. D. (1989). Orientation specificity in spatial memory: What makes a path different from a map of a path? *Journal of Experimental Psychology: Learning, Memory, and Cognition, 15*, 887-897.

Presson, C. C. & Hazelrigg, M. D. (1984). Building spatial representations through primary and secondary learning. *Journal of Experimental Psychology: Learning, Memory, and Cognition, 10*, 716-722.

Presson, C. C. & Montello, D. R. (1994). Updating after rotational and translational body movements: Coordinate structure of perspective space. *Perception, 23*, 741-750.

Richardson, A. E., Montello, D. R., & Hegarthy, M. (1999). Spatial knowledge acquisition from maps and from navigation in real and virtual environments. *Memory and Cognition, 27*, 741-750.

Rieser, J. J. (1989). Access to knowledge of spatial structure at novel points of observation. *Journal of Experimental Psychology: Learning, Memory, and Cognition, 15*, 1157-1165.

Roskos-Ewoldsen, B., McNamara, T. P., Shelton, A. L., & Carr, W. (1998). Mental representations of large and small spatial layouts are orientation dependent. *Journal of Experimental Psychology: Learning, Memory, and Cognition, 24*, 215-226.

Ruggiero, G. & Iachini, T. (2006). The effect of familiarity on egocentric and allocentric spatial representations of the environment. *Cognitive Processing, 7, supplement 5*, 88-89.

Ruggiero, G., Sergi, I., & Iachini, T. (2008). Gender differences in remembering and inferring spatial distances. *Memory, 16,* 821-835.

Schmitz, S. (1999). Gender differences in acquisition of environmental knowledge related to wayfinding behavior, spatial anxiety, and self-estimated environmental competencies. *Sex Roles, 41*, 71–93.

Shelton, A. L. & McNamara, T. P. (1997). Multiple views of spatial memory. *Psychonomic Bulletin & Review, 4,* 102–106.

Shelton, A. L. & McNamara, T. P. (2001). Systems of spatial reference in human memory. *Cognitive Psychology, 43*, 274-310.

Sholl, M. J. (1987). Cognitive maps and orientation schemata. *Journal of Experimental Psychology: Learning, Memory, and Cognition, 13*, 615-628.

Sholl, M. J. & Nolin, T. L. (1997). Orientations specificity in representations of place. *Journal of Experimental Psychology: Learning, Memory and Cognition, 23,* 1494–1507.

Siegel, A. W., Kirasic, K. C., & Kail, R. V. (1979). Stalking the elusive cognitive map: the developmental of children's representations of geographic space. In J. F. Wohlwill, & I. Altman (Eds.) *Human behavior and environment*. New York: Plenum.

Siegel, A. W. & White, S. H. (1975). The development of spatial representations of large-scale environments. In Reese, H. W. (Eds.) *Advances in child development and behaviour* (37-55). New York Academic Press.

Thorndyke, P. W. & Hayes-Roth, B. (1982). Differences in spatial knowledge acquired from maps and navigation. *Cognitive Psychology, 14*, 560-589.

Ungerleider, L. G. & Mishkin, M. (1982). Two cortical visual systems. In D.J. Ingle, M.A. Goodale & R. J. W. Mansfield (Eds.) *Analysis of visual behavior* (549-586). Cambridge, MA: MIT Press.

Waller, D., Montello, D. R., Richardson, A. E., & Hegarthy, M. (2002). Orientation specificity and spatial updating of memories for layouts. *Journal of Experimental Psychology: Learning, Memory, and Cognition, 28*, 1051-1063.

Werner, S. & Schmidt, K. (1999). Environmental reference systems for large scale spaces. *Spatial Cognition and Computation, 1*, 447-473.

In: Learning and Memory Developments...
Editors: L. C. Eklund, A. S. Nyman, pp. 209-224
ISBN: 978-1-60876-397-9

Chapter 9

DOES DISREGARD OF TRANSIENT CHANGES IN THE ENVIRONMENT DIFFERENTIATE BEHAVIOUR OF CHILDREN WITH AUTISM FROM TYPICALLY DEVELOPING CHILDREN AND THOSE WITH DOWN SYNDROME AND IDIOPATHIC INTELLECTUAL DISABILITY?

Nahal Goharpey, Robin Laycock[1], David P. Crewther, and Sheila G. Crewther*

[1] School of Psychological Science, La Trobe University, Victoria, Australia, 3086.
[2]Brain Sciences Institute, Swinburne University of Technology, Hawthorn, Australia, 3122.

ABSTRACT

In the research literature, Intellectual Disability (ID) is conceptualised as a set of unique cognitive deficits associated with particular genetic causes rather than simply low IQ. We add to this literature by exploring social/communication features that differentiate ID of three different etiologies: Low Functioning (LF) Autism, Down Syndrome (DS) and Idiopathic ID. A body of research suggests that slow shifting and/or disengaging visual attention in Autism is likely to be a major contributing factor to their impaired social and cognitive development. We propose that slow visual orienting ability in Autism is due to impairment in magnocellular processing of the visual system. Thus, we suggest that individuals with Autism are delayed in shifting and/or disengaging attention as evidenced by a disregard for transient stimuli in their environment, where as individuals with DS and Idiopathic ID show the opposite pattern, in that they appear to be unable to maintain attention to a task, being easily distracted by transient stimuli in their environment. The implications of this visual orienting deficit are discussed in terms of

* Corresponding author: E-mail: screwther@latrobe.edu.au; Tel: +613 9214 5877; Fax: +613 9214 5525

conceptualisation of Autism, visual orienting research in Autism and evidence based educational practice for children with Autism, DS and Idiopathic ID.

Keywords: Attention, intellectual disability, Autism, Down Syndrome, Idiopathic Intellectual Disability, shifting attention, disengaging attention, visual orienting, The Magnocellular Advantage.

INTRODUCTION

Intellectual Disability (ID) is defined as an IQ score below 70 on the Wechsler Intelligence Scale for Children- Fourth Edition (WISC-IV; Wechsler, 2003) and an inability to adapt to the local environment during the developmental period (AAMR, 2002; Katz & Lazcano-Ponce, 2008; WHO, 1993). Currently in the research literature, cognitive impairments among individuals with ID of different etiologies, such as Autism and Down Syndrome (DS) have often been attributed to brain abnormalities characteristic of the particular etiology rather than ID *per se* (Vicari, 2004). This approach has supported the theoretical position that ID is not equivalent to low intelligence (Goharpey, Bello, Crewther & Crewther, under review), but a set of cognitive profiles associated with distinct brain pathology. Greater understanding of the cognitive profiles of different groups of ID may reveal common cognitive and neurological impairments in all individuals with ID regardless of genetic cause.

Autism is one of a number of neurodevelopmental disorders on the Autism Spectrum, characterised by abnormal social and communication development and the presence of repetitive behaviour (American Psychiatric Association, 2000), and is diagnosed four times more in males than females (Christian et al., 2008). According to prevalence studies in the past 20 years, there has been a rise in cases of Autism (Barbaresi, Katusic & Voigt, 2006). According to Crewther et al. (2003), an estimated 27 in every 10,000 children in Victoria, Australia are diagnosed with severe Autism. Fifty to 70% of all children with Autism Spectrum Disorder also have an ID (referred to as Lower Functioning; Matson & Shoemaker, 2009) and it has been suggested that etiology of Autism may vary with IQ (Szaimari & Jones, 1991). Despite this, the cognitive profile of Low Functioning (LF) Autism is rarely investigated.

In this chapter, we will investigate how LF Autism and High Functioning (HF) Autism compare to DS and Idiopathic ID in terms of one important aspect of the attentional system: ability to shift and/or disengage visual attention from stimuli in the environment. We will argue that shifting and/or disengaging visual attention is delayed in both LF and HF children and adults with Autism in comparison to DS, Idiopathic ID and Typically Developing (TD) individuals matched for mental age (MA) and/or chronological age (CA). We will report research that suggests that this deficit in ability to rapidly shift visual attention could contribute to the impaired social development in Autism. We propose that this visual orienting deficit in Autism may be due to impaired processing and activation of attention by the magnocellular pathway of the visual system. The magnocellular system dominates the dorsal visual pathway and is reported to contribute to attentional processing (Laycock, Crewther & Crewther, 2007; Pammer, Hansen & Cornelissen, 2006; Vidyasagar, 1999). Thus, individuals with Autism could be delayed in shifting and/or disengaging visual attention because they fail to activate to transient stimuli in their environment and therefore are unlikely to shift their visual attention to new stimuli, especially socially relevant activity such as changes in facial expression, like TD individuals of the same MA. We explore this theory in greater detail and briefly explain the theoretical and practical implication of this theory in our understanding of ID and its implication for the methods by which children with Autism, DS and Idiopathic ID are educated.

1. Impaired Shifting and/or Disengaging of Attention in High Functioning Autism

What essentially characterises and differentiates Autism from Idiopathic ID and DS as well as TD individuals is a marked deficit in social development. Interestingly, it has been suggested in the literature that this might be due to a delay in rapidly shifting visual attention (orienting attention to a different location in space) and/or disengaging attention (termination of the visual information processing at a certain location in space) as this hinders an infant's ability to engage in joint attention early in life and as a result leads to impaired social understanding, communication, imitation, turn-taking, symbolic play and the ability to exchange experiences and emotions with others (Courchesne et al., 1994; Landry & Bryson, 2004; Tronick, 1982). Tronick suggested that a slow orienting of visual attention to stimuli in the environment may derail the infant with Autism from the typical developmental trajectory and presumably lead to social and cognitive developmental abnormalities. Thus, an infant with Autism who is unable to rapidly shift his/her visual attention from one stimulus to another, is unlikely to be able to keep up with the rapidly changing social responses in the environment, and as a result the social world of these children may only be made up of fragments of information that lack context and temporal continuity (Courchesne et al.).

Research shows that voluntary (endogenous) shifts of visual attention are influenced by cognitive factors (e.g. one's current goals, knowledge and expectations) and involuntary (exogenous) shifts of visual attention are influenced by sensory properties of stimuli in the environment (e.g. level of object saliency and novelty; Corbetta & Shulman, 2002). It is the interaction of these cognitive and sensory factors at any one time that is central to determining how, where and to what object in the environment visual attention is oriented. Neurophysiological studies indicate that exogenous and endogenous visual attention is controlled by two partially segregated neuronal pathways. Corbetta and Shulman have argued that endogenous or top-down attentional modulation is controlled by a dorsal frontoparietal network (not to be confused with the dorsal visual stream), a system that appears to be bilateral. This system interacts with a more ventral frontoparietal network which is reported to be largely lateralized to the right hemisphere and is exogenously driven by behaviourally relevant stimuli. In particular this ventro-frontoparietal network may be recruited to redirect visual attention to unexpected or salient visual events.

Endogenous and exogenous orienting in Autism have been widely studied using Posner's visual orienting task (Burack, 1994; Casey, Gordon, Mannheim & Rumsey, 1993; Courchesne et al., 1994; Posner, Walker, Freidrich & Rafal, 1984; 1987; Townsend, Courchesne & Egaas, 1996; Wainwright-Sharp & Bryson, 1993), which is usually presented as a series of three boxes located in the centre, right and left side of a computer screen. A visual cue is presented in one of the boxes, followed by a visual target that is presented either at the same location or at a different location as the cue. Cues that validly direct attention to the target location are used as a measure of ability to engage attention on the target location, where as cues that invalidly direct attention serve as a measure of ability to disengage attention from the cued location, then shift attention from the cued location to the target location and engage attention at the target location (Posner, 1988; Posner & Dehaene, 1994). Reaction times to targets vary depending on the nature of the cues. Cues that provide information regarding a target's location (e.g. an arrow) elicit endogenous shifts of attention which result in faster reaction times at valid than invalid cued locations. Cues which are characterised by a sudden change in luminance or movement in the periphery elicit exogenous shifts of attention that result in faster reaction times to targets within 150 ms following a valid than invalid cue. Reaction times are slower to targets presented 300ms after a valid cue than an invalid cue (Rosen et al., 1999).

It has been widely reported in the literature that children and adults with HF Autism are slower to disengage and/or shift exogenous and endogenous visual attention compared to TD individuals matched for CA and/or MA (Casey et al., 1993; Courchesne, Akshoomoff & Townsend, 1990; Courchesne et al., 1994; Landry & Bryson, 2004; Rinehart, Bradshaw, Moss, Brereton & Tonge, 2001; Townsend, Courchesne & Egaas, 1996; Townsend, Harris & Courchesne, 1996; Wainwright & Bryson, 1996; Wainwright-Sharp & Bryson, 1993). A study by Wainwright-Sharp and Bryson found that adults with HF Autism or Asperger's disorder were delayed in shifting and/or disengaging attention to the target location on a visual orientation task compared to TD individuals of the same CA and handedness. TD adults were faster to detect the target at valid than invalid endogenously cued locations, regardless of the cue to target delay. However, adults with HF Autism or Asperger's disorder showed no cue effect for 100 ms cue to target delay, but a faster reaction time to targets at 800 ms cue delay to valid than invalid cues. The findings are consistent with past research which suggests that individuals with HF Autism are delayed in shifting and/or disengaging their visual attention compared to TD individuals of the same MA and/or CA (Casey et al; Courchesne et al; Landry & Bryson; Rinehart et al; Townsend, Courchesne & Egaas; Townsend, Harris & Courchesne; Wainwright & Bryson; Wainwright-Sharp & Bryson). The authors of the study suggested that the HF Autism and Asperger's disorder group may not have shown the reaction time advantage to valid cues in the 100ms cue to target delay because they did not have sufficient time to process the centrally (arrow) presented cue, which indicated the targets location symbolically. However a study by Townsend, Courchesne and Egaas employed a visual orientation task in which the exogenous cue (brightening of one of the boxes) was presented for 50ms and then covered by a visual mask, before the target appeared in either the central or peripheral locations and found that adults with HF Autism were still less accurate and slower to detect targets at the 100ms cue to target delay than the 800ms cue to target delay compared to age matched TD adults, whose performance did not differ between the two conditions. In this study, the authors concluded that individuals with HF Autism failed to orient to 100ms cue to target delay because they were slow to orient to new stimuli and not because they did not process the cue. All the participants with HF Autism in their study previously had magnetic resonance imaging (MRI) which confirmed the presence of bilateral cerebellar abnormalities. Thus, the authors attributed slow visual orienting deficit in the HF Autism group to cerebellar abnormality. The cerebellum is the most consistently reported neurological abnormality in Autism and this is consistent with evidence suggesting that the cerebellum is involved in the modulation of attention (Courchesne et al; Townsend, Harris & Courchesne).

A study by Courchesne and colleagues (1994), found that like patients with acquired cerebellar damage, individuals with HF Autism were impaired in their ability to rapidly shift attention (within 2.5 seconds or less) between visual and auditory stimulus modalities. However, when the time between stimuli presentation was increased, HF Autistic and cerebellar patients were comparable to TD individuals in their speed and accuracy of target detection. Therefore, the authors suggested that the cerebellum may act to optimize the neural signal-to-noise conditions in the systems involved in processing up-coming stimuli. Thus, acquired damage to the cerebellum may not inhibit shifts of attention entirely but merely make attentional shifts slow and inaccurate. In addition to cerebellar abnormalities, parietal lobe abnormalities have also been implicated in visual orienting deficits in individuals with Autism. One study found that individuals with HF Autism showed difficulty disengaging and shifting visual attention from the right to the left side of space, a pattern that is also seen in patients with hemi-spatial neglect, which is typically associated with damage to the right parietal cortex (Bryson, Wainwright-Sharp & Smith, 1990). Using MRI, Townsend, Courchesne and Egaas noted that cerebellar abnormalities alone were associated with deficits in shifting attention, whereas cerebellar plus parietal abnormalities were associated with deficits in both shifting and disengaging visual attention in Autism.

Even though neurological abnormalities have been implicated in the deficit to shift and/or disengage attention in Autism, level of intelligence has been consistently ruled out as being related to the extent of the deficit in shifting and/or disengaging attention in Autism (Landry & Bryson, 2004; Rinehart et al., 2001; Wainwright & Bryson, 1996). Interestingly, many studies have combined individuals with HF Autism with those with Asperger's disorder in the same clinical group, and concluded that they are comparable in their deficit in shifting and/or disengaging attention without any direct comparison in performance. For example, Wainwright and Bryson compared exogenously driven visual orienting performance of 4 individuals with HF Autism and 7 individuals with Asperger's disorder matched to one sample of TD individuals on CA (*M*= 20:6) and to another sample of TD individuals on handedness and receptive language ability as measured by the Peabody Picture Vocabulary Test-Revised (PPVT-R; Dunn & Dunn, 1981). Participants were required to press the space bar whenever they detected a target appear either centrally (at the location of the fixation cross) or on the left or right side of the fixation cross. Results showed that adults with a HF Autism or Asperger's disorder diagnosis responded faster to centrally located targets than lateralised targets compared to TD individuals matched either on CA or receptive language ability and handedness. Despite their small sample size, the authors concluded based on observation of the data, that adults with HF Autism and those with Asperger's disorder both show a deficit in shifting and/or disengaging attention. However, findings in a more recent study (Rinehart et al.) found that children with HF Autism were delayed in their ability to shift attention compared to TD children matched on sex, CA and MA, where as a group of children with Asperger's disorder of similar age who were matched to another control group on sex, CA and MA did not show this same visual orienting deficit. The authors suggested that individuals with HF Autism but not Asperger's disorder exhibit a delay in shifting attention, which further suggest that impaired shifting and/or disengaging visual attention may be related to the Autism diagnosis and not MA.

2. Impaired Shifting/ and or Disengaging of Visual Attention Could Differentiate Low Functioning Autism from Down Syndrome, Idiopathic Intellectual Disability and Typical Development

Difficulties shifting and/or disengaging visual attention in Autism are consistent with claims that attention in these individuals is overly focused on local rather than global scenarios (Lovaas, Schreibman, Koegal & Rehm, 1971; Rincover & Ducharme, 1987; Wainwright-Sharp & Bryson, 1993). Individuals with Autism typically focus on one aspect of their environment and are not easily distracted. Interestingly, Landry and Bryson (2004) found the opposite pattern in children with DS. Very little research on visual orientation has been conducted on children with LF Autism. However in this one study (Landry & Bryson) visual orienting was compared in 15 children with LF Autism/ pervasive developmental disorder (PDD), 13 with DS and 13 with TD matched on non-verbal and verbal MA, as measured by the Leiter International Performance Scale (Leiter, 1948) and the Test of Auditory Comprehension of Language (TACL-R; Carrow-Woolfolk, 1985). Two conditions on the task provided independent measures of disengaging and shifting visual attention exogenously. All groups were faster to shift than disengage attention, except for the DS group who showed no reaction time difference between these two conditions. The LF Autism group displayed a subtle impairment in executing rapid shifts of attention and was slower to disengage their visual attention compared to the other groups. The DS group however, was faster to disengage their visual attention than the other groups. The findings indicated that visual attention is more randomly distributed in space in children with DS and overly focused in space in children with LF Autism. Therefore, children with LF Autism and DS are both presenting with impairments in visual orientation but at opposite poles from one another. It is also important to note that the ability to disengage attention was not related to verbal or non-verbal intelligence, which has been consistently shown in previous studies (Landry & Bryson; Rinehart et al., 2001; Wainwright & Bryson, 1996).

Individuals with Idiopathic ID showed a similar pattern of visual orientation to those with DS. Previous studies have shown that individuals with Idiopathic ID have difficulty focusing on relevant information and their learning and memory formation are disrupted more by irrelevant information compared to individuals without Idiopathic ID (Hagen & Huntsman, 1971). Merrill and O'Dekirk (1994) tested 16 individuals with ID (8 with DS and 8 with Idiopathic ID) and 16 TD individuals on a target detection task, where targets were flanked by one distracter either from the same category or a different category as the target. The spatial degree of separation between targets and distracters was also varied. Results showed that both individuals with DS and Idiopathic ID experienced a larger degree of interference for lower target- distracter separation than TD individuals and unlike the TD group, those with DS did not show more interference for same-category distracters than different-category distracters. These findings suggest that both individuals with DS and those with Idiopathic ID are more distractible than the TD group. This suggests that DS and Idiopathic ID may be impaired in their ability to sustain attention. Despite these findings, other studies have found that sustained attention in individuals with Idiopathic ID may be delayed in childhood (Kirby, Nettelbeck & Thomas, 1979; Semmel, 1965) but then become comparable to TD individuals in the adolescence and adulthood (Kirby et al; Ware, Baker & Sipowicz, 1962; Warm & Berch, 1985).

Tomporowski and Allison (1988) suggested that comparable findings between TD individuals and those with Idiopathic ID, on sustained attention may have been due to ceiling effects because the tasks were not sufficiently demanding on participants' attention and/or cognition. Therefore, in their study they increased the working memory load on a sustained attention task and found that individuals with Idiopathic ID performed worse than TD individuals. Their impaired performance was attributed to their impaired working memory and not necessarily an impaired ability to sustain attention (Tomporowski, Hayden & Applegate, 1990). However, many neuroscientists researching memory consider that the laying down of memory traces is not possible without learning and that learning first requires attention to the task information (Bear, Connors & Paradiso, 2006). Thus, this study further supports the findings that individuals with Idiopathic ID and DS have difficultly sustaining visual attention compared to TD individuals. This suggests that individuals with Autism may be differentiated from Idiopathic ID and those with DS by an over focused sustained attention, which has been associated with delayed shifting and/or disengaging attention in the literature (Lovaas et al., 1971; Rincover & Ducharme, 1987; Wainwright-Sharp & Bryson, 1993).

3. New Biological Explanations for Impaired Shifting and/or Disengaging Attention in Autism

Psychophysiological studies have demonstrated repeatedly that children and adults with Autism show a deficit in shifting and/or disengaging visual attention which is thought to behaviourally manifest as an over-focused and narrow "spotlight" of attention (Lovaas et al., 1971; Rincover & Ducharme, 1987; Wainwright-Sharp & Bryson, 1993). Studies have also shown that this is the opposite for children with Idiopathic ID and DS who are very easily distracted and do not sustain attention readily (Hagen & Huntsman, 1971; Landry and Bryson, 2004; Merrill and O'Dekirk, 1994; Tomporowski & Allison, 1988). It has consistently been shown that this pattern of findings is not related to MA (Landry & Bryson) and therefore may distinguish Autism from Idiopathic ID and DS. We suggest a new biological explanation for this pattern of findings. As the magnocellular stream of the visual cortex is associated with activation of visual perception to transient stimuli, we suggest that activation of this magnocellular pathway may be impaired in individuals with Autism, thus leading to impaired shifting and/or disengaging of visual attention. Thus, we suggest that individuals with Autism have difficulty shifting attention because they apparently show a disregard for transient visual stimuli in the environment. Thus, individuals with Autism are unlikely to shift their attention to transient stimuli as readily as TD individuals, making it difficult to distract them from the current focus of their attention. We suggest that the opposite is true for individuals with Idiopathic ID and DS, who respond very readily to transient stimuli in their environment, and can not sufficiently sustain their attention in comparison to individuals with TD and individuals with Autism. Thus, individual with Idiopathic ID or DS are very easily distractible.

3.1. What is The Magnocellular Advantage?

The Magnocellular and Parvocellular streams are the two major subcortical visual projections that convey information from the retina to the primary visual cortex (V1). Magnocellular neurons have been shown to be sensitive to motion and luminance contrast at higher temporal and lower spatial frequencies, along with providing rapid signal transmission. In comparison, parvocellular neurons code for colour and have greater spatial sensitivity at lower temporal frequencies and do not saturate with higher contrast (Callaway, 2005; Kaplan & Shapley, 1982; Merigan, Bryne & Maunsell, 1991; Merigan & Maunsell, 1993; Schiller & Logothetis, 1990). The magnocellular pathway provides the major visual input to the dorsal cortical stream through to primate parietal cortex (Maunsell, 1992; Maunsell, Nealey & DePriest, 1990; Merigan et al.). Magnocellular processing has consistently been associated with visual search and particularly transient attentional processing (Li, Sampson & Vidyasagar, 2007; Pammer et al., 2006; Steinman, Steinman & Lehmkuhle, 1997; Wijers, Lange, Mulder & Mulder, 1997). In addition, the dorsal cortical stream leading to the parietal cortex is also responsible for visuo-motor control, while perception and object recognition is contingent on the ventral stream (Goodale & Milner, 1992). Both magnocellular and parvocellular signals contribute to the ventral stream projecting through to the inferotemporal cortex (Merigan & Maunsell). Essentially, the inferotemporal cortex and in particular regions within the lateral occipital complex in extrastriate cortex provide a neural centre of object representation (Malach et al., 1995), whereas the parietal cortex and its dorsal cortical projections are more commonly associated with the spatial representation of objects (Livingstone & Hubel, 1987) or with visuo-motor action (Goodale, 2008).

Traditional feed-forward neurobiological models of the visual system describe the hierarchical passage of visual information from lower to higher visual areas via two visual streams: the dorsal and ventral visual streams. Specifically, signals travel from the retina to the lateral geniculate nucleus (LGN) and then pass on to areas V1/V2. From there processing proceeds dorsally through regions including V3, the middle temporal area (MT), V6 and through to parietal cortical regions before continuing on to frontal regions such as the Frontal Eye Fields and dorsolateral prefrontal cortex (DLPFC). On the other hand a ventral stream signal proceeds from primary visual cortical areas to V4, LOC and through to inferotemporal cortex and onto the ventrolateral prefrontal cortex (VLPFC).

However, it is now more commonly understood that many feedforward connections are reciprocated by feedback connections from higher to lower order areas. According to Bullier's (2001) visual processing model, visual information is rapidly transmitted by feed-forward and feed-back cortical projections of the magnocellular dominated dorsal pathway to V1 to provide for global processing and figure-ground segregation which could not otherwise be handled by horizontal connections within V1/V2. The feedforward-feedback loop is completed prior to parvocellular inputs to V1 which is used as an active 'blackboard' to continue more fine-tuned detailed processing. This type of model has been elaborated more recently (Laycock et al., 2007; Laycock, Crewther & Crewther, 2008), such that magnocellular inputs arrive in V1 up to 20 milliseconds prior to the parvocellular signals. This timing advantage of the magnocellular system allows rapid activation of exogenously driven attention mechanisms in parietal cortex to influence detailed processing in V1 and object recognition through the ventral stream. In this way, even processing normally associated with the ventral stream is assisted by a rapid activation of exogenously driven attention through the dorsal stream. An impairment in the subcortical magnocellular system, or in the cortical dorsal stream feedforward/feedback loop (though not synonymous with the magnocellular pathway, it is largely driven by such inputs) could thus affect ones ability to engage and disengage visual attention to new salient events.

4. Implications for Understanding Visual Orienting in Autism, Down Syndrome and Idiopathic Intellectual Disability

4.1. Inhibition of Return Research in Autism

Posner and Cohen (1984) first noticed that visually presented targets that appeared 150 ms before the cue were detected faster at cued than un-cued locations (facilitation of return). However, targets that appeared 200 ms or more after the cue were detected faster at invalid than valid cued locations. They termed this detection pattern Inhibition of Return (IOR) and suggested that it reflects an attentional orienting mechanism that facilitates search behaviour by inhibiting attention from returning to previously inspected locations (Klein, 2000). However, according to the perceptual theory of IOR, search is facilitated because attention is drawn to processing novel stimuli rather than being inhibited from returning to previously inspected locations and objects (Lupiáñez et al., 2004). The authors suggested that when a target is presented shortly after a cue, these two events may be encoded as the same perceptual event, which explains facilitation of return effect. However, when the target is presented after a long delay (i.e. 200 ms +) after the cue, it is perceived as a new and separate event from the cue. Assuming novelty biases attention, it is then drawn faster to the target at the un-cued location than at the cued location, because it is "novel". This explains the IOR effect, whilst making the distinction from the attentional hypothesis that IOR does not occur from an inhibition at the cued location. This is supported by Lupiáñez and colleagues who examined the pattern of reaction times for targets that proceeded non-informative cued locations (50% of trials were valid cued locations) compared to reaction times for targets that appeared in informative cue trials (80% of trials were valid cued locations). The authors found that for TD individuals, the IOR effect occurred for both non-informative and informative cue trials, where targets were expected to appear in cued locations most of the time and hence attention was not usually orientated away from the cued location. This finding suggests that IOR can occur even when attention is not removed from the cued location.

It has been widely reported in the literature that children and adults with HF Autism show superior visual search ability as evidenced by faster target detection rates on feature and conjunctive visual search tasks, compared to TD individuals of comparable MA and/or CA (Brenner, Turner & Müller, 2007; O'Riordan, 2000;,2004; O'Riordan & Plaisted, 2001; O'Riordan, Plaisted, Driver & Baron-Cohen, 2001; Plaisted, O'Riordan & Baron-Cohen, 1998). In feature visual search tasks the target differs on all properties from the surrounding distracters (e.g. a red R target among yellow T distracters), whereas it shares at least one property from each distracter in a conjunctive search task (e.g. a red R target among yellow R and red T distracters). Therefore, the target is thought to "pop out" in feature search tasks, whereas each distracter must be serially attended to in conjunctive search tasks until the target is located (O'Riordan & Plaisted). In addition, individuals with HF Autism have a faster target detection rate in the embedded figures task (Jarrold, Gilchrist & Bender, 2005; Jolliffe & Baron-Cohen, 1997; Keehn et al., 2009; Shah & Frith, 1993), which requires the participants to search and find a hidden figure that is embedded in a larger figure, as well as faster performance on the block design task of the Wechsler scales (Shah & Frith; Tymchuk, Simmons & Neafsey, 1977).

It has been suggested in the literature that if the role of IOR is to facilitate search, superior visual search in HF Autism may be due to a larger IOR effect (Rinehart, Bradshaw, Moss, Brereton & Tonge, 2008). However, neurological investigations of IOR have implicated the superior colliculus as a neural structure that is especially important in IOR effect (Posner, Rafal, Choate & Vaughan, 1985; Rafal, Posner, Friedman, Inhoff & Bernstein, 1988; Sapir, Soroker, Berger & Henik, 1999). The superior colliculus has projections to the Left Frontal Eye Fields and V5 within the dorsal visual stream. Thus, we suggest that if visual orienting is delayed in Autism due to a deficit in the magnocellular projections' ability to activate attention mechanisms, then we would expect a delayed onset of IOR in Autism compared to TD individuals of the same MA.

Surprisingly, very little research has been conducted on IOR in individuals with Autism and thus far the findings have been mixed. A study by McConnell (2004) found excessive facilitation of return and delayed IOR in adolescents and adults with HF Autism compared to Typically Developing individuals matched on CA. However, a study by Brian (2001) found excessive IOR in a mixed sample of adults with HF Autism and Asperger's disorder in comparison to chronologically age matched TD individuals, which supported the predication that the IOR mechanism may account for superior visual search in Autism. These findings were only partially supported in a more recent study by Rinehart and colleagues (2008) who found who found a borderline significant trend towards a greater IOR effect in a group of children with Asperger's disorder than a group of children with HF Autism or TD, matched on sex, CA and full-scale IQ. However, the group of children with Asperger's disorder did have a borderline significant trend towards showing greater IOR effect than the HF Autism group and TD participants. It is difficult to compare findings across studies due to methodological differences across studies such as differences in tasks used as well as the diagnoses and MA of participants. In order to test the magnocellular impairment hypothesis in Autism and its effect on IOR, future research will need to compare IOR as well as visual search performance in individuals with HF and LF Autism.

4.2. Theoretical and Educational Implications

If a deficient magnocellular advantage was the biological mechanism behind impaired shifting and/or disengaging visual attention in Autism, it would have serious implications for the way we conceptualise ID as well as the way we educate children with Autism, DS and Idiopathic ID. Learning can not occur without attention, therefore from a practical perspective, educational material will need to be presented differently to children with Autism compared to children with DS and Idiopathic ID. Given that children with Autism are slow to orient their attention and are not easily distracted, we suggest the use of therapies which follow the child's line of attention rather than attempting to constantly shift the child's attention onto a pre-selected stimulus. If begun very early, infants with HF Autism may come back onto the typical social developmental trajectory and prevent the social and cognitive developmental deficits occurring later on. On the other hand, given that children with DS and Idiopathic ID have difficulty sustaining attention and are easily distracted, we suggest the need to minimize distractions (particularly of a transient nature) in the teaching environment. In addition, teaching should occur over short periods of time and with the use of new and variable objects in an attempt to sustain the attention and motivation of such children. Furthermore, as already described, a major implication of a deficient magnocellular system is a delayed IOR effect, which is likely to disrupt the normal pattern of eye movements needed for reading (Hammad, 2005). Indeed, a delayed IOR may contribute to some of the reading deficits reported by individuals with Autism. Future research is needed to investigate this possibility.

On a theoretical level, impairments in magnocellular driven attention in all individuals with ID whether it be slow shifting of attention in individuals with Autism and over activated shifting of attention in those with Idiopathic ID and DS would contribute to their respective deficiencies in sustained attention, and is essentially closely associated with the etiology of their intellectual disabilities. More specifically, it suggests that sustained attention may be a common impairment in ID regardless of genetic etiology, as either way, the necessity of sustained attention for learning is going to be impaired. This collection of research adds to the differentiation of the cognitive profiles of HF and LF Autism compared to DS and Idiopathic ID. This further contributes to the growing conceptualisation of ID as having different sets of problem solving strategies and information processing abilities associated with different brain pathologies rather than simply low IQ. The finding of visual orienting differences between Autism compared to DS and Idiopathic ID brings us a step closer to understanding which features are different and which features are common in these three forms of ID.

REFERENCES

American Association of Mental Retardation (2002). *Mental retardation: definition, classification, and systems of support* (10th ed.). Washington, DC: American Association on Mental Retardation.

American Psychiatric Association. Diagnostic and statistical manual of mental disorders (4th ed.) (2000). Text revision: DSM IV-TR. 4th edition. Washington, DC: American Psychiatric Association.

Barbaresi, W. J., Katusic, S. K., & Voigt, R. G. (2006). Autism: A review of the state of the science for pediatric primary health care clinicians. *Archives of Pediatrics & Adolescent Medicine, 160,* 1167-1175.

Bear, M. F., Connors, B. W., & Paradiso, M. A. (Eds.). (2006). *Neuroscience: Exploring the brain,* (3rd Ed.). Baltimore, MD: Lippincott Williams & Wilkins.

Brenner, L. A., Turner, K. C., & Müller, R. (2007). Eye movement and visual search: Are there elementary abnormalities in autism? *Journal of Autism and Developmental Disabilities, 37,* 1289-1309.

Brian, J. A. (2001). Inhibition in autism: evidence of excessive inhibition-of-return. *Dissertation Abstracts International: Section B: The Sciences and Engineering, 65*(12-B), 6733.

Bryson, S. E., Wainwright-Sharp, J. A., & Smith, I. M. (1990). Autism: A developmental spatial neglect syndrome? In J. Enns (Ed.), *The development of attention: Research and theory* (pp. 405-427). Amsterdam: Elsevier.

Bullier, J. (2001). Integrated model of visual processing. *Brain Research Reviews, 36*(2-3), 96-107.

Burack, J. A. (1994). Selective attention deficits in persons with autism: Preliminary evidence of an inefficient attentional lens. *Journal of Abnormal Psychology, 103,* 535-543.

Callaway, E. M. (2005). Structure and function of parallel pathways in the primate early visual system. *Journal of Physiology, 566,* 13-19.

Casey, B. J., Gordon, C. T., Mannheim, G. B., & Rumsey, J. (1993). Dysfunctional attention in autistic savants. *Journal of Clinical and Experimental Neuropsychology, 15,* 933-946.

Carrow-Woolfolk, E. (1985). *Test of Auditory Comprehension of Language-Revised.* TX: DLM Teaching Resources.

Christian, S. L., Brune, C. W., Sudi, J., Kumar, R. A, Liu, S., KaraMohamed, S., et al. (2008). Novel Submicroscopic chromosomal abnormalities detected in autism spectrum disorder. *Biological Psychiatry, 63*(12), 1111-1117.

Corbetta, M., & Shulman, G. L. (2002). Control of goal-directed and stimulus-driven attention in the brain. *Nature Review Neuroscience, 3,* 201-215.

Courchesne, E., Akshoomoff, N., & Townsend, J. (1990). Recent advances in autism. *Current Opining In Pediatrics, 2,* 685-693,

Courchesne, E., Townsend, J., Akshoomoff, N. A., Saitoh, O., Yeung- Courchesne., R., Lincoln, A. J., James, H. E., Haas, R. H., Schreibman, L., & Lau, L. (1994). Impairment in shifting attention in autistic and cerebellar patients. *Behavioural Neuroscience, 108*(5), 848-865.

Crewther, S. G., Goodyear, M. J., Bavin, E. L., Lawson, M. L., Wingenfield, S. A., & Crewther, D. P. (2003). *Autism in Victoria: An investigation of prevalence and servicedelivery for children aged 0-6 years.* Victorian Government Department of Human Services, Melbourne, Victoria.

Dunn, L., & Dunn, L. M. (1981). *The Peabody Picture Vocabulary Test- Revised.* Circle Pines, MN: American Guidance Service.

Goharpey, N., Bello, K., Crewther, S., & Crewther, D. (under review). Similar mental age does not mean similar problem solving strategy in children with intellectual disability and typical development.

Goodale, M. A. (2008). Action without perception in human vision. *Cognitive Neuropsychology, 25,* 891-919.

Goodale, M. A., & Milner, A. D. (1992). Separate visual pathways for perception and action. *Trends Neuroscience, 15,* 20-25.

Hagen, J. W., & Huntsman, N. (1971). Selective attention and mental retardation. *Developmental Psychology, 5,* 151-160.

Hammad, S. T. M. (2005). The left-to-right bias in inhibition of return is due to the direction of reading. *Psychological Science, 16,* 15-18.

Jolliffe, T., & Baron-Cohen, S. (1997). Are people with autism and aspergers syndrome faster than normal on the embedded figures test? *Journal of Child Psychology and Psychiatry, 38,* 527-534.

Jarrold, C., Gilchrist, I. D., & Bender, A. (2005). Embedded figures detection in autism and typical development: Preliminary evidence of a double dissociation in relationships with visual search. *Developmental Science, 8*(4), 344-351.

Kaplan, E., & Shapley, R. M. (1982). X and Y cells in the lateral geniculate nucleus of macaque monkeys. *Journal of Physiology, 330,* 125-143.

Katz, G., & Lazcano-Ponce, E. (2008). Intellectual disability: Definition, etiological factors, classification, diagnosis, treatment and prognosis. *Salud pública de México, 50 suppl(2),* 132-141.

Keehn, B., Brenner, L. A., Ramos, A. I., Lincolin, A. J., Marshall, S. P., & Müller, R. (2009). Brief report: eye-movement patterns during an embedded figures test in children with ASD. *Journal of Developmental Disorders, 39,* 383-387.

Kirby, N. H., Nettelbeck, T., & Thomas, P. (1979). Vigilance performance of mildy mentally retarded children. *American Journal of Mental Deficiency, 84,* 184-187.

Klein, R. (2000). Inhibition of return. *Trends in Cognitive Science, 4,* 138-147.

Landry, R., & Bryson, S. E. (2004). Impaired disengagement of attention in young children with autism. *Journal of Child Psychology and Psychiatry, 45*(6), 1115-1122.

Laycock, R., Crewther, S. G., & Crewther, D. P. (2007). A role for the 'magnocellular advantage' in visual impairments in neurodevelopmental and psychiatric disorders. *Neuroscience Biobehavioral Reviews, 31,* 363-376.

Laycock, R., Crewther, S. G., & Crewther, D. P. (2008). The advantage in being magnocellular: A few more remarks on attention and the magnocellular system. *Neuroscience and Biobehavioral Reviews, 32,* 1409-1415.

Leiter, R. G. (1948). *Leiter International Performance Scale.* Chicago: Stoelting Co.

Li, J. C., Sampson, G. P., & Vidyasagar, T. R. (2007). Interactions between luminance and colour channels in visual search and their relationship to parallel neural channels in vision. *Experimental Brain Research, 176,* 510-518.

Livingstone, M. S., & Hubel, D. H. (1987). Psychophysical evidence for separate channels for the perception of form, color, movement, and depth. *Journal of Neuroscience, 7,* 3416-3468.

Lovaas, O. I., Schreibman, L., Koegal, R., & Rehm, R. (1971). Selective responding by autistic children to multiple sensory input. *Journal of Abnormal Psychology, 77,* 211-222.

Lupiáñez, J., Decaiz, C., Siéroff, E., Chokron, S., Milliken, B., & Bartolomeo, P. (2004). Independent effects of endogenous and exogenous spatial cueing: Inhibition of return at endogenously attended target locations. *Experimental Brain Research, 159,* 447-457.

Malach, R., Reppas, J. B., Benson, R. R., Kwong, K. K., Jiang, H., Kennedy, W. A., et al. (1995). Object-related activity revealed by functional magnetic resonance imaging in human occipital cortex. *Proceedings of the National Academy of Sciences of the United States of America, 92,* 8135-8139.

Matson, J. L., & Shoemaker, M. (2009). Intellectual disability and its relationship to autism spectrum disorders. *Research in Developmental Disabilities.*

Maunsell, J. H. R. (1992). Functional visual streams. *Current Opinion in Neurobiology, 2,* 506-510.

Maunsell, J. H., Nealey, T. A., & DePriest, D. D. (1990). Magnocellular and parvocellular contributions to responses in the middle temporal visual area (MT) of the macaque monkey. *The Journal of Neuroscience, 10,* 3323-3334.

McConnell, B. A. (2004). Inhibition of return in individuals with autism spectrum disorders: Evidence for excessive facilitation and delayed inhibition. *Dissertation Abstracts International: Section B: The Sciences and Engineering, 65*(1-B), 468.

Merigan, W. H., Byrne, C. E., & Maunsell, J. H. (1991). Does primate motion perception depend on the magnocellular pathway? *Journal of Neuroscience, 11,* 3422-3429.

Merigan, W. H., & Maunsell, J. H. (1993). How parallel are the primate visual pathways? *Annual Review of Neuroscience, 16,* 369-402.

Merrill, E. C., & O'Dekirk, J. M. (1994). Visual selective attention and mental retardation. *Cognitive Neuropsychology, 11*(2), 117-132.

O'Riordan, M. (2000). Superior modulation of activation levels of stimulus representations does not underlie superior discrimination in autism. *Cognition, 77,* 81-96.

O'Riordan, M. (2004). Superior visual search in adults with autism. *Autism, 8*(3), 229-248.

O'Riordan, M., & Plaisted, K. (2001). Enhanced discrimination in autism. *The Quarterly Journal of Experimental Psychology, 54A*(4), 961-979.

O'Riordan, M. A., Plaisted, K., Driver, J., & Baron-Cohen, S. (2001). Superior visual search in autism. *Journal of Experimental Psychology: Human Perception and Performance, 27*(3), 719-730.

Pammer, K., Hansen, P., Holliday, I., & Cornelissen, P. (2006). Attentional shifting and the role of the dorsal pathway in visual word recognition. *Neuropsychologia, 44*(14), 2926-36.

Plaisted, K., O'Riordan, M. A., & Baron-Cohen, S. (1998). Enhanced discrimination of novel, highly similar stimuli by adults with autism during a perceptual learning task. *Journal of Child Psychology and Psychiatry, 39,* 765-775.

Posner, M. I. (1988). Structures and functions of selective attention. In T. Boll & B. Bryant (Eds.), *Clinical neuropsychology and brain function: Research, measurement and practice* (pp. 169-202). Washington, D.C: American Psychological Association.

Posner, M. I., & Cohen, Y. (1984). Components of visual orienting. In H. Bouma & D. Bowhuis (Eds.), *Attention and Performance X* (pp. 531- 556). Hillsdale, N. J: Erlbaum.

Posner, M. I., & Dehaene, S. (1994). Attentional networks. *Trends in Neuroscience, 17,* 75-79.

Posner, M. I., Rafal, R. D., Choate, L. S., & Vaughan, J. (1985). Inhibition of return: Neural basis and function. *Cognitive Neuropsychology, 2,* 211-228.

Posner, M. I., Walker, J. A., Freidrich, F. A., & Rafal, R. D. (1984). Effects of parietal injury on covert orienting of attention. *Journal of Neuroscience, 4,* 1863-1874.

Posner, M. I., Walker, J. A., Freidrich, F. A., & Rafal, R. D. (1987). How do parietal lobes direct covert attention? *Neuropsychologia, 25,* 135-145.

Rafal, R. D., Posner, M. I., Friedman, J. H., Inhoff, A. W. & Bernstein, E. (1988). Orienting of visual attention in progressive supranuclear palsy. *Brain, 111,* 267-280.

Rincover, A., & Ducharme, J. M. (1987). Variables influencing stimulus overselectivity and "tunnel vision" in developmentally delayed children. *American Journal of Mental Deficiency, 91,* 422-430.

Rinehart, N. J., Bradshaw, J. L., Moss, S. A., Brereton, A. V., & Tonge, B. J. (2001). A deficit in shifting attention present in high-functioning autism but not asperger's disorder. *Autism, 5(1),* 67-80.

Rinehart, N. J., Bradshaw, J. L., Moss, S. A., Brereton, A. V., & Tonge, B. J. (2008). Brief report: Inhibition of return in young people with autism and asperger's disorder. *Autism, 5*(1), 67-80.

Rosen, A. C., Rao, S. M., Caffarra, P., Scaglioni, A., Bobholz, A. A., Woodley, S. J., et al. (1999). Neural basis of endogenous and exogenous spatial orienting: a functional MRI study. *Journal of Cognitive Neuroscience, 11*(2), 135-152.

Sapir, A., Soroker, N., Berger, A., & Henik, A. (1999). Inhibition of return in spatial attention: Direct evidence for collicular generation. *Nature Neuroscience, 2,* 1053-1054.

Schiller, P. H., & Logothetis, N. K. (1990). The color-opponent and broad-band channels of the primate visual system. *Trends in Neuroscience, 13,* 392-398.

Semmel, M. I. (1965). Arousal theory and vigilance behaviour of educable mentally retarded and average children. *American Journal of Mental Deficiency, 70,* 38-47.

Shah, A., & Frith, U. J. (1993). Why do autistic individuals show superior performance on the block design task? *Child Psychology and Psychiatry, 34,* 1351-1364.

Steinman, B. A., Steinman, S. B., & Lehmkuhle, S. (1997). Transient visual attention is dominated by the magnocellular stream. *Vision Research, 37,* 17-23.

Stomme, P., & Diseth, T. H. (2000). Prevalence of psychiatric diagnoses in children with mental retardation: Data from a population based study. *Developmental Medicine and Child Neurology, 42,* 266-270.

Szaimari, P., & Jones, M. B. (1991). IQ and the genetics of autism. *Journal of Child Psychology and Psychiatry, 23,* 897-908.

Tomporowski, P. D., & Allison, P. (1988). Sustained attention of adults with mental retardation. *American Journal on Mental Retardation, 92*(6), 525-530.

Tomporowski, P. D., Hayden, A. M., & Applegate, B. (1990). Effects of background event rate on sustained attention of mentally retarded and nonretarded adults. *American Journal on Mental Retardation, 94*(5), 499-508.

Townsend, J., Courchesne, E., & Egaas, B. (1996). Slowed orienting of covert visual-spatial attention in autism: Specific deficits associated with cerebellar and parietal abnormality. *Development and Psychopathology, 8,* 563-584.

Townsend, J., Harris, N. S., & Courchesne, E. (1996). Visual attention abnormalities in autism: Delayed orienting to location. *Journal of International Neuropsychological Society, 2,* 541-550.

Tronick, E. Z. (1982). Affectivity and sharing. In E. Z. Tronick (Ed.), *Social interchange in infancy: Affect, cognition and communication* (pp. 1-6). Baltimore, MD: University Park Press.

Tymchuck, A. J., Simmons, J. Q., & Neafsey, S. (1977). Intellectual characteristics of adolescent childhood psychotics with high verbal ability. *Journal of Mental Deficiency Research, 21,* 133-138.

Vicari, S. (2004). Memory development and intellectual disabilities. *Acta Paediatrics Supplements, 445,* 60-64.

Vidyasagar, T. R. (1999). A neuronal model of attentional spotlight: parietal guiding the temporal. *Brain Research Reviews, 30,* 66-76.

Wainwright, J. A., & Bryson, S. E. (1996). Visual-spatial orienting in autism. *Journal of Autism and Developmental Disorders, 26*(4), 423-438.

Wainwright-Sharp, J. A., & Bryson, S. E. (1993). Visual orienting deficits in high-functioning people with autism. *Journal of Autism and Developmental Disorders, 23,* 1-13.

Ware, J. R., Baker, R. A., & Sipowicz, R. R. (1962). Performance of mental deficients on a simple vigilance task. *American Journal of Mental Deficiency, 66,* 647-650.

Warm, J. S., & Berch, D. B. (1985). Sustained attention in the mentally retarded: The vigilance paradigm. In N. R. Ellis & N. W. Bray (Eds.), *International review of research in mental retardation* (Vol. 13, pp. 1-41). New York: Academic Press.

Wechsler, D. (2003). *Wechsler Intelligence Scale for Children- Fourth Edition.* San Antonio, TX: Psychological Corporation.

Wijers, A. A., Lange, J. J., Mulder, G., & Mulder, L. J. (1997). An ERP study of visual spatial attention and letter target detection for isoluminant and nonisoluminant stimuli. *Psychophysiology, 34,* 553-565.

World Health Organization (1993). Mental disorders: glossary and guide to their classification in accordance with the the tenth revision of the International Classification of Diseases. Geneva (Switzerland).

In: Learning and Memory Developments...
Editors: L. C. Eklund, A. S. Nyman, pp. 225-238
ISBN: 978-1-60876-397-9

Chapter 10

STUDYING MEMORY: FROM THE FRONTAL TO THE TEMPORAL LOBE AND VICE-VERSA

Orlando Francisco Amodeo Bueno*
Department of Psychobiology of Universidade Federal de São Paulo/UNIFESP, São Paulo, Brazil.
Rua Napoleão de Barros, 925, Vila Clementino, São Paulo, SP, Brazil, Zip code: 04024-002.

ABSTRACT

Lesions of hippocampal formation structures produce a severe global amnesia, encompassing verbal as well as non-verbal material. Since the first studies with medial temporal lobe amnesic patients, it was noted that they do not exhibit deficits of short-term memory despite the severe long-term memory impairment and this was taken as a strong evidence in favor of a subdivision of memory, that between long-term and short-term memory. The continuing studies with H.M. and other amnesic patients have led to an important discovery that gave rise to the notion of multiple memory systems. The crucial finding was that, in spite of their profound amnesia, amnesic patients usually are able to learn and retain a number of tasks. This has led to the important subdivision of memory between explicit (or declarative) episodic memory and implicit (or non-declarative memory. Implicit memory refers to retrieval independent of consciously processes. Explicit memory can be defined as the ability to store and consciously retrieve facts and events. Other fundamental finding was that the prefrontal cortex is involved with short-term memory, a concept that developed to a larger scope framework, that of working memory. The prefrontal cortex plays a crucial role in working memory, and, in particular, contributes to the functioning of the working memory episodic buffer in which multimodal information is maintained for a short time allowing for the binding of information to create integrated episodes. It has been traditionally accepted that the hippocampal system is not necessary for working memory, but, recently, this widely accepted neuroanatomic dissociation has been challenged by a number of studies that

* Corresponding author: Telephone number: + 55 11 2149 0155, E-mail: ofabueno@psicobio.epm.br

have disclosed a relationship between long-term memory and working memory. Working memory has been shown to contribute to episodic memory formation, and the reverse also seems to occur, that is, long-term memory contributing to working memory as well. The relativelly small deficit of episodic memory in the healthy elderly can be explained by a decline in the working memory capacity and executive functions that is observed in this age. Episodic memory impairment caused by haloperidol, an antagonist of D2 dopamine receptors widely used as an antipsychotic drug, can be fully explained by the drug's action in the working memory capacity but not in the central executive. Other line of evidence can be found in the increasing number of work employing neuroimaging and electrophysiological recording that reveals a relationship between the prefrontal cortex activity and the temporal lobe memory system. These studies lend support to the notion of large scale connection pathways between frontal and posterior brain regions underlying and linking the functioning of the multiple memory subsystems instead of independent modules for each type of memory.

Studying Memory: From the Frontal to the Temporal Lobe and Vice-Versa

Despite early suggestions that the hippocampus is related to memory (e.g., Bechterew, 1900, cited by Finger, 1994; Zola-Morgan et al., 1986), it was quite a surprise, at the time, what happened to the patient H.M. He underwent a surgical procedure in which a large part of his medial temporal lobe (MTL) was resected bilaterally, including the hippocampus and surrounding cortex, in order to relieve an intractable MTL epilepsy. Several reports of other amnesic patients bearing hippocampal formation lesions have appeared since then (e.g., Damasio et al., 1985; Hirst, 1982; Penfield and Milner, 1958).

The finding that lesions of hippocampal formation structures produce a severe global amnesia, encompassing verbal as well as non-verbal material, had a tremendous impact in all fields of neuroscience and gave rise to the new area of neuropsychology of memory. One of the consequences is that, nowadays, hippocampal resection is limited to unilateral medial temporal lobe epileptic patients with severe and intractable seizures. Soon after the first reports on human beings, researchers tried to produce animal models of amnesia by placing experimental lesions in laboratory animals, including monkeys and rodents (Cohen and Eichenbaum, 1993). But they failed to replicate the human findings: animals bearing hippocampal lesions could learn the usual tasks employed to study learning in animals.

Two lines of evidence helped to explain this initial failure, one derived from the continuing experimentation with amnesic patients, and the other from animal experimentation itself. The animal evidence dates back to Tolman's work (1948) on cognitive maps which pointed that learning cannot be thoroughly explained by a unique set of principles, namely Pavlovian and instrumental (or operant) conditioning, but instead required a new concept applied to place learning, nowadays known as spatial memory. In addition to the capacity for learning stimuli-response contingencies, rodents are able to learn location-specific stimuli based on spatially distributed distal cues (O'Keefe and Nadel, 1978). The cognitive map theory gained strong support with the discovery of place-firing cells in the rat hippocampus suggesting that its fundamental function is to build and maintain spatial maps of the environment (O'Keefe and Nadel, 1978). Interestingly, lesions on this structure impair completely spatial learning while sparing response and discriminative learning (Oliveira et al., 1997; Xavier et al., 1990). This is why the hippocampal lesions in animals failed to mimic the severe deficits of memory that have been reported in the human being: people was searching in the wrong place, or better, with the wrong tasks.

Meanwhile, the continuing studies with H.M. and other amnesic patients have led to a parallel discovery in humans that gave rise to the notion of multiple memory systems. The crucial finding was that, in spite of their profound amnesia, amnesic patients usually are able to learn and retain a number of tasks, ranging from motor and cognitive skills to pattern-analysing skills, and also demonstrate preserved priming (Brooks and Baddeley, 1976; Cohen, 1984; Cohen and Squire, 1980; Corkin, 1968; Graf et al., 1984; Milner et al., 1968; Schacter, 1987). This has led to the important subdivision of memory between explicit (or declarative) memory and implicit (or non-declarative memory). Non-declarative or implicit memory refers to retrieval independent of conscious processes. Explicit memory can be defined as the ability to store and consciously retrieve facts and events (Saint-Cyr et al., 1988; Squire and Zola-Morgan, 1991). It corresponds quite closely to William James' (1890) secondary memory in which the information gained before is brought back to consciousness. A further subdivision comprising two components of declarative memory, that between episodic and semantic memory, is widely accepted. Episodic memory refers to the memory for events experienced by an individual and stored in specific spatial-temporal contexts, and semantic memory is a system that stores general knowledge (Tulving, 1983). The medial temporal complex is crucially involved in the processes of episodic memory while the lateral portions of the temporal lobe and other associative areas are thought to store semantic memory information. Therefore, in humans, as in animals, it was disclosed that some memories are hippocampal-dependent while others are hippocampal-independent (Squire, 1994). By hippocampal-dependent we mean a system centered on this structure and extending to regions around it in the medial temporal lobe and closed connected diencephalic structures such as the mammilary bodies and dorsomedial thalamus. The hippocampal-independent memories are more heterogeneous in nature, encompassing procedural memory which refers to cognitive and motor habits build up with the repetition of information, in addition to perceptual priming, classical and operant conditioning, and non-associative learning (see Squire, 1991; 1994, for a general taxonomy of memory, inaccurate as it may be but with heuristic value). Given the variety of nondeclarative memories, the neural systems involved are widespread throughout the brain, from the basal nuclei, neocortex, MTL, to cerebellar areas (Gabrieli et al., 1998; Knowlton, 2002; Saint-Cyr et al., 1988; Thompson, 1990). Much has to be learned yet on the neural basis of these several memory types (e.g., Ferreira et al., 2008; Lee et al., 2008).

The precise functions of the hippocampus remains controversial, with some authors insisting that its main role is linked to spatial memory (e.g., Kumaran and Maguire, 2005) and others considering it to be relational memory (e.g., Finke et al., 2008; Giovanello et al., 2004), and still others trying to reconciliate the two divergent positions (e.g., Bird and Burgess, 2008; Eichenbaum et al., 1999). Many authors consider the hippocampus a place where binding of previously unrelated items occur (for reviews, see Eichenbaum, 2006).

Summarizing, one can say that the main consequence of these pioneering studies has been that the memory phenomenon begun to be more amenable to study because it was realized that it can be fractionated in types and subtypes.

Since the first studies, it was noted that MTL-lesioned patients do not exhibit deficits of short-term memory despite the severe long-term memory impairment (Cave and Squire, 1992;

Milner et al., 1968; Spiers et al., 2001) and this was taken as a strong evidence in favor of a subdivision of memory, that between long-term and short-term memory, which dates back to as early as William James (1890) time. However, a role for the frontal lobe in short-term memory has been assigned since the 1930s in lesion studies with monkeys in which the animals performed poorly on delayed response tasks (Jacobsen, 1931; 1935, cited by Finger, 1994). Work on this theme with man and monkeys employed many other techniques, such as electrocortical stimulation during the early period of a two-choice delayed response trial (Stamm, 1969), single-unit recording (Funahashi et al., 1989; Fuster and Alexander, 1971; Niki, 1974), and more recently PET and fMRI (Narayanan et al., 2005; Swartz et al., 1994) neuroimaging. The behavioral techniques were based mainly on variants of delayed response tasks, such as delayed-matching- (or nonmatching-) to-sample. The fundamental finding of a large number of such studies was the demonstration of a network of brain areas centered in the prefrontal cortex involved with short-term memory, a concept that soon developed to a larger scope model, that of working memory.

In contrast with MTL lesions that have devastating effects in long-term memory, even massive frontal lesions provoke only modest effects or even no effect at all as the case of Phineas Gage demonstrated, as far as it could be detected at the time (Harlow, 1848; cited in Macmillan, 1996). With the arrival of the neuroimaging techniques the prefrontal cortex (PFC) was shown to be involved in the processes underlying both acquisition and retrieval of episodic memory (Cabeza and Nyberg, 2000).

Nonetheless, PFC lesions can induce subtle and differential effects on memory attributed to specific deficits in several executive functions such as proactive interference, inhibition, perseveration, attention or organization in thought and behavior (Milner and Petrides, 1984; Passingham, 1985; Turner et al., 2007). Among the frontal functions, working memory, in particular, that is truly memorial in nature, is the recent focus of attention of researchers. A number of studies have established the crucial contribution of prefrontal cortex to working memory and most of the early work implicating frontal areas with short-term memory can be reinterpreted as so.

Working memory is a limited capacity system that simultaneously hold and manipulates information during a short period of time for reasoning, comprehending, learning or retrieval (Baddeley, 2003). The original Baddeley and Hitch's multi-component model of working memory comprised three components, two of them responsible for short-term maintenance of visual/ spatial or verbal information (the visuospatial sketchpad and the phonological loop, respectively), an important departure from early unimodal models of short-term memory (e.g., Atkinson and Shiffrin, 1968; Waugh and Norman, 1965) and an attentional control system (the central executive), responsible for the manipulation of information and for controlling the other subsystems (Baddeley and Hitch, 1974). More recently, Baddeley (2000) added other component, the episodic buffer which is a store capable of multi-dimensional coding, allowing for the binding of information and thus to create integrated episodes. A number of recent studies dealing with working memory and prefrontal cortex succeeded in corroborating the view that the prefrontal cortex plays a crucial role in working memory, and in particular in the functioning of the episodic buffer encompassing (maintenance and binding of currently relevant information), as assessed by many neuropsychological techniques (e.g., Carlesimo et al., 2001; D'Esposito et al., 1998; 1999; Levy and Goldman-Rakic, 2000; Sala and Courtney, 2007).

The episodic buffer helped to acommodate the notion of working memory capacity within the same framework. Working memory capacity deals with the limitations of the working memory system, and, more precisely, of the relative incapacity of actively retain and use relevant information in face of interference or distraction (Engle et al., 1999). The episodic buffer concept accounts precisely for such human ability. Working memory capacity tasks combine storage and processing, requiring, for example, that the subject carry out arithmetical operations (processing) and simultaneously read words that must be subsequently recalled (storage) (Turner and Engle, 1989). This task demands storage processes that exceed the capacity of the phonological loop and the visuospatial sketchpad. Thus, working memory capacity is assumed to reflect the storage capacity of the episodic buffer, together with the efficiency with which the central executive can use this capacity (Baddeley, 2007). People who has high working memory capacity can hold a greater number of items at the same time (e.g., Rissman et al., 2008) or, as an alternative view, is more able to select appropriate stimuli or responses for the moment (e.g., Awh, 2008; Towse et al., 2008).

As working memory thought to be involved in the temporary maintenance of multi-modal information (episodic buffer) and controlled attentional allocation (central executive), tasks that can separate these functions are needed, to further our understanding oh those cognitive processes.

The capacity for generating sequences of random numbers or letters can be used to evaluate the central executive of working memory (Guarnieri et al., submitted; Jahanshahi et al., 2006) while working memory capacity tasks are used to measure the episodic buffer (De Luccio et al., 2005).

Beginning with the work of Daneman and Carpenter (1980), several tasks were devised to evaluate the working memory capacity. These authors developed a task that combines processing and maintainance of information: the subject is required to read a set of unrelated sentences and remember the final word of each one. The largest set size in which the subject can recall perfectly all the final words is the measure of working memory capacity. This test is called the reading span task. A variant of this test is the operation span task in which the subject has to make arithmetical operations instead of reading phrases (Turner and Engle, 1989). A high correlation between these measures with reading comprehension, intelligence and reasoning was found (Conway et al. 2005; Merikle and Daneman, 1996). Considering that the amount of words is recalled in a situation in which the subject solves a mathematical operation and concurrently hold words in mind, we are measuring how many items can be actively maintained while attention is directed to some other activity.

A clear separation between the neural substrates of long-term declarative memory and working memory appeared to be warranted by the available experimental and clinical findings, with long-term memory relying primarily on the MTL and diencephalic structures (Squire and Zola-Morgan, 1991) and working memory on a network of PFC and parietal areas (Jonides et al., 1993; Paulesu et al., 1993; Petrides et al., 1993; Smith and Jonides, 1997). It has been traditionally accepted that the hippocampal system is not necessary for working memory (Axmacher et al., 2007; Campo et al., 2005; Ranganath and Blumenfeld, 2005; Wagner et al, 2009) but, recently, this widely accepted neuroanatomic dissociation has been challenged by a number of studies that have disclosed a relationship between long-term memory and working memory (Axmacher et al., 2008a; b; Ranganath and Blumenfeld; 2005). Working memory has been shown to contribute to episodic memory formation, and the reverse also seems to occur, that is, long-term memory contributing to working memory as well.

An event is composed by the combination of multiple features, e.g. information about the place and time at which it has occurred; items parameters such as color and size; modality of presentation; and so forth (Chalfonte and Johnson, 1996). Creating associations between the elementary features of an experience is critical for establishing episodic memories (Quinette et al., 2006). The hippocampal system appears to be critical for the formation of new associations between previously non-related items. The inclusion of the episodic buffer "assumed to be a temporary storage system that is able to combine information from the loop, the sketchpad, long-term memory, or indeed from perceptual input, into a coherent episode" (Baddeley, 2007) opened the way to theoretical predictions concerning the relationships between working memory and long-term memory, and, in particular, raised the possibility of associations between the features of an event being established in the early stage of encoding, that is, in working memory (Chalfonte & Johnson, 1996). At the neuroanatomical level, a connection between PFC and the hippocampal formation would warrant such relationship at the cognitive level.

Behavioral evidence for a relationship between episodic memory and working memory comes also from work with amnesic patients, Alzheimer's disease patients, normal healthy elderly and pharmacological studies. Binding and maintenance of multimodal information were spared in transient global amnesia patients with storage disorders but were impaired in patients with encoding deficits, a finding the authors interpreted as the episodic buffer representing an interface between working memory and episodic memory (Quinette et al., 2006). Post-surgical right MTL lesions led to impairment in delayed-matching-to-sample tasks requiring visual-spatial associations (Finke et al., 2008). Left hippocampal resection was found to influence the episodic buffer evaluated by the operation span task (Tudesco, 2008), a finding that is consonant with the suggestion of Berlingeri et al. (2008) that the left anterior hippocampus contributes to the episodic buffer based on Alzheimer's patients performance on immediate prose recall. These authors also suggest that the episodic buffer and the central executive of working memory are, to some extent, independent from each other.

It is well established in the literature that normal elderly people, when compared to young adults, present an impairment in working memory (Fisk and Warr, 1996; Light, 1991) and in episodic memory (Light, 1991; Salthouse, 1996), with spared semantic memory (Hedden and Gabrieli, 2004; Nilsson, 2003). Comparison between younger and older adults has shown that the latter present less lateralization of PFC activity during recall of a verbal task, a finding that was interpreted as a functional compensation for cognitive difficulties of the elderly (Cabeza, 2002). Some authors have suggested that the impairment of episodic memory can be explained by the decline of working memory (Hertzog, *et al.*, 2003; Light, 1991). De Luccia *et al.* (2005) studied the relationship between episodic and working memory in healthy young and elderly people. The evaluation of episodic memory was done by the free recall of wordlists test in which semantically related words were inserted in the middle of the lists and compared to all-unrelated wordlists. The episodic buffer of working memory was evaluated by the operation span test. Semantically related words inserted in the middle of the lists were recalled more than nonrelated words in both groups but, compared to young people, the recall of the elderly was impaired. A positive correlation between the decline of episodic memory and working memory was observed. A decrease in the magnitude of semantic facilitation was observed in healthy elderly, which was completely reversed when the scores of the working memory capacity task were parceled out (De Luccia et al., 2005). Therefore, a decrease in semantic facilitation takes place only in the elder people who also show reduced working memory capacity. We argue that, beyond the semantic network integrity of the healthy elder, working memory is involved in the semantic facilitation effect because it helps to bind the related words chunks to contextual features.

When compared to the healthy elderly, Alzheimer's patients present cognitive deficits in working memory (Germano and Kinsella, 2005), in episodic memory and also in semantic memory (Giffard et al., 2001). Alzheimer's patients in the moderate stage did not benefit from midlist semantic relatedness to enhance free recall in lists containing 15 words finding that would be in agreement with a semantic knowledge degradation in these patients, except for the fact that they show a benefit when the lists are shortened to 9 words, although in a lesser extent than controls (Bueno et al., 2008). That is, in smaller sets of material to be recalled, semantic facilitation still occurs, suggesting that a reduced episodic buffer capacity in these patients preclude the accessibility of the semantic information brought about by larger number of to-be-remembered related items (Bueno et al., 2008). This finding was replicated by Covre et al. (in preparation) but, it was seen that the reduced working memory capacity can explain only partially the episodic memory impairment of Alzheimer's patients.

Episodic memory impairment caused by haloperidol, an antagonist of D2 dopamine receptors widely used as an antipsychotic drug, can be fully explained by the drug's action in the working memory capacity but not in the central executive component of working memory because when the operation span measured was factored out of the correlation with episodic memory the impairment of the latter was no longer seen. The same did not happen with the random generation of numbers, suggesting that the central executive impairment is not responsible for the deficit caused by haloperidol administration (Guarnieri et al., submitted).

The episodic buffer is conceived as a working memory device that promotes the binding of separate elements to give rise to coherent episodes. Thus, the binding of features during short delays can be attributed to structures other than the hippocampus, namely the PFC. In fact, the participation of PFC has been attested not only in relational encoding but also in item-specific encoding. Dorsolateral PFC was found to contribute to long-term memory formation by the reinforcement of associations between separate elements organized in the working memory (Blumenfeld and Ranganath, 2006; Murray and Ranganath, 2007), that is, during relational encoding but not during item-specific encoding, while the ventrolateral PFC is involved in both, relational and item-specific encoding (Murray and Ranganath, 2007). Nonetheless, the involvement of hippocampal and MTL related areas in making conjunctions of visual stimuli over as delays as short as 1-8 s (Olson et al., 2006a; b; Hannula and Ranganath, 2008) were observed. Finally, it has been shown that activity in both, hippocampus and PFC, during the initial stages of working memory maintenance predicts subsequent long-term performance (Ranganath et al., 2005; see also Fernández and Tendolkar, 2001; Kirchhoff et al., 2000). Work with EEG recording also demonstrates interaction of electrical brain activity between frontal and temporal/parietal regions according to Weiss and Rappelsberger (2000), who have shown a long-range enhanced synchronization in several frequency bands that correlates with successful memory performance. Using electrophysiological techniques, Axmacher et al. (2007) reported that the MTL is specifically activated during performance of a Sternberg paradigm. A combined intracranial EEG and functional magnetic resonance study demonstrated that working memory for multiple items depends on control of activity by MTL (Axmacher et al., 2008 a). Interaction of long-term and working memory was observed in the MTL by functional magnetic resonance (Axmacher et al., 2008 b). Moreover, the same group (Axmacher et al., 2009) found that maintenance impairment of multiple items in working memory deteriorates simultaneous long-term memory encoding, and that high working memory load increased hippocampal activation, while, in contrast, hippocampal activation related to long-term memory encoding was stronger with low working memory load. These finding suggest that working memory demands affects long-term memory encoding by an interacting processes with the MTL. In summary, an increasing number of work employing neuroimaging and electrophysiological recording reveals a relationship between the prefrontal cortex activity and the temporal lobe memory system. These studies lend support to the notion that large scale connection pathways between frontal and posterior brain regions exist (e.g., Buckner et al., 2000), underlying and linking the functioning of the multiple memory subsystems, instead of independent modules for each type of memory. Dual pathways linking the dorsolateral PFC with hippocampal formation and parahippocampal cortex (Goldman-Rakic et al., 1984) turn this relationship feasible from the neuroanatomical point-of- view.

One of the present issues is to investigate how the subsystems interact with each other to compose what was once named the faculty of memory and today must of the investigators acknowledge that presents multiple interlinked aspects.

REFERENCES

Atkinson RC; Shiffrin RM. Human memory: a proposed system and its control processes. In: Spence KW and Spence JT, editors, *The Psychology of Learning and Motivation: Advances in Research and Theory, vol. 2.* New York: Academic Press; pp. 89-195; 1968.

Awh E. (2008). The bouncer in the brain. *Nature Neuroscience, 11: 5-6.*

Axmacher N; Mormann F; Fernandez G; Cohen MX; Elger CE; Fell J. (2007). Sustained neural activity patterns during working memory in the human medial temporal lobe. *Journal of Neuroscience, 27:* 7807-7816.

Axmacher N, Schmitz DP, Wagner T, Elger CE; Fell J. (2008a). Interactions between medial temporal lobe, prefrontal cortex, and inferior temporal regions during visual working memory: a combined intracranial EEG and functional magnetic resonance study. *Journal of Neuroscience, 28:* 7304-7312.

Axmacher N, Schmitz DP, Weinreich I, Elger CE; Fell J. (2008b). Interaction of working memory and long-term memory in the medial temporal lobe. *Cerebral Cortex,18:* 2868-2878.

Axmacher N, Haupt S; Cohen MX; Elger CE; Fell J. (2009). Interference of working memory load with long-term memory formation. *European Journal of Neuroscience, 29:* 1501-1513.

Baddeley A. (2003). Working memory: looking back and looking forward. *Nature Reviews Neuroscience, 4:* 829-839.

Baddeley A. *Working Memory, Thought, and Action.* Oxford: Oxford University Press; 2007.

Baddeley AD. (2000). The episodic buffer: a new component of working memory? *Trends in Cognitive Sciences, 4:* 417-423.

Baddeley AD; Hitch GJ. Working memory. In: Bower GA, editor. *Recent Advances in Learning and Memory, vol. 8:* 47-90; 1974; pp. 47-89.

Berlingeri M; Bottini G; Basilico S; Silani G; Zanardi G; Sberna M; Colombo N; Sterzi R; Scialfa G; Paulesu E. (2008). Anatomy of the episodic memory: a voxel-based morphometry study in patients with dementia. *Behavioural Neurology, 19:* 29-34.

Bird CM; Burgess N. (2008). The hippocampus and memory: insights from spatial processing. *Nature Reviews Neuroscience, 9:* 182-194.

Blumenfeld RS; Ranganath C. (2006). Dorsolateral prefrontal cortex promotes long-term memory through its role in working memory organization. *Journal of Neuroscience, 18:* 916-925.

Brooks DN; Baddeley AD. (1976). What can amnesic patients learn ? *Neuropsychologia, 14:* 111-122.

Buckner RI; Logan J; Donaldson DI; Wheeler ME. (2000). Cognitive neuroscience of episodic memory encoding. *Acta Psychologica, 105,* 127-139.

Bueno OFA; Bertolucci PH; Oliveira MGM; Abrisqueta-Gomez J. (2008).Effects of semantic relations, repetition of words and list length in verbal free recall of Alzheimer's patients. *Arquivos de Neuropsiquiatria, 66, 2B:* 312-317.

Cabeza R. (2002). .Hemispheric asymmetry reduction in older adults: the HAROLD model. *Psychology and Aging, 17:* 85-100.

Cabeza R; Nyberg L. (2000). Imaging cognition II: an empirical review of 275 PET and fMRI studies. *Journal of Cognitive Neuroscience, 12:* 1-47.

Campo P; Maestú F; Ortiz T; Capilla A; Fernández S; and Fernández A. (2005). Is medial temporal lobe activation specific for encoding long-term memory? *Neuroimage, 25:* 34-42.

Carlesimo GA; Perri R; Turriziani P; Tomaiuolo F; Caltagirone C. (2001). Remembering what but not where: independence of spatial and visual working memory in the human brain. *Cortex, 37:* 519-534.

Cave CB, Squire LR. (1992). Intact verbal and nonverbal short-term memory following damage to the human hippocampus. *Hippocampus, 2:* 151-164.

Chalfonte BL; Johnson MK. (1996). Feature memory and binding in young and older adults. *Memory and Cognition, 24:* 403-416.

Cohen NJ. Preserved learning capacity in amnesia: evidence for multiple memory systems. In: Squire LR and Butters N, editors. *The Neuropsychology of Memory.* New York: Guilford Press; 1984, pp. 83-103.

Cohen NJ; Eichenbaum H. *Memory, Amnesia, and the Hippocampal System.* Cambridge, MA: MIT Press; 1993.

Cohen NJ; Squire LR. (1980). Preserved learning and retention of pattern-analysing skill in amnesia: dissociation of knowing how and knowing that. *Science, 210:* 207-210.

Conway AR; Kane MJ; Bunting MF; Hambrick DZ; Wilhelm O; Engle RW. (2005). Working memory span tasks: a methodological review and user's guide. *Psychonomic Bulletin Reviews, 12:* 769-786.

Corkin S. (1968). Acquisition of motor skill after bilateral medial temporal lobe excisions. *Neuropsychologia, 6:* 255-265.

Covre P; Bertolucci PHF; Bueno OFA. Relationship of working memory capacity to the binding of features in episodic memory in patients with mild Alzheimer's disease. *Manuscript in preparation.*

Damasio AR; Eslinger PJ; Damasio H; van Hoesen GW; Cornell S. (1985). Multimodal amnesic syndrome following bilateral temporal and basal forebrain damage. *Archives of Neurology, 42:* 252-259.

Daneman M and Carpenter PA. (1980). Individual differences in working memory and reading. *Journal of Verbal Learning and Verbal Behavior, 19:* 450-466.

De Luccia GCP; Bueno OFA; Santos RF. (2005). Recordação livre de palavras e memória operacional em idosos. *Distúrbios da Comunicação, 17:* 347-358.

D'Esposito M; Aguirre GK; Zarahn E; Ballard D; Shin RK; Lease J. (1998).Functional MRI studies of spatial and nonspatial working memory. *Cognitive Brain Research, 7:* 1-13.

D'Esposito M; Postle BR; Ballard D; Lease J. (1999).Maintenance versus manipulation of information held in working memory: an event-related fMRI study. *Brain and Cognition, 41:* 66-86.

Eichenbaum H. Memory binding in hippocampal relational networks. In: Zimmer HD, Mecklinger A and Lindenberger U. *Handbook of binding and memory: perspectives from cognitive neuroscience.* Oxford: University Press, 2006: 25-51.

Eichenbaum H; Dudchenko P; Wood E; Shapiro M; Tanila H. 1999The hippocampus, memory, and place cells: is it spatial memory or a memory space? *Neuron, 23:* 209-226.

Engle RW; Tuholski SW; Laughlin JE; Conway ARA. (1999). Working memory, short-term memory and general fluid intelligence: a latent-variable approach. *Journal of Experimental Psychology: General, 128:* 309-331.

Ferreira TL; Shammah-Lagnado SJ; Bueno OFA; Moreira KM; Fornari RV; Oliveira MGM. (2008). The indirect amygdala-dorsal striatum pathway mediates conditioned freezing: insights on emotional memory networks. *Neuroscience 153:* 84-94.

Fernández G; Tendolkar I. (2001). Integrated brain activity in medial temporal and prefrontal areas predicts subsequent memory performance: human declarative memory formation at the system. *Brain Research Bulletin, 55:* 1-9.

Finger, S. *Origins of Neuroscience. A History of Explorations into Brain Functions.* New York: Oxford University Press; 1994.

Finke C; Braun M; Ostendorf F; Lehmann T-N; Hoffmann K-T; Kopp U; Ploner CJ. (2008). The human hippocampal formation mediates short-term memory of colour-location associations. *Neuropsychologia, 46:* 614-623.

Fisk JE; Warr P. (1996). Age and working memory: the role of perceptual speed, the central executive, and the phonological loop. *Psychology and Aging,* 11:316-23.

Funahashi S; Bruce CJ; Goldman-Rakic PS. (1989). Mnemonic coding of visual space in the monkey's dorsolateral prefrontal cortex. *Journal of Neurophysiology, 61:* 331-349.

Fuster JM; Alexander GE. (1971). Neuron activity related to short-term memory. *Science, 173:* 652-654.

Gabrieli JDE; Brewer JB; Poldrack RA. (1998). Images of medial temporal lobe functions in human learning and memory, *Neurobiology of Learning and Memory, 70:* 275-283.

Gabrieli JDE; Poldrack RA; Desmond JE. (1998). The role of the left prefrontal cortex in language and memory. *Proceedings of the National Academy of Sciences of the United States of America, 95:* 906-913.

Germano C; Kinsella GJ. (2005). Working memory and learning in early Alzheimer's disease. *Neuropsychology Review, 15:* 1-10.

Giffard B; Desgranges B; Nore-Mary F; Lalevee C;;de la Sayette V, Pasquier F; Eustache F. (2001). The nature of semantic memory deficits in Alzheimer´s disease: new insights from hyperpriming effects. *Brain, 124:* 1522-1532.

Giovanello KS; Schnyer DM; Verfaellie M. (2004). A critical role for the anterior hippocampus in relational memory: evidence from an fMRI study comparing associative and item recognition. *Hippocampus, 14:* 6-6.

Goldman-Rakic PS; Selemon LD; Schwartz ML. (1984).Dual pathways connecting the dorsolateral prefrontal cortex with the hippocampal formation and parahippocampal cortex in the rhesus monkey. *Neuroscience, 12:* 719-743.

Graf P; Squire LR; Mandler G. 1984The information that amnesic patients do not forget. *Journal of Experimental Psychology: Learning, Memory, and Cognition, 10:* 164-178.

Guarnieri RV; Nogueira AML; Galduroz JC; Bueno OFA. Effects of haloperidol on memory of healthy young volunteers: relationships between episodic and working memory. *Submitted to publication.*

Hannula DE; Ranganath C. 2008Medial temporal lobe activity predicts successful relational memory binding. *Journal of Neuroscience, 28:* 116-124.

Hannula DE; Tranel D; Cohen NJ. (2006). The long and the short of it: relational memory impairments in amnesia, even at short lags. *Journal of Neuroscience, 26:* 8352-8359.

Harlow JM. (1848). Passage of an iron rod bar through the head. *Boston Medical and Surgical Journal, 39:* 389-393; cited by Macmillan M. (1996). Phineas Gage: a case for all reasons. In: Code C, Wallesch C-W, Joanette Y and Lecours AR, editors. *Classic Cases in Neuropsychology,* Hove: Psychology Press; 1996; 243-262.

Hedden T; Gabrieli JD. (2004). Insights into the ageing mind: a view from cognitive neuroscience. *Nature Reviews Neuroscience, 5:* 87-96.

Hertzog C; Dixon RA; Hultsch DF; MacDonald SWS. (2003). Latent changes models of adult cognition: are changes in processing speed and working memory associated with changes in episodic memory? *Psychology and Aging, 18:* 755-769.

Hirst W. (1982). The amnesic syndrome: descriptions and explanations. *Psychological Bulletin, 91:* 435-460.

Jahanshahi M; Saleem T; Ho AK; Dimberger G; Fuller R. (2006). Random number generation as an index of controlled processes. *Neuropsychology, 20:* 391-399.

James W. *The Principles of Psychology (vol.1).* New York: Holt; 1890.

Jonides J; Smith EE; Koeppe RA; Awh E; Minoshima S; Mintun MA. (1993). Spatial working memory in humans as revealed by PET. *Nature, 363:* 623-625.

Knowlton B. The role of basal ganglia in learning and memory. *In:* Squire LR and Schacter DL (eds). *Neuropsychology of Memory,* 3rd edition. New York: Guilford, 2002.

Kirchhoff BA; Wagner AD; Maril A; Stern CE. (2000). Prefrontal-temporal circuitry for episodic encoding and subsequent memory. *Journal of Neuroscience, 20:* 6173-6180.

Kumaran D; Maguire EA. (2005). The human hippocampus: cognitive maps or relational memory? *Journal of Neuroscience, 25:* 7254-7259.

Lee AS; Duman RS; Pittenger C. (2008). A double dissociation revealing bidirectional competition between striatum and hippocampus during learning. *Proceedings of the National Academy of Sciences of the United States of America, 105:* 17163-17168.

Levy R; Goldman-Rakic PS. (2000). Segregation of working memory functions within the dorsolateral prefrontal cortex. *Experimental Brain Research, 133:* 23-32.

Light LL. (1991). Memory and aging: four hypotheses in search of data. *Annual Review of Psychology, 42:* 333-376.

Macmillan M. (1996). Phineas Gage: a case for all reasons. In: Code C, Wallesch C-W, Joanette Y and Lecours AR, editors. *Classic Cases in Neuropsychology,* Hove: Psychology Press; 1996; 243-262.

Marklund P; Fransson P; Cabeza R; Petersson KM; Ingvar M; Nyberg L. (2007). Sustained and transient neural modulations in prefrontal cortex related to declarative long-term memory, working memory, and attention. *Cortex, 43:* 22-37.

Merikle PM; Daneman M. (1996). Working memory and language comprehension: a meta-analysis. *Psychonomic Bulletin Reviews, 3:* 422-433.

Milner B; Corkin S; Teuber HL. (1968). Further analysis of the hippocampal amnesic syndrome: 14-year follow-up study of H.M. *Neuropsychologia, 6:* 215-234.

Milner B; Petrides M. (1984). Behavioural effects of frontal-lobe lesions in man. *Trends in Neuroscience, 7:* 403-407.

Murray LJ; Ranganath C. (2007). The dorsolateral prefrontal cortex contributes to successful relational memory encoding. *Journal of Neuroscience, 27:* 5515-5522.

Narayanan NS; Prabhakaran V; Bunge SA; Christoff K; Fine EM; Gabrieli JDE. (2005). The role of the prefrontal cortex in the maintenance of verbal working memory: an event-related fMRI analysis. *Neuropsychology, 19,* 223-232.

Niki H. (1974). Differential activity of prefrontal units during right and left delayed response trials. *Brain Research, 70:* 346-349.

Nilsson LG. (2003). Memory function in normal aging. *Acta Neurologica Scandinavica, 107:* 7-13.

O'Keefe J; Nadel L. *The Hippocampus as a Cognitive Map.* Oxford: Clarendon; 1978.

Oliveira MGM; Bueno OFA; Pomarico AC; Gugliano EB. (1997). Strategies used by hippocampal- and caudate-putamen-lesioned rats in a learning task. *Neurobiology of Learning and Memory, 68:* 32-41.

Olson IR; Moore KS; Stark M; Chatterjee A. (2006a). Visual working memory is impaired when the medial temporal lobe is damaged. *Journal of Cognitive Neuroscience, 18:* 1087-1097.

Olson IR; Page K; Moore KS; Chaterjee A; Verfaellie M. (2006b). Working memory for conjunctions relies on the medial temporal lobe. *Journal of Neuroscience, 26:* 4596-4601.

Passingham R.E. (1985). Memory of monkeys (*Macaca mullata*) with lesions in prefrontal cortex. *Behavioral Neuroscience, 99:* 3-21.

Paulesu E; Frith CD; Frackowiak RSJ. (1993). The neural correlates of the verbal component of working memory. *Nature, 362:* 342-345.

Penfield W; Milner B. (1958). Memory deficit produced by bilateral lesions in the hippocampal zone. *Archives of Neurology and Psychiatry, 79:* 475-497.

Petrides M; Alivisatos B; Meyer E; Evans AC. (1993). Functional activation of the human frontal cortex during the performance of verbal working memory tasks. *Proceedings of the National Academy of Sciences of the United States of America, 90:* 878-882.

Piekema C; Fernández G; Postma A; Hendriks MPH; Wester AJ; Kessels RPC. (2007).Spatial and non-spatial contextual working memory in patients with diencephalic or hippocampal dysfunction. *Brain Research, 1172:* 103-109.

Quinette P; Guillery-Giscard B; Noel A; de la Sayette V; Viader F; Desgranges B; Eustache F. (2006). The relationship between working memory and episodic memory disorders in transient global amnesia *Neuropsychologia, 44:* 2508-.2519.

Ranganath C; Blumenfeld RS. (2005). Doubts about double dissociations between short- and long-term memory. *Trends in Cognitive Sciences, 9:* 374-380.

Ranganath C; Cohen MX; Brozinsky CJ. (2005). Working memory maintenance contributes to long-term memory formation: neural and behavioral evidence. *Journal of Cognitive Neuroscience, 17:* 994-1010.

Repovs G; Baddeley A. (2006). The multi-component model of working memory: explorations in experimental cognitive psychology. *Neuroscience, 139:* 5-21.

Rissman J; Gazzaley A; D'Esposito M. (2008). Dynamic adjustments in prefrontal, hippocampal, and inferior temporal interactions with increasing visual working memory load. *Cerebral Cortex, 18:* 1618-1629.

Rosen AC; Gabrieli JDE; Stoub T; Prull MW; O'Hara R; Yesavage J; deToledo-Morrell. (2005). Relating medial temporal lobe volume to frontal fMRI activation for memory encoding in older adults. *Cortex, 41:* 595-602.

Saint-Cyr JA; Taylor AE; Lang AE. (1988). Procedural learning and neostriatal dysfunction in man. *Brain, 111:* 941-959,.

Sala JB; Courtney SM. (2007). Binding of what and where during working memory maintenance. *Cortex, 43:* 5-21.

Salthouse TA. (1996). The processing-speed theory of adult age differences in cognition. *Psychology and Aging, 103:* 403-428.

Scoville WB; Milner B. (1957). Loss of recent memory after bilateral hippocampal lesions. *Journal of Neurology, Neurosurgery and Psychiatry, 20,* 11-21.

Schacter DL. (1987). Implicit memory: history and current status. *Journal of Experimental Psychology: Learning, Memory and Cognition, 13:* 501-518.

Smith EE; Jonides J. (1997). Working memory: a view from neuroimaging. *Cognitive Psychology, 33:* 5-42.

Spiers HJ, Maguire EA, Burgess N. (2001). Hippocampal amnesia. *Neurocase, 7:* 357-382.

Squire LR. Declarative and nondeclarative memory: multiple brain systems supporting learning and memory. *In:* Schacter DL and Tulving E. *Memory Systems 1994.* Cambridge, MA: MIT Press; 1994; pp. 203-231.

Squire LR; Zola-Morgan S. (1991). The medial temporal lobe memory system. *Science, 253:* 1380-1386.

Squire LR; Zola-Morgan S; Chen KS. (1988). Human amnesia and animal models of amnesia: performance of amnesic patients on tests designed for the monkey. *Behavioral Neuroscience, 102*: 210-221.

Stamm JS. (1969). Electrical stimulation of monkey's prefrontal cortex during delayed response performance. *Journal of Comparative and Physiological Psychology, 67:* 535-546.

Swartz BE; Halgren E; Fuster J; Mandelkern M. (1994). An FDG-PET study of cortical activation during a short-term visual memory task in humans. *Neuroreport, 5:* 925-928.

Thompson RF. (1990). Neural mechanisms of classical conditioning in mammals. *Philosophical Transactions of the Royal Society of London, Series B, 329:* 161-170.

Tolman EC. Cognitive maps in rats and men. (1948). *Psychological Review, 55:* 189-208.

Towse JN; Cowan N; Hitch GJ; Horton NJ. (2008). The recall of information from working memory: insights from behavioural and chronometric perspectives. *Experimental Psychology, 55:* 371-383.

Tudesco ISS (2008). Memória episódica, memória semantic e memória operacional em pacientes com epilepsia do lobo temporal mesial antes e após a corticoamigdalohipocamp ectomia. *Master thesis,* Universidade Federal de São Paulo.

Tulving E. *Elements of Episodic Memory.* Oxford, UK: Clarendon Press; 1983.

Turner ML; Engle RW. (1989). Is working memory task dependent? *Journal of Memory and Language, 28:* 127-154.

Turner M.S; Cipolotti; L, Yousry T; Shallice, T. (2007). Qualitatively different memory impairments across frontal lobe subgroups. *Neuropsychologia, 45*: 1540-1552.

Unworth N; Engle RW. (2007). The nature of individual differences in working memory capacity: active maintenance in primary memory and controlled search from secondary memory. *Psychological Review, 114:* 104-132.

Wagner DD; Sziklas V; Garver KE; Jones-Gotman M (2009). Material-specific lateralization of working memory in the medial temporal lobe. *Neuropsychologia, 47:* 112-122.

Waugh NC; Norman DA. (1965). Primary memory. *Psychological Review, 72:* 89-104.

Weiss S; Rappelsberger P. (2000). Long-range EEG synchronization during word encoding correlates with successful memory performance. *Cognitive Brain Research, 9:* 299-312.

Xavier GF; Stein C; Bueno OFA. (1990). Rats with dorsal hippocampal-lesions do react to new stimuli but not to spatial changes of known stimuli. *Behavioral and Neural Biology, 54:* 172-183.

Zola-Morgan S; Squire LR. (1985). Medial temporal lesions in monkeys impair memory on a variety of tasks sensitive to human amnesia. *Behavioral Neuroscience, 99:* 22-34.

Zola-Morgan S; Squire LR; Amaral DG. (1986). Human amnesia and the medial temporal region: enduring memory impairment following a bilateral lesion limited to field CA1 of the hippocampus. *Journal of Neuroscience, 6:* 2950-2967.

In: Learning and Memory Developments...
Editors: L. C. Eklund, A. S. Nyman, pp. 239-253

ISBN: 978-1-60876-397-9

Chapter 11

LEARNING AND MEMORY DEVELOPMENTS LEARNING DEFICITS IN PRESENILIN MUTANT MICE

R. Lalonde[1,*] and C. Strazielle[2]

[1]CHUM/St-Luc, Neuroscience Research Unit, 1058 St. Denis St, University of Montreal, Faculty of Medicine, Montreal, Canada H2X 3J4 and University of Rouen, Faculty of Sciences.

[2]University of Nancy, INSERM U954, Faculty of Medicine, 54500 Vandoeuvre-les-Nancy France.

ABSTRACT

When inserted into mouse brain by transgenic or knockin methods, *PS1* mutations responsible for hereditary Alzheimer's disease, despite the absence of Aβ plaques, cause anomalies in calcium homeostasis, potentiate excitotoxicity, and alter the electrophysiologic properties of neurons. Transgenic and knockin mice with presenilin mutations are slower than age-matched controls in acquisition of spatial learning in the Morris water maze, as well as non-spatial learning in object recognition and Pavlovian trace conditioning. These detrimental effects are likely mediated either by increased $A\beta_{42}$ concentrations or by the direct action of mutated *PS1*.

Keywords: Alzheimer's disease; PS1; PS2; Spatial learning; Motor coordination; Motor activity

1. BEHAVIORALLY CHARACTERIZED *PS1* AND *PS2* MUTANTS

Mutations of *APP*, *PS1,* and *PS2* genes [Campion et al, 1999; De Jonghe and Van Broeckhoven, 1999; Larner and Doran, 2006; Tanzi and Bertram, 2001] and duplication of

* Corresponding author: Email: robert.lalonde@umontreal.ca; Tel.: +1 (514) 890-8000; ext 35739; Fax: +1 (514) 412-7314.

the *APP* locus [Rovelet-Lecrux et al, 2006] have been identified as causes of autosomal dominant Alzheimer's disease. For some *PS1* mutations, dementia is diagnosed as early as the twenties [Campion et al, 1996; De Jonghe and Van Broeckhoven, 1999]. But presumably because of species differences in life span, no normal or genetically modified mouse for *PS1* or *PS2* genes develops Aβ plaques. Despite this limitation, these models offer the possibility of examining the effects of presenilin mutations on neurobehavioral function prior to plaque formation. Behaviorally characterized transgenic or knockin (KI) models with human *PS1* and *PS2* mutations are presented in Table 1.

Mice with *PS1*/M146L and *PS1*/M146V transgenes driven by the *PDGFβ2* promoter are characterized by higher $A\beta_{42}$ but not $A\beta_{40}$ concentrations [Duff et al, 1996]. A second *PS1*/M146L line, together with a *PS1*/L286V one, was generated by cDNA insertion into a hamster *PrP* expression vector, enhancing $A\beta_{42}$ concentrations when bred with transgenics for human wild-type APP_{695} [Citron et al, 1997]. A third *PS1*/M146L transgene was generated with the *HMGCR* (hydroxy-methyl-glutaryl-coenzyme A reductase) promoter [Blanchard et al, 2003]. In addition, a *PS1*/L235P transgenic line was reported and, as with the first line described above, $A\beta_{42}$ but not $A\beta_{40}$ concentrations increased relative to wild-type [Huang et al, 2003]. Moreover, a *PS1*/ΔE9 transgene driven by the endogenous *PrP* promoter has been generated [Jankowsky et al, 2005]. *PS1*/A246E and *PS1*/wild-type transgenes driven by the human *THY1* promoter have been generated on a murine *PS1* knockout background, the former with elevated $A\beta_{42}$ concentrations relative to the latter [Qian et al, 1998].

Two *PS1* KI models are available. The insertion of human *PS1* with the Japanese I213T mutation on the chromosomal site normally occupied by the endogenous gene augmented $A\beta_{42}$ concentrations relative to normal wild-type [Nakano et al, 1999]. The second KI model contains the M146L mutation [Guo et al, 1999a,b].

With respect to *PS2* models, a transgenic mouse with the N141I Volga-German mutation is available, driven by the *NSE* (neuron-specific enolase) promoter [Hwang et al, 2002]. As with *PS1* mutants, *PS2*/N141I mutants have elevated $A\beta_{42}$ concentrations relative to non-transgenic controls.

Table 1. Description of behaviorally characterized transgenic or knockin (KI) mice expressing mutated *PS1* or *PS2*

Mutation	Type	Promoter	References
PS1/M146L *PS1*/M146V	transgenic	*PDGFβ2*	Duff et al, 1996
PS1/M146L *PS1*/L286V	transgenic	hamster *PrP*	Citron et al, 1997
PS1/M146L	transgenic	*HMGCR*	Blanchard et al, 2003
PS1/L235P	transgenic	not mentioned	Huang et al, 2003
PS1/ΔE9	transgenic	murine *PrP*	Jankowsky et al, 2005
PS1/A246E	transgenic	human *THY1*	Qian et al, 1998
PS1/M146L	knockin	endogenous control	Guo et al,1999a,b
PS1/I213T	knockin	endogenous control	Nakano et al, 1999
PS2/N141I	transgenic	*NSE*	Hwang et al, 2002

2. Neurochemical Characteristics

2. 1 Calcium Homeostasis and Neurodegeneration

The potential neurotoxic effect of *PS1* mutations has been examined in KI mice. Kainate injections into the hippocampus caused more severe neuronal death in *PS1*/M146L KI mice than wild-type [Guo et al, 1999a]. In hippocampal cell cultures, the mutant form was more vulnerable to glutamate-induced toxicity. One possible reason for this potentiation of excitatory amino acid-linked neurodegeneration is through alteration in calcium homeostasis. Despite equivalent basal Ca^{2+} concentrations, glutamate-induced Ca^{2+} increases inside neurons were greater in the KI mice than in those of controls, as well as cellular peroxides, mitochondrial reactive oxygen species (ROS), and lipid peroxidation [Guo et al, 1999a]. Moroever, dietary restriction decreased lipid peroxidation and protected neurons from kainate-induced excitotoxicity [Zhu et al, 1999]. Under basal conditions in hippocampal cell cultures, growth and survival were normal in the KI mice [Guo et al, 1999b]. But when exposed to Aβ, their neurons were more susceptible to degeneration, presumably because of increased ROS and lipid peroxidation, as amyloid-induced neurotoxicity was counteracted by an antioxidant. Likewise, neuronal apoptosis was more pronounced in KI hippocampal cells than that of controls after glucose deprivation [Xie et al, 2001]. The same KI mutant was evaluated for neural responses in prefrontal cortex slices to inositol triphosphate (IP_3), a secondary messenger binding to receptors on the endoplasmic reticulum membrane to release sequestered Ca^{2+} into the cytosol [Stutzmann et al, 2004]. The IP_3-evoked but not the spike-evoked transient rise in intracellular Ca^{2+} levels was enhanced in the KI mice.

Similar results have been obtained in transgenic models. Despite normal basal levels, KCl- and Aβ-induced Ca^{2+} increases in synaptosomes from *PS1*/M146L/*PDGFβ2* and from *PS1*/M146V transgenic mice were elevated related to non-transgenic controls [Begley et al, 1999]. Moreover, cells from hippocampal slices of the former responded with higher Ca^{2+} levels to K^+-induced depolarization than those of controls [Barrow et al, 2000]. The calcium-related anomalies may be responsible for altered electrophysiologic properties noted in mutant brains. In particular, hippocampal long-term potentiation (LTP) was enhanced in *PS1*/M146L/*PDGFβ2* [Barrow et al, 2000], *PS1*/ΔE9 [Zaman et al, 2000], and *PS1*/A246E [Parent et al, 1999] transgenic mice. In contrast, an age-related decline in LTP was found in *PS1*/M146L/ *HMGCR* transgenic mice [Gruart et al, 2008], a discrepancy which may be due either to the nature of the mutation or to methodologic factors related to measuring LTP.

The effects of *PS1* mutations on the unfolded protein response (UPR), as defined by reduced expression or phosphorylation of chaperone proteins facilitating protein folding, have been studied in response to endoplasmic reticulum stress. The UPR response was disturbed in fibroblasts cultured from *PS1*/I213T KI mouse embryos [Yasuda et al, 2002] and in SK-N-SH neuroblastoma cells transfected with complementary DNA containing *PS1*/A246E or *PS1*/ΔE9 mutations [Katayama et al, 2001]. But primary neocortical neurons from *PS1*/P264L KI mice were not more prone than controls to apoptosis after exposure to three pro-apoptotic agents including $A\beta_{42}$ [Siman et al, 2000]. In addition, the UPR of primary neocortical neurons derived from the mutant mice did not differ from that of controls in response to endoplasmic reticulum stressors [Siman et al, 2001], both results indicating the possibility of mutation-specific effects.

PS1/H163R and *PS1*/L286V transgene insertions driven by the *PDGFβ2* promoter contained more neurons with $A\beta_{42}$ but not $A\beta_{40}$ than non-transgenic controls [Chui et al, 1999]. Despite the lack of extracellular Aβ deposits, the two mutants had lower neuronal counts in frontal cortex and hippocampus. Other anomalies with potential behavioral significance include deficient adult neurogenesis in the dentate gyrus of the hippocampal formation of *PS1*/P117L transgenic mice [Wen et al, 2004].

2. 2 Cholinergic System

Degeneration of the basal forebrain cholinergic system is one of the most prominent aspects in Alzheimer brain, playing a central role in cognitive deterioration [Whitehouse et al, 1982]. In Alzheimer cortex, there is decreased activity of the specific acetylcholine-producing enzyme, choline acetyltransferase (ChAT) [Coyle et al, 1983; Efange et al, 1997; Gil-Bea et al, 2005; Hardy et al, 1985; Minger et al, 2001] and of the non-specific catabolizing enzyme, acetylcholinesterase (AChE), in postmortem samples [Blusztajn and Berse, 2000; Coyle et al, 1983; Gil-Bea et al, 2005; Hardy et al, 1985], for the latter particularly the tetrameric isoform related to enzymatic activity [Atack et al, 1983; Sberna et al, 1998] and on PET scans [Herholz et al, 2004; Kuhl et al, 1999; Okamura et al, 2008; Rinne et al, 2003]. In addition, vesicular acetylcholine transporter (VAChT) binding declined [Efange et al, 1997], at least partly due to neurodegeneration in basal forebrain [Coyle et al, 1983; Hardy et al, 1985; Lyness et al, 2003; Wu et al, 2005]. However, AChE staining is sometimes enhanced in hippocampal subregions [Hyman et al, 1987], either as a compensatory response or because of its link with Aβ plaques [Kalaria et al, 1992; Moran et al, 1993].

No such widespread degeneration seems prevalent in *PS1* mutants. Indeed, VAChT density was unchanged in frontal and parietal cortex of *PS1*/M146L mutants [Wong et al, 1999], as well as ChAT activity in frontoparietal cortex, hippocampus, and dorsomedial striatum of *PS1*/L286V mutants [Vaucher et al, 2002] and in hippocampus of *PS1*/L235P mutants [Huang et al, 2003]. A more detailed cartography of the cholinergic system was reported with respect to AChE activity in *PS1*/A246E mutants relative *PS1*/wild-type controls [Jazi et al, 2009]. Similar to Alzheimer hippocampus [Hyman et al, 1987] and murine models overexpressing C99 [Dumont et al, 2006] or C100 [Sberna et al, 1998] fragments of APP, AChE staining increased in pyramidal cell layers of CA1 and CA2-3 subregions of *PS1*/A246E mice, as well as in granule and polymorphic cell layers of dentate gyrus and subiculum. This upregulation extended to several neocortical regions, striatum, thalamus, and areas containing cholinergic cell bodies, including medial septum, vertical diagonal band, substantia inominata, and pedunculopontine nuclei. No ongoing cell degeneration was detected in these and other areas based on FluoroJade labelling [Jazi et al, 2009]. These results indicate that mutated *PS1* overexpression or increased $A\beta_{42}$ concentrations is sufficient to upregulate AChE activity in early stages of Alzheimer-like pathology.

3. Myoclonus and Epilepsy

Two neurological symptoms liable to appear in Alzheimer's disease are myoclonus and epileptic seizures [Chen et al, 1991; Förstl et al, 1992], particularly in its hereditary form [Campion et al, 1996]. Unlike the sporadic form, Aβ plaques accumulate in cerebellum of patients with autosomal dominant Alzheimer's disease and myoclonus [Ishino et al, 1984; Lemere et al, 1996].

In transgenic *PS1*/A246E but not *PS1*/wild-type mice, jumping myoclonus was reported, consisting of repetitive jumping against the walls of their home cage [Lalonde et al, 2003]. It is possible that this sign is triggered by the effects of $A\beta_{42}$ on 5-hydroxytryptamine (5HT)-related pathways, since myoclonus was observed in normal animals injected with 5HT precursors [Pappert et al, 1998]. However, myoclonic jumping was not detected in *PS1*/I213T KI mice [Lalonde and Strazielle, 2005], either because of different mutations or genetic backgrounds.

4. Sensorimotor Learning

Alzheimer's disease is characterized by deficient posture and gait even in its early stage [Pettersson et al, 2002], perhaps due to vermal Purkinje cell atrophy [Sjöbeck and Englund, 2001]. There is therefore interest in determining sensorimotor learning in animals with amyloid pathology.

One of the most frequently used test is the rotorod, requiring balance and coordination synchronized to beam movement. *PS1*/A246E mice were impaired relative to *PS1*/wild-type controls on a constant-speed rotorod [Lalonde et al, 2003], but not in comparison with non-transgenic controls on a more difficult accelerating version [Dineley et al, 2002]. Likewise, *PS1*/L286V transgenic mice performed worse than human wild-type *PS1* on the accelerated rotorod but no worse than non-transgenic controls [Vaucher et al, 2002]. Moreover, *PS1*/I213T KI mice performed normally on the accelerating rotorod relative to non-transgenic controls [Lalonde and Strazielle, 2005]. The overall evidence seems so far to indicate only mild or no detrimental impact of *PS1* transgenesis on sensorimotor learning.

5. Spatial Learning

One of the earliest features of Alzheimer dementia is anterograde amnesia, defined as a difficulty in acquiring new information [Jacobs et al, 1995], including visuospatial material, exemplied in line drawings [Graham et al, 2004]. Constructional apraxia is also manifested in the form of copying drawings and reproducing geometric figures with building blocks [Graham et al, 2004; Helmes and Ostbye, 2002; Henderson et al, 1989; Nielson et al, 1996]. As a result, Alzheimer patients are more liable to be disoriented in a maze [Rainville et al, 2002a], a hospital ward [Monacelli et al, 2003], and in the streets while driving a motored vehicle [Uc et al, 2004]. Possible reasons underlying spatial deficits include impairments in flow perception [Tetewsky and Duffy, 1999], visual search [Parasuraman et al, 2000; Tales et al, 2004], abstract reasoning [Helmes and Ostbye, 2002], and executive functions [Collette et al, 1999; Graham et al, 2004; Rainville et al, 2002b].

One of the main methods used for screening spatial function in Alzheimer-like models is the Morris water maze, in which mice are trained to escape by reaching a platform [Morris et al, 1982]. In the hidden platform condition, mice reach the goal on the basis of spatial landmarks (place learning). In the visible platform subtask, mice may swim directly to the goal thanks to local cues (visuomotor guidance). To maximize mouse performances, special care must be taken to avoid water-induced hypothermia by using a suitably long intertrial interval. For water temperatures ranging between 20° and 24°C, body temperatures returned to normal with a 13 min but not a 30 s intertrial interval [Iivonen et al, 2003]. After acquisition, a probe trial is often conducted, with the submerged platform removed from the pool, causing the mice to float or swim in the vicinity of where the platform used to be. Spatial learning in the Morris water maze is sensitive to lesions in rat extrastriate [Espinoza et al, 1999], parietal [DiMattia and Kesner, 1988; Hoh et al, 2003], prefrontal [Hoh et al, 2003], posterior cingulate [Vann and Aggleton, 2002], and entorhinal/perirhinal [Nagahara et al, 1995] cortex, as well as large [Brun et al, 2002; Morris et al, 1982] and CA1-restricted [Stubley-Weatherly et al, 1996] parts of the hippocampus.

The effects of *PS1* mutations on this test are presented in Table 2. Relative to age-matched non-transgenic controls at 8 months, acquisition of the hidden platform condition was deficient in *PS1*/M146L/*PDGFβ2* mutants [Sadowski et al, 2004]. However, both groups had equivalent acquisition rates at 6 and 9 [Holcomb et al, 1999] or 22 [Sadowski et al, 2004] months of age. The lack of an effect in the oldest group may be due to poorer performance in controls, causing an inverted ceiling effect, but the negative outcome at 6 and and 9 months is more difficult to explain, possibly a result of methodologic factors such as sex distribution or pool size. Nevertheless, three other transgenic models had normal place learning, namely *PS1*/L235P [Huang et al, 2003], *PS1*/A246E [Lalonde et al, 2003], and a mixed group consisting of two *PS1*/M146L/*Prp* lines and *PS1*/L286V [Janus et al, 2000]. However, the mixed group had poorer probe trial performances relative to non-transgenic controls, indicating impaired long-term memory. Although a probe trial deficit was also reported in *PS2*/N141I transgenic mice [Hwang et al, 2002], this was obtained with the unusual procedure of measuring distance travelled in the pool with the missing platform and not time spent in the target quadrant.

Further mild deficits in spatial learning have also been described in two KI models. Indeed, acquisition of the hidden platform task was slowed down in *PS1*/I213T KI mice relative to wild-type [Lalonde and Strazielle, 2005]. However, no detrimental action was found in the probe trial. Conversely, probe trial performance was impaired despite normal acquisition in *PS1*/M146L KI mutants [Sun et al, 2005]. Neither mutation affected swimming towards the visible platform, indicating cognitive as opposed to visuomotor or motivational deficits. It remains to be determined whether other KI models are deficient and whether this is due to increased $A\beta_{42}$ concentrations, since intracerebroventricular injections of soluble $A\beta_{25-35}$ impaired spatial learning in the Morris water maze in rats [Sun and Alkon, 2002].

6. NON-SPATIAL LEARNING

6. 1 Object Recognition

Non-spatial memory can be evaluated by form recognition, in which the length of time mice explore a novel as opposed to a previously presented object is measured. In one version [Huang et al, 2003; Vaucher et al, 2002], mice first explore two objects and then one of them is replaced by a new one. In a second version [Dewachter et al, 2002; Howlett et al, 2004], a single object is presented, followed by this object together with a new one. In either version, retention is evaluated by the novel/total time preference ratio, dependent on the recognition of visual and tactile features of familiar objects.

The sensivity of object recognition memory to Alzheimer-like pathology was demonstrated in *PS1*/L235P transgenic mice [Huang et al, 2003]. However, object recognition memory was similar in *PS1*/L286V mice relative either to human wild-type *PS1* or to non-transgenic mice [Vaucher et al, 2002].

6. 2 Shock Avoidance and Fear Conditioning

In contextual fear conditioning, mice are given footshocks in a compartment and removed, then placed back in the same compartment while time spent in an immobile posture (freezing) is measured [Dineley et al, 2002]. In cued fear conditioning, mice are given footshocks during presentation of an auditory tone (or other cue). Afterwards, the mice are placed in the same compartment or in a different one and the immobility time during presentation of the auditory tone is measured. In comparison to non-transgenic controls, neither contextual nor cued fear conditioning tasks were altered in *PS1*/A246E transgenic mice [Dineley et al, 2002]. The same negative result was reported in *PS1*/M146L KI mice relative to wild-type, although the former had poorer contextual learning when one wild-type allele was removed by interbreeding with a *PS1* knockout [Wang et al, 2004].

6. 3 Eyeblink Conditioning

In Pavlovian eyeblink conditioning, mice receive contingent pairings between the conditioned stimulus (CS) and the unconditioned stimulus (US), so that the CS alone produces the conditioned response. The CS may be a sound and the US an electric shock to the upper eyelid muscle, or else stimulating electrodes are placed in the supraorbitary nerve for presentation of weak and strong pulses, respectively, as the CS and US. In delay eyeblink conditioning, the CS begins before the US, but both terminate at the same time. In trace conditioning, there is a time gap between the end of the CS and the start of the US. As found in Alzheimer dementia [Woodruff-Pak and Papka, 1996], trace conditioning was impaired in *PS1*/M146L/*HMGCR* transgenic mice relative to wild-type [Gruart et al, 2008]. The deficiency was found at 12 but not 3 months of age.

Table 2. Behavioral performances of *PS1* transgenic or knockin (KI) mutants and a transgenic *PS2* mutant relative to normal controls or to human *PS1* wild-type for *PS1*/A246E in hidden and visible platform versions as well as the probe trial in the Morris water maze.

Mutant	Hidden platform	Probe trial	Visible platform	References
PS1/M146L/PDGFβ2	normal	normal	normal	Holcomb et al, 1999
PS1/M146L/PDGFβ2	↓	untested	untested	Sadowski et al, 2004
PS1/M146L/Prp + PS1/L286V/Prp	normal	↓	normal	Janus et al, 2000
PS1/A246E	normal	normal	normal	Lalonde et al, 2003
PS1/L235P	normal	normal	untested	Huang et al, 2003
PS1/I213T KI	↓	normal	normal	Lalonde and Strazielle, 2005
PS1/M146L KI	normal	↓	normal	Sun et al, 2005
PS2/N141I	unreported	↓	untested	Hwang et al, 2002

↓=deficit
normal=not impaired vs controls

6. 4 Conditioned Taste Aversion

In conditioned taste aversion, a novel-tasting solution, such as saccharin, is paired with an aversive stimulus, such as an injection of nausea-causing LiCl, so that saccharin becomes aversive. Conditioned taste aversion was not affected in *PS1*/ΔE9 transgenic mice in comparison to wild-type [Pistell et al, 2008].

6. 5 Habituation of the Startle Response and Prepulse Inhibition

Mice are placed in a chamber with a weak background noise while a loud auditory stimulus is presented to cause a startle response, which decreases after successive trials. In prepulse inhibition, an auditory stimulus weaker than the original stimulus but stronger than the background noise is presented, so that the startle response is inhibited. Though Alzheimer patients were impaired in a similar test [Ueki et al, 2006], prepulse inhibition was equivalent in *PS1*/M146L/*HMGCR* transgenic mice relative to wild-type [Gruart et al, 2008].

7. Conclusion

Though seemingly of a mild nature, spatial deficits have been described in *PS1* mutants relative to controls. Deficits in object recognition memory and trace conditioning of the eyeblink response have also been documented, though only in a single model on each task. These detrimental effects may be mediated by increased $A\beta_{42}$ concentrations or by the direct action of mutated *PS1*. Although behavioral deficits appear subtle, further experimentation on mutated presenilin models seems worth pursuing.

REFERENCES

Atack, J. R., Perry, E. K., Bonham, J. R., Perry, R. H., Tomlinson, B. E., Blessed, G. & Fairbairn, A. (1983). Molecular forms of acetylcholinesterase in senile dementia of Alzheimer type: selective loss of the intermediate (10S) form. *Neurosci. Lett., 40*, 199-204.

Barrow, P. A., Empson, R. M., Gladwell, S. J., Anderson, C. M., Killick, R., Yu, X., Jefferys, J. G. R. & Duff, K. (2000). Functional phenotype in transgenic mice expressing human mutant *presenilin-1. Neurobiol. Dis., 7*, 119-126.

Begley, J. G., Duan, W., Chan, S., Duff, K. & Mattson, M. P. (1999). Altered calcium homeostasis and mitochondrial dysfunction in cortical synaptic compartments of presenilin-1 mutant mice. *J. Neurochem., 72*, 1030-1039.

Blanchard, V., Moussaoui, S., Czech, C., Touchet, N., Bonici, B., Planche, M., Canton, T., Jedidi, I., Gohin, M., Wirths, O., Bayer, T. A., Langui, D., Duyckaerts, C., Tremp, G. & Pradier, L. (2003). Time sequence of maturation of dystrophic neurites associated with Aβ deposits in APP/PS1 transgenic mice. *Exp. Neurol., 184*, 247-263.

Blusztajn, J. K. & Berse, B. (2000). The cholinergic neuronal phenotype in Alzheimer's disease. *Met. Brain Dis., 15*, 45-64.

Brun, V. H., Otnaess, M. K., Molden, S., Steffenach, H. -A., Witter, M. P., Moser, M. -B. & Moser, E. I. (2002). Place cells and place recognition maintained by direct entorhinal-hippocampal circuitry. *Science, 296*, 2243-2246.

Campion, D., Brice, A., Dumanchin, C., Puel, M., Baulac, M., De la Sayette, V., Hannequin, D., Duyckaerts, C., Michon, A., Martin, C., Moreau, V., Penet, C., Martinez, M., Clerget-Darpoux, F., Agid, Y. & Frébourg, T. (1996). A novel presenilin *1* mutation resulting in familial Alzheimer's disease with an onset age of 29 years. *NeuroReport, 7*, 1582-1584.

Campion, D., Dumanchin, C., Hannequin, D., Dubois, B., Bellliard, S., Puel, M., Thomas-Anerion, C., Michon, A., Martin, C., Charbonnier, F., Raux, G., Camuzat, A., Penet, C., Mesnage, V., Martinez, M., Clerget-Darpoux, F. & Frebourg, T. (1999). Early-onset autosomal dominant Alzheimer disease, prevalence, genetic heterogeneity, and mutation spectrum. *Am. J. Hum. Genet., 65*, 664-670.

Chen, J. -Y., Stern, Y., Sano, M. & Mayeux, R. (1991). Cumulative risks of developing extrapyramidal signs, psychosis, or myoclonus in the course of Alzheimer's disease. *Arch. Neurol., 48*, 1141-1143.

Chui, D. -H., Tanahashi, H., Ozawa, K., Ikeda, S., Checler, F., Ueda, O., Suzuki, H., Araki, W., Inoue, H., Shirotani, K., Takahashi, K., Gallyas, F. & Tabira, T. (1999). Transgenic mice with Alzheimer presenilin 1 mutations show accelerated neurodegeneration without amyloid plaque formation. *Nature Med., 5*, 560-564.

Citron, M., Westway, D., Xia, W., Carlson, G., Diehl, T., Levesque, G., Johnson-Wood, K., Lee, M., Seubert, P., Davis, A., Kholodenko, D., Motter, R., Sherrington, R., Perry, B., Yao, H., Strome, R., Lieberburg, I., Rommens, J., Kim, S., Schenk, D., Fraser, P., St George Hyslop, P. & Selkoe, D. J. (1997). Mutant presenilins of Alzheimer's disease increase production of 42-residue amyloid β-protein in both transfected cells and transgenic mice. *Nature Med., 3*, 67-72.

Collette, F., Van der Linden, M. & Salmon E. (1999). Executive dysfunction in Alzheimer's disease. *Cortex, 35*, 57-72.

Coyle, J. T., Price, D. L. & DeLong, M. R. (1983). Alzheimer's disease: a disorder of cortical cholinergic innervation. *Science, 219*, 1184-1190.

De Jonghe, C. & Van Broeckhoven, C. (1999). Identification and functional analysis of genes and genetic risk factors in Alzheimer's disease. In: Crusio W., Gerlai R. (Eds) Handbook of Molecular-Genetic Techniques for Brain and Behavior Research, Techniques in the Behavioral and Neural Sciences, Vol. 13, 841-862, Amsterdam, Elsevier.

Dewachter, I., Reversé, D., Caluwaerts, N., Ris, L., Kuipéri, C., Van den Haute, C., Spittaels, K., Umans, L., Serneels, L., Thiry, E., Moechars, D., Mercken, M., Godaux, E. & Van Leuven, F. (2002). Neuronal deficiency of presenilin 1 inhibits amyloid plaque formation and corrects hippocampal long-term potentiation but not a cognitive defect of amyloid precursor protein [V717I] transgenic mice. *J. Neurosci., 22*, 3445-3453.

DiMattia, B. D. & Kesner, R. P. (1988). Spatial cognitive maps, differential role of parietal cortex and hippocampal formation. *Behav. Neurosci., 102*, 471-480.

Dineley, K. T., Xia, X., Bui, D., Sweatt, J. D. & Zheng, H. (2002). Accelerated plaque accumulation, associative learning deficits, and up-regulation of α7 nicotinic receptor protein in transgenic mice co-expressing mutant human presenilin 1 and amyloid precursor proteins. *J. Biol. Chem., 277*, 22768-22780.

Duff, K., Eckman, C., Zehr, C., Yu, X., Prada, C. -M., Perez-tur, J., Hutton, J., Buee, L., Harigaya, Y., Yager, D., Morgan, D., Gordon, M. N., Holcomb, L., Refolo, L., Zenk, B., Hardy, J. & Younkin, S. (1996). Increased β-amyloid42(43) in brains of mice expressing mutant presenilin 1. *Nature, 383*, 710-713.

Dumont, M., Lalonde, R., Ghersi-Egea, J. -F., Fukuchi, K., Strazielle, C. (2006). Regional acetylcholinesterase activity and its correlation with behavioral performances in 15-month old transgenic mice expressing the human C99 fragment of *APP. J. Neural Transm., 113*, 1225-1241.

Efange, S. M., Garland, E. M., Staley, J. K., Khare, A. B. & Mash D. C. (1997). Vesicular acetylcholine transporter density and Alzheimer's disease. *Neurobiol. Aging, 18*, 407-413.

Espinoza, S., Pinto-Hamuy, T., Passig, C., Carreno, F., Marchant, F., Urzua, C. (1999). Deficit in the water-maze after lesions in the anteromedial extrastriate cortex in rats. *Physiol. Behav., 66*, 493-496.

Förstl, H., Burns, A., Levy, R., Cairns, N., Luthert, P. & Lantos, P. (1992). Neurologic signs in Alzheimer's disease: results of a prospective clinical and neuropathologic study. *Arch. Neurol., 49*, 1038-1042.

Gil-Bea, F. J., Garcia-Alloza, M., Dominguez, J., Marcos, B. & Ramirez, M. J. (2005). Evaluation of cholinergic markers in Alzheimer's disease and in a model of cholinergic deficit. *Neurosci. Lett., 375*, 37-41.

Graham, N. L., Emery, T. & Hodges, J. R. (2004). Distinctive cognitive profiles in Alzheimer's disease and subcortical vascular dementia. *J. Neurol. Neurosurg. Psychiatry, 75*, 61-71.

Gruart, A., Lopez-Ramos, J. C., Munoz, M. D. & Delgado-Garcia, J. M. (2008). Aged wild-type and APP, PS1, and APP+PS1 mice present similar deficits in associative learning and synaptic plasticity independent of amyloid load. *Neurobiol. Dis., 30*, 439-450.

Guo, Q., Fu, W., Sopher, B. L., Miller, M. W., Ware, C. B., Martin, G. M. & Mattson, M. P. (1999a). Increased vulnerability of hippocampal neurons to excitotoxic necrosis in presenilin-1 mutant knock-in mice. *Nature Med., 5*, 101-106.

Guo, Q., Sebastian, L., Sopher, B. L., Miller, M. W., Ware, C. B., Martin, G. M. & Mattson, M. P. (1999b). Increased vulnerability of hippocampal neurons from presenilin-1 mutant knock-in mice to amyloid β-peptide toxicity: central roles of superoxide production and caspase activation. *J. Neurochem., 72*, 1019-1029.

Hardy, J., Adolfsson, R., Alafuzoff, I., Bucht, G., Marcusson, J., Nyberg, P., Perdahl, E., Wester, P. & Winblad, B. (1985). Transmitter deficits in Alzheimer's disease. *Neurochem. Int., 7*, 545-563.

Helmes, E. & Ostbye, T. (2002). Beyond memory impairment: cognitive changes in Alzheimer's disease. *Arch. Clin. Neuropsychol., 17*, 179-193.

Henderson, V. W., Mack, W. & Williams, B. W. (1989). Spatial disorientation in Alzheimer's disease. *Arch. Neurol., 46*, 391-394.

Herholz, K., Weisenbach, S., Zundorf, G., Lenz, O., Schroder, H., Bauer, B., Kalbe, E. & Heiss, W. D. (2004). *In vivo* study of acetylcholine esterase in basal forebrain, amygdala, and cortex in mild to moderate Alzheimer disease. *NeuroImage, 21*, 136-143.

Hoh, T. E., Kolb, B., Eppel, A., Vanderwolf, C. H. & Cain, D. P. (2003). Role of the neocortex in the water maze task in the rat: a detailed behavioral and Golgi-Cox analysis. *Behav. Brain Res., 138*, 81-94.

Holcomb, L. A., Gordon, M. N., Jantzen, P., Hsiao, K., Duff, K. & Morgan, D. (1999). Behavioral changes in transgenic mice expressing both amyloid precursor protein and presenilin-1 mutations: lack of association with amyloid deposits. *Behav. Genet., 29*, 177-185.

Howlett, D. R., Richardson, J. C., Austin, A., Parsons, A. A., Bate, S. T., Davies, D. C. & Gonzalez, M. I. (2004). Cognitive correlates of Aβ deposition in male and female mice bearing amyloid precursor protein and presenilin-1 mutant transgenes. *Brain Res., 1017*, 130-136.

Huang, X. G., Yee, B. K., Nag, S., Chan, S. T. H. & Tang, F. (2003). Behavioral and neurochemical characterization of transgenic mice carrying the human presenilin-1 gene with or without the leucine-to-proline mutation at codon 235. *Exp. Neurol., 183*, 673-681.

Hwang, D. Y., Chae, K. R., Kang, T. S., Hwang, J. H., Lim, C. H., Kang, H. K., Goo, J. S., Lee, M. R., Lim, H. J., Min, S. H., Cho, J. Y., Hong, J. T., Song, C. W., Paik, S. G., Cho, J. S. & Kim, Y. K. (2002). Alterations in behavior, amyloid β-42, caspase-3, and Cox-2 in mutant *PS2* transgenic mouse model of Alzheimer's disease. *FASEB J., 16*, 805-813.

Hyman, B. T., Kromer, L. J. & Van Hoesen, G. W. (1987). Reinnervation of the hippocampal perforant pathway zone in Alzheimer's disease. *Ann. Neurol., 21*, 259-267.

Iivonen, H., Nurminen, L., Harri, M., Tanila, H. & Puoliväli, J. (2003). Hypothermia in mice tested in Morris water maze. *Behav. Brain Res., 141*, 207-213.

Ishino, H., Higashi, S., Chuta, M. & Ohta, H. (1984). Juvenile Alzheimer's disease with myoclonus: amyloid plaques and grumose alteration in the cerebellum. *Clin. Neuropathol., 3*, 193-198.

Jacobs, D. M., Sano, M., Dooneief, G., Marder, K., Bell, K. L. & Stern, Y. (1995). Neuropsychological detection and characterization of preclinical Alzheimer's disease. *Neurology*, *45*, 957-962.

Jankowsky, J. L., Melnikova, T., Fadale, D. J., Xu, G. M., Slunt, H. H., Gonzales, V., Younkin, L. H., Younkin, S. G., Borchelt, D. R. & Savonenko, A. V. (2005). Environmental enrichment mitigates cognitive deficits in a mouse model of Alzheimer's disease. *J. Neurosci.*, *25*, 5217-5224.

Janus, C., D'Amelio, S., Amitay, O., Chishti, M. A., Strome, R., Fraser, P., Carlson, G. A., Roder, J. C., St. George-Hyslop, P. & Westaway, D. (2000). Spatial learning in transgenic mice expressing presenilin 1 (*PS1*) transgenes. *Neurobiol. Aging*, *21*, 541-549.

Jazi, R., Lalonde, R. & Strazielle, C. (2009). Regional brain evaluation of acetylcholinesterase activity in PS1/A246E transgenic mice. *Neurosci. Res.*, *63*, 106-114.

Katayama, T., Imaizumi, K., Honda, A., Yoneda, T., Kudo, T., Takeda, M., Mori, K., Rozmahel, R., Fraser, P., St. George-Hyslop, P. & Tohyama, M. (2001). Disturbed activation of endoplasmic reticulum stress transducers by familial Alzheimer's disease-linked presenilin-1 mutations. *J. Biol. Chem.*, *276*, 43446-43454.

Kalaria, R. N., Kroon, S. N., Grahovac, I. & Perry, G. (1992). Acetylcholinesterase and its association with heparan sulphate proteoglycans in cortical amyloid deposits of Alzheimer's disease. *Neuroscience*, *51*, 177-184.

Kuhl, D. E., Koeppe, R. A., Minoshima, S., Snyder, S. E., Ficaro, E. P., Foster, N. L., Frey, K. A., Kilbourn, M. R., Frey, K. A. & Kilbourn, M. R. (1999). *In vivo* mapping of cerebral acetylcholinesterase activity in aging and Alzheimer's disease. *Neurology*, *52*, 691-699.

Lalonde, R. & Strazielle, C. (2005). *PS1* knockin mice with the Japanese I213T mutation: effects on exploratory activity, motor coordination, and spatial learning. *Behav. Brain Res.*, *162*, 182-190.

Lalonde, R., Qian, S. & Strazielle, C. (2003). Transgenic mice expressing the *PS1*-A246E mutation: effects on spatial learning, exploration, anxiety, and motor coordination. *Behav. Brain Res.*, *138*, 71-79.

Larner, A. J. & Doran, M. (2006). Clinical phenotypic heterogeneity of Alzheimer's disease associated with mutations of the presenilin-1 gene. *J. Neurol.*, *253*, 139-158.

Lemere, C. A., Lopera, F., Kosik, K. S., Lendon, C. L., Ossa, J., Saido, T. C., Yamaguchi, H., Ruiz, A., Martinez, A., Madrigal, L., Hincapie, L., Arango, J. C. L., Anthony, D. C., Koo, E. H., Goate, A. M., Selkoe, D. J. & Arango, J. C. V. (1996). The E280A presenilin 1 Alzheimer mutation produced increased Aβ42 deposition and severe cerebellar pathology. *Nature Med.*, *2*, 1146-1150.

Lyness, S. A., Zarow, C. & Chui, H. C. (2003). Neuron loss in key cholinergic and aminergic nuclei in Alzheimer's disease: a meta-analysis. *Neurobiol. Aging*, *24*, 1-23.

Minger, S. L., Honer, W. G., Esiri, M. M., McDonald, B., Keene, J., Nicoll, J. A., Carter, J., Hope, T. & Francis, P. T. (2001). Synaptic pathology in prefrontal cortex is present only with severe dementia in Alzheimer disease. J. Neuropathol. *Exp. Neurol.* 60, 929-936.

Monacelli, A. M., Cushman, L. A., Kavcic, V. & Duffy, C. J. (2003). Spatial disorientation in Alzheimer's disease: the remembrance of things passed. *Neurology*, *61*, 1491-1497.

Moran, M. A., Mufson, E. J. & Gomez-Ramos, P. (1993). Colocalization of cholinesterases with β amyloid protein in aged and Alzheimer's brain. *Acta Neuropathol.*, *85*, 362-369.

Morris, R. G. M., Garrud, P., Rawlins, J. N. P. & O'Keefe, J. (1982). Place navigation impaired in rats with hippocampal lesions. *Nature*, *292*, 681-683.

Nagahara, A. H., Otto, T. & Gallagher, M. (1995). Entorhinal-perirhinal lesions impair performance of rats on two versions of place learning in the Morris water maze. *Behav. Neurosci.*, *109*, 3-9.

Nakano, Y., Kondoh, G., Kudo, T., Imaizumi, K., Kato, M., Miyazaki, J., Tohyama, M., Takeda, J. & Takeda, M. (1999). Accumulation of murine amyloidβ42 in a gene-dosage-dependent manner in *PS1* 'knock-in' mice. *Eur. J. Neurosci.*, *11*, 2577-2581.

Nielson, K. A., Cummings, B. J. & Cotman, C. W. (1996). Constructional apraxia in Alzheimer's disease correlates with neuritic neuropathology in occipital cortex. *Brain Res.*, *741*, 284-293.

Okamura, N., Funaki, Y., Tashiro, M., Kato, M., Ishikawa, Y., Maruyama, M., Ishikawa, H., Meguro, K., Iwata, R. & Yanai, K. (2008). *In vivo* visualization of donepezil binding in the brain of patients with Alzheimer's disease. *Br J. Clin. Pharmacol.*, *65*, 472-479.

Pappert, E. J., Goetz, C. J., Stebbins, M., Belden, M. & Carvey, P. M. (1998). 5-Hydroxytryptamine-induced myoclonus in guinea pigs: mediation through $5\text{-HT}_{1/2}$ receptor subtypes. *Eur. J. Pharmacol.*, *347*, 51-56.

Parasuraman, R., Greenwood, P. M., Alexander, G. E., Parasuraman, R., Greenwood, P. M. & Alexander, G. E. (2000). Alzheimer disease constricts the dynamic range of spatial attention in visual search. *Neuropsychologia*, *38*, 1126-1135.

Parent, A., Linden, D. J., Sisodia, S. S. & Borchelt, D. R. (1999). Synaptic transmission and hippocampal long-term potentiation in transgenic mice expressing FAD-linked presenilin 1. *Neurobiol. Dis.*, *6*, 56-62.

Pettersson, A. F., Engardt, M. & Wahlund, L. -O. (2002). Activity and balance in subjects with mild Alzheimer's disease. *Dement. Geriatr. Cogn. Dis.*, *13*, 213-216.

Pistell, P. J., Zhu, M. & Ingram, D. K. (2008). Acquisition of conditioned taste aversion is impaired in the amyloid precursor protein/presenilin 1 mouse model of Alzheimer's disease. *Neuroscience*, *152*, 594-600.

Qian, S., Jiang, P., Guan, X. -M., Singh, G., Trumbauer, M. E., Yu, H., Chen, H. Y., Van der Ploeg, L. H. T. & Zheng, H. (1998). Mutant human presenilin-1 protects presenilin 1 null mouse against embryonic lethality and elevates Aβ1-42/43 production. *Neuron*, *20*, 611-617.

Rainville, C., Marchand, N. & Passini, R. (2002a). Performances of patients with a dementia of the Alzheimer type in the Standardized Road-Map test of Direction Sense. *Neuropsychologia*, *40*, 567-573.

Rainville, C., Amieva, H., Lafont, S., Dartigues, J. F., Orgogozo, J. M. & Fabrigoule, C. (2002b). Executive function deficits in patients with dementia of the Alzheimer's type: a study with a Tower of London task. *Arch. Clin. Neuropsychol.*, *17*, 513-530.

Richards, J. G., Higgins, G. A., Ouagazzal, A. -M., Ozmen, L., Kew, J. N. C., Bohrmann, B., Malherbe, P., Brockhaus, M., Loetscher, H., Czech, C., Huber, G., Bluethmann, H., Jacobsen, H. & Kemp, J. A. (2003). PS2APP transgenic mice, coexpressing hPS2mut and hAPPswe, show age-related cognitive deficits associated with discrete brain amyloid deposition and inflammation. *J. Neurosci.*, *23*, 8989-9003.

Rinne, J. O., Kaasinen, V., Jarvenpää, T., Nagren, K., Roivainen, A., Yu, M., Oikonen, V. & Kurki, T. (2003). Brain acetylcholinesterase activity in mild cognitive impairment and early Alzheimer's disease. *J. Neurol. Neurosurg. Psychiatry*, *74*, 113-115.

Rovelet-Lecrux, A., Hannequin, D., Raux, G., Le Meur, N., Laquerriere, A., Vital, A., Dumanchin, C., Feuillette, S., Brice, A., Vercelletto, M., Dubas, F., Frébourg, T. & Campion, D. (2006). APP locus duplication causes autosomal dominant early-onset Alzheimer disease with cerebral amyloid angiopathy. *Nature Genet.*, *38*, 24-26.

Sadowski, M., Pankiewicz, J., Scholtzova, H., Ji, Y., Quartermain, D., Jensen, C. H., Duff, K., Nixon, R. A., Gruen, R. J. & Wisniewski, T. (2004). Amyloid-β deposition is associated with decreased hippocampal glucose metabolism and spatial memory impairment in APP/PS1 mice. *J. Neuropathol. Exp. Neurol.*, *63*, 418-428.

Sberna, G., Saez-Valero, J., Li, Q-X., Czech, C., Beyruther, K., Masters, C. L., McLean, C. A. & Small, D. H. (1998). Acetylcholinesterase is increased in the brains of transgenic mice expressing the C-terminal fragment (CT100) of the β-amyloid protein precursor of Alzheimer's disease. *J. Neurochem.*, *71*, 723-731.

Siman, R., Flood, D. G., Thinakaran, G. & Neumar, R. W. (2001). Endoplasmic reticulum stress-induced cysteine protease activation in cortical neurons. *J. Biol. Chem.*, *276*, 44736-44743.

Siman, R., Reaume, A. G., Savage, M. J., Trusko, S., Lin, Y. -G., Scott, R. W. & Flood, D. G. (2000). Presenilin-1 P264L knock-in mutation: differential effects on Aβ production, amyloid deposition, and neuronal vulnerability. *J. Neurosci.*, *20*, 8717-8726.

Sjöbeck, M. & Englund, E. (2001). Alzheimer's disease and the cerebellum: a morphologic study on neuronal and glial changes. *Dement. Geriatr. Cogn. Disord.*, *12*, 211-218.

Stubley-Weatherly, L., Harding, J. W. & Wright, J. W. (1996). Effects of discrete kainic acid-induced hippocampal lesions on spatial and contextual learning and memory in rats. *Brain Res.*, *716*, 29-38.

Stutzmann, G. E., Caccamo, A., LaFerla, F. M. & Parker, I. (2004). Dysregulated IP_3 signaling in cortical neurons of knock-in mice expressing an Alzheimer's-linked mutation in presenilin1 results in exaggerated Ca^{2+} signals and altered membrane excitability. *J. Neurosci.*, *24*, 508-513.

Sun, M. K. & Alkon, D. L. (2002). Impairment of hippocampal CA1 heterosynaptic transformation and spatial memory by β-amyloid$_{25\text{-}35}$. *J. Neurophysiol.*, *87*, 2441-2449.

Sun, X., Beglopoulos, V., Mattson, MP. & Shen, J. (2005). Hippocampal spatial memory impairments caused by the familial Alzheimer's disease-linked presinilin 1 M146V mutation. *Neurodegenerative Dis.*, *2*, 6-15.

Tales, A., Muir, J., Jones, R., Bayer, A. & Snowden, R. J. (2004). The effects of saliency and task difficulty on visual search performance in ageing and Alzheimer's disease. *Neuropsychologia*, *42*, 335-345.

Tanzi, R. E; & Bertram, L. (2001). New frontiers in Alzheimer's disease genetics. *Neuron*, *32*, 181-184.

Tetewsky, S. J. & Duffy, C. J. (1999). Visual loss and getting lost in Alzheimer's disease. *Neurology*, *52*, 958-965.

Uc, E. Y., Rizzo, M., Anderson, S. W., Shi, Q. & Dawson, J. D. (2004). Driver route-following and safety errors in early Alzheimer disease. *Neurology*, *63*, 832-837.

Ueki, A., Goto, K., Sato, N., Iso, H. & Morita, Y. (2006). Prepulse inhibition of acoustic startle response in mild cognitive impairment and mild dementia of Alzheimer type. *Psychiatry Clin. Neurosci.*, *60*, 55-62.

Vann, S. D. & Aggleton, J. P. (2002). Extensive cytotoxic lesions of the rat retrosplenial cortex reveal consistent deficits on tasks that tax allocentric spatial memory. *Behav. Neurosci.*, *116*, 85-94.

Vaucher, E., Fluit, P., Chishti, M. A., Westaway, D., Mount, H. T. J. & Kar, S. (2002). Object recognition memory and cholinergic parameters in mice expressing human presenilin 1 transgenes. *Exp. Neurol.*, *175*, 398-406.

Wang, R., Dineley, K. T., Sweatt, J. D. & Zheng, H. (2004). Presenilin 1 familial Alzheimer's disease mutation leads to defective associative learning and impaired adult neurogenesis. *Neuroscience*, *126*, 305-312.

Wen, P. H., Hof, P. R., Chen, X., Gluck, K., Austin, G., Younkin, S. G., Younkin, L. H., DeGasperi, R., Gama Sosa, M. A., Robakis, N. K., Haroutunian, V. & Elder, G. A. (2004). The presenilin-1 familial Alzheimer disease mutant P117L impairs neurogenesis in the hippocampus of adult mice. *Exp. Neurol.*, *188*, 224-237.

Whitehouse, P. J., Price, D. L., Struble, R. G., Clark, A. W., Coyle, J. T. & Delong, M. R. (1982). Alzheimer's disease and senile dementia: loss of neurons in the basal forebrain. *Science*, *215*, 1237-1239.

Wong, T. P., Debeir, T., Duff, K. & Cuello, A. C. (1999). Reorganization of cholinergic terminals in the cerebral cortex and hippocampus in transgenic mice carrying mutated presenilin-1 and amyloid precursor protein transgenes. *J. Neurosci.*, *19*, 2706-2716.

Woodruff-Pak, D. S. & Papka, M. (1996). Alzheimer's disease and eyeblink conditioning: 750 ms trace vs. 400 ms delay paradigm. *Neurobiol. Aging*, *17*, 397-404.

Wu, C. -K., Thal, L., Pizzo, D., Hansen, L., Masliah, E. & Geula, C. (2005). Apoptotic signals within the basal forebrain cholinergic neurons in Alzheimer's disease. *Exp. Neurol.*, *195*, 484-496.

Xie, J., Chang, X., Zhang, X. & Guo, Q. (2001). Aberrant induction of Par-4 is involved in apoptosis of hippocampal neurons in presenilin-1 M146V mutant knock-in mice. *Brain Res.*, *915*, 1-10.

Yasuda, Y., Kudo, T., Katayama, T., Imaizumi, K., Yatera, M., Okochi, M., Yamamori, H., Matsumoto, N., Kida, T., Fukumori, A., Okumura, M., Tohyama, M. & Takeda, M. (2002). FAD-linked presenilin-1 mutants impede translation regulation under ER stress. *Biochem. Biophys. Res. Comm.*, *296,* 313-318.

Zaman, S. H., Parent, A., Laskey, A., Lee, M. K., Borchelt, D. R., Sisodia, S. S. & Manilow, R. (2000). Enhanced synaptic potentiation in transgenic mice expressing presenilin 1 familial Alzheimer's disease mutation is normalized with a benzodiazepine. *Neurobiol. Dis.*, *7*, 54-63.

Zhu, H., Guo, Q. & Mattson, M. P. (1999). Dietary restriction protects hippocampal neurons against the death-promoting action of presenilin-1 mutation. *Brain Res.*, *842*, 224-229.

In: Learning and Memory Developments…
Editors: L. C. Eklund, A. S. Nyman, pp. 255-269
ISBN: 978-1-60876-397-9

Chapter 12

ASSESSING ALERTNESS IN CHILDREN WITH PROFOUND INTELLECTUAL AND MULTIPLE DISABILITIES

Carla Vlaskamp and Vera Munde
University of Groningen, Department of Special Education.

ABSTRACT

Assessment of cognitive, motor, sensory, and communicative functions in children with profound intellectual and multiple disabilities (PIMD) is still in its infancy. There is a lack of standardized instruments, with the instruments mainly used being checklists and observation scales. Although these lists often fail to meet the requirements of validity and reliability, they nevertheless often prove a helpful tool to determine how the person involved can best be supported.

One very specific factor entailed in assessment that is related to the complexity and severity of their disabilities is the level of alertness in a child with PIMD. The assessors are often not sure when the "best moment" to start an assessment is. In addition, they are often unaware of which conditions can help provoke and maintain optimal alertness levels for assessment. Alertness, however, is not just a way to optimize the assessment process; it can also be the objective of the assessment process itself.

An observation list has been developed to assess the level of alertness in children with PIMD in order to 1. establish the optimal period or periods during the day to offer a stimulus or an activity; and 2. to establish the pattern of alertness in a child and the contextual influences on this pattern. In the chapter, the meaning of the concept 'alertness' will be discussed. Furthermore, a description of the content of the list and its use will be presented. For this list, inter-observer and intra-observer reliability were determined by comparing the scores of three (groups of) observers: teachers, an external observer who had received additional information about the clients, and an external observer who did not know the clients at all. The results of the reliability scores for 78 situations will be presented.

The observation list seems to be a functional and sensitive instrument that provides direct support staff with the opportunity to discern individual differences in alert moments and the impact that different stimuli have on alertness. This information can be useful in clinical practice.

1. Introduction

A key objective of assessment is to determine the progress a child is making either developmentally or with regard to the goals of parents and professionals. There is, however, a category of children for whom progress or development in the generally accepted sense is lacking. Children with profound intellectual and multiple disabilities (PIMD) certainly do progress as they get older, although not always towards goals that are generally seen as crucial or important in our society. Some children with PIMD even have such profound cerebral lesions that, based on neurological evidence, no functional adaptation is said to be possible (Robertson & Murre, 1999). On the other hand, most parents and most direct support persons (DSPs) believe firmly in the abilities of children with PIMD, even when these seem to run counter to clinical or educational assessment (Vlaskamp, 2005).

In this chapter, the characteristics of children with PIMD will be described in brief. The importance of alertness for making an assessment, both as a means and as an objective, will subsequently be explained. The implications of such a complex pattern of disabilities as PIMD entails for the assessment of alertness will be considered. We will then describe the content and use of an observation list that was developed in order to: 1) establish the optimal period or periods during the day to offer a stimulus; and 2) to establish the pattern of alertness and the contextual influences on this pattern. Results of the inter-observer reliability and intra-observer reliability of this list will be given, and its practical use will be illustrated by an example. Though the list seems sufficiently useful and reliable, its actual use may still be problematic. We will therefore conclude this chapter with some remarks on the use of this list in clinical practice.

2. Children with Profound Intellectual and Multiple Disabilities

A profound intellectual disability is almost always the consequence of neurological impairments arising from trauma or from genetic influences (Arvio & Sillanpää, 2003) that have implications for overall functioning. Central nervous system (CNS) damage results in profound intellectual disorders, severe or profound motor disorders (e.g., spastic quadriplegia), and in sensory disorders. Characteristically, children with PIMD will be at the preverbal stage of communication, though some will have limited spoken or signed expressive language, and limited communicative comprehension. Understanding of causality and space will be limited and adaptive: self-help abilities will be at a level where the support they require will be pervasive. Other consequences of such CNS damage are that most children with PIMD are wheelchair users, frequently have limited use of hands and arms, and have difficulties in maintaining postural balance. Both gross motor and fine motor functions, then, are profoundly disturbed. In fact, sensory impairments are common: recent studies show that at least 85% of people with profound intellectual disabilities experience visual impairments. In most cases these are caused by damage to the visual cortex in the occipital lobe (cortical blindness) (Evenhuis, Theunissen, Denkers, Verschuure, & Kemme, 2001; van Splunder, Stilma, Bernsen, & Evenhuis, 2006). Between 25% and 33% of children with profound intellectual disabilities have auditory impairments, but it is suspected that a substantial number of cases may actually remaine unidentified (Evenhuis et al., 2001). In addition, dysfunctions of taste and smell are relatively common (Bromley, 2000) but usually ignored. The tactile and coetaneous senses that include the receptors of touch, pressure, temperature, and pain are frequently thought to be impaired to some degree as well (Dunn, 1991; Oberlander, Gilbert, Chambers, O'Donnell, & Craig, 1999). In addition to the intellectual, motor, and sensory disabilities just noted, further concomitant impairments should also be mentioned as they, too, have significant implications for assessment. Extensive "additional" impairments include seizure disorders, chronic pulmonary infections, and skeletal deformations (e.g., Evenhuis et al., 2001; Hogg, 1992; Janicki & Dalton, 1998; van Splunder et al., 2006; Warburg, 2001; Woodhouse, Griffiths, & Gedling, 2000). Since each child with PIMD represents a unique configuration of abilities and constraints in regard to functioning, children with PIMD form a heterogeneous group in terms of central nervous system integrity, physical growth, development and behavioral repertoires (Zijlstra & Vlaskamp, 2005). Notwithstanding this huge diversity, children with PIMD are comparable in terms of the degree of profound intellectual, along with severe or profound motor disabilities, and may be considered as constituting the most disabled group of people in the populations of individuals with intellectual disabilities. They form a very vulnerable group with heavy or total dependence on personal assistance for their physical care, education, stimulation, and recreation.

3. Assessing Children with Profound Intellectual and Multiple Disabilities

Assessment of children with PIMD presents special challenges. Even though a child with PIMD cannot be understood as just a simple combination of assessment results for different impairments, it is still necessary to ascertain what his or her disabilities and potential entail so as to understand how these factors affect the overall functioning of the child (Vlaskamp, 2005). However, assessing intellectual, motor, or sensory functioning comes up against a wide range of barriers to conventional types of assessment that are quite feasible with more able individuals. These barriers are partly due to the multiplicity of the disabilities involved and because of the fact that each child with PIMD represents a unique configuration of abilities and constraints to functioning; however, the problem of assessment is also due to the fact that there are not many suitable designed instruments available (Vlaskamp, 2005). Since there are as yet insufficient research data relating to the way these profoundly disabled children develop (or can develop), it is indeed no an easy task to design and develop reliable and valid instruments. This lack of valid and reliable instruments for determining a child's abilities vis-à-vis on the various developmental domains is most likely what has contributed to the development of situation-based observation lists and the use of observations in everyday life situations. In cases such as these, hoewever, validity and reliability are often considered to be limited. To remedy this, formulating observation regulations and ascertaining targeted areas for observation prior to the start of the observation would be a good start. The reliability of the observations is determined not just by setting requirements for inter- and intra-assessment reliability. The inclusion or exclusion of environmental factors may also play a role in terms of factors such as the extent of the reliability of the direct staff, the occurrence of audible noises in the background during observation, the presence of other persons, and the position and posture of the child under observation (Lohrmann-O'Rourke & Browder, 1998). Moreover, children with PIMD may have specific, idiosyncratic thresholds for stimuli: some children react in a hypersensitive way and subsequently try to ignore certain stimuli or parts of stimuli while others may need very strong stimuli before they can actually respond. Selecting the focus and maintaining attention to sensory stimuli may be hampered. In addition, understanding behavioral responses is difficult because of the complexity of the behavior of children with PIMD. The same expression, sound, or movement may have different meanings in different situations (Grove, Bunning, Porter, & Olsson, 1999). Therefore, ascribing meaning to an behavior is at least partly based on the assessor's interpretation, which is a potential threat to reliability. To overcome this threat, some researchers use physiological reactions (e.g., muscle tone) or measurements of brain activity to study the reactions that children with PIMD are having to sensory stimuli (Chaney, Givens, Aoki, & Gombiner, 1989). However, these types of instruments are difficult to use in practice as they may be intrusive. Furthermore, one might question how practical such methods are, since specialized equipment and technicians are necessary to measure the children's physiological reactions and, even more importantly, since the results obtained in this way do not elucidate the meaning that the measured behavior actually has for the children themselves.

4. Alertness

As stated in the previous paragraph, we encounter a wide range of barriers to the conventional types of assessment that are feasible with more able individuals who lack these complex disabilities. One of the barriers that we may experience is timing. In children with PIMD, the focus on the environment is irregularl, and changes rapidly (Mudford, Hogg, & Roberts, 1997). Moreover, these short moments are often difficult to detect because of individual differences in how "being focused on the environment" is expressed. Based on these difficulties, we face recurring questions when assessing children in the target group. What is the best moment to assess the cognitive, motor, and sensory abilities of a child with PIMD? How can we determine this "best moment" and what is the duration of such a moment? Only if we know that the stimuli that are presented in the assessment are able to enter the consciousness of the child, can we expect the assessment to be unbiased (Nelson, van Dijk, McDonnell, & Thompson, 2002). Consequently, it is very important to take these "best moments" into account during the assessment, even though they may only lat for a short time.

Looking at the "best moments" more closely in the literature, we encounter various terms and descriptions (Munde, Vlaskamp, Ruijssenaars, & Nakken, 2009). Authors employ terms such as "behavior state", "alertness", "involvement" and "on-task behavior." From this, we see that mainly two types of descriptions can be found. One group of given terms is linked to the internal state of the individual that becomes manifest and visible in the individual's behavior. In contrast, other authors shift the focus from the individual alone to the individual in his or her environmental context. These authors emphasize interaction and engagement with the environment, which can then be observed on different levels with the highest level equaling "best moments." This differentiation aside, all the descriptions consider the "best moment" for individuals with PIMD to be observable through the individual's behavior.

Since the term "alertness" is the one most used in behavioral observations with individuals of the target group, we will be using this term in this chapter from here on out.

5. Observing Alertness

Since alertness is not only considered a precondition for assessment but an objective of it as well, a number of instruments for observing alertness in individuals with PIMD are presented in the literature (Munde et al., 2009). All the instruments are based on observations to detect the subtle alertness expressions of individuals with PIMD. Since the meaning of one signal may differ for different situations, DSPs need to register the behavior of their client and interpret the signal based on their knowledge about the client and the situation, all at the same time. Individual differences in expressions of alertness as well as contextual factors can, as a result, have an impact on the interpretations (Hogg, Reeves, Roberts, & Mudford, 2001). Because the subjectivity of the interpretations is a potential threat to validity and reliability (Vlaskamp, 2005), physiological measurements might be considered as possible alternatives. However, these do not reveal detailed information about the complex behavior of individuals in this target group, while at the same time it is observation that is the most obvious method for determining alertness in individuals in the target group (Mudford et al., 1997; Vlaskamp & Cuppen-Fonteine, 2007).

The instruments described in the literature differ in the number of alertness levels they measure (Munde et al., 2009). This said, the observation system of Guess and his colleagues (1993) can be described as the standard scale. Nine alertness levels are differentiated here: Asleep-Inactive, Asleep-Active, Drowsy, Daze, Awake Inactive-Alert, Awake Active-Alert, Awake-Active/Stereotypy, Crying/Agitated, and Seizures. In other studies, authors have modified this scale and used a different number of levels with the number of levels for these analyses always reduced to a maximum of six (e.g., Mudford et al., 1997). In determining the number of observation levels, several authors have discussed the position of self-injuring behavior. Whereas Woodyatt and colleagues (2004) expect this behavior to occur in all states, Siegel-Causey and Bashinski (1997) classify self-injurious behavior as a form of communication, not as an alertness level.

Scoring is another aspect of alertness observation in individuals with PIMD that is discussed in the studies mentioned above. Two problems have been described in the literature: the frequency with which observations are measured, and whether or not to include the context in the observations. As for the frequency, various authors mention that in order to register the quick changes and reveal the maximum amount of information, short scoring intervals or continuous scoring would seem to be necessary (Mudford et al., 1997). For continuous observations, hand-held registration systems may be used: these allow for a new score after a three-second minimum (Guess, Roberts, & Rues, 2002; Mellstrom, Saunders, Saunders, & Olswang, 2005). However, since continuous scoring is time-consuming and registration systems are expensive, most studies use interval scoring with ten-second intervals (e.g., Arthur, 2004; Belfiore, Browder, & Mace, 1993; Lancioni, O'Reilly, & Mantini, 1999). For scoring in real time, these intervals of observations are alternated with ten-second intervals for scoring the behavior (Arthur, 2004; Parsons, Rollyson, & Reid, 2004). To prevent information loss, other authors first videotape the situations. Then, in a second step, they looked at the tapes for intervals of ten seconds and stop the videotapes for scoring (Guess et al., 2002; Guess et al., 1993). The size and impact of loss of information when interval scores are used instead of continuous scores is, as yet, unclear. Even more important is the fact that continuous scoring is just about impossible to realize in clinical practice. Observations are very time-consuming (Petry & Maes, 2006) and continuous scoring is found to be difficult to integrate into daily routines.

The second problem is related to the context. Contextual information will influence observational judgments. Although the context does not seem to have an influence on the judgment per se, expectations and experiences about the way context might influence things can make the observers' judgment more extreme (Hogg et al., 2001). As a result, when the client is not expected to appreciate the situation, DSPs tend to interpret the expressions more negatively. In addition, scoring of the context is itself another challenge. In real-time observations, registration of behavior and context at the same time is only possible by employing two observers. For observations with only one observer, videotapes can solve the problem of information loss. Observers can then register behavior the first time they look at the videotapes and note contextual factors the second time (Arthur, 2004; Guess et al., 1993). However, obtaining observations in this way is again difficult to carry out in clinical practice.

Taking both thse problems into account, it is clear that to be able to attune to the client's "best moment", practice requires an instrument that is, on the one hand, easy to use and not too time consuming, while being reliable on the other.

6. The Alertness Observation List

Analogously, just as an assessor can conduct the assessment optimally when the child is alert, DSPs are better off beginning an activity when the child with PIMD is most likely to be susceptible to the stimulus (Arthur-Kelly, Bochner, Center, & Mok, 2007; Richards & Richards, 1997). In general, DSPs offer stimuli in order to promote learning and development in their clients. However, timing and the choice of stimulus are recurrent issues in the care for children in this target group.

Based on the need of DSPs to be able todetermine the "best moment" to begin an activity, Vlaskamp, Fonteine and Tadema (2005) developed the Alertness Observation List (AOL). This list was developed for use by DSPs and its aim is to formulate an individual alertness profile in five steps.

As part of step one, and before actually starting the observations, DSPs need to decide whether or not the day agreed upon for observation is a representative day for the child with PIMD. Only if the child is "feeling good" (e.g,. has not had any seizures prior to the observation) and has not received any unusual medication may observations reveal a representative picture of alertness. When the first step reveals that the selected day is an "ordinary" day for the client who is to be observed, the agreed-upon observation can then take place. For this second step, alertness levels are noted every fiteen minutes in order to determine the best moment in terms of alertness during the day. The first and second steps require three days to be carried out, which translates as not necessarily three days in a row but as at least within a one-week period. In the next two steps (3 and 4), the relationship between an activity and alertness is determined. Based on the previous observations, the best moment in terms of alertness during the day is determined. At that selected "best moment", the DSP then offers a stimulus to the child with PIMD. In this way, we are able to distinguish between three sorts of stimuli: visual, auditory, and tactile, although combinations of these three are also possible. When offering the stimulus, DSPs need to take into account the following. Only if the stimulus is considered to have an impact on the alertness of this particular child with PIMD, can we expect to see changes. Consequently, the choice of a stimulus has to be made based on the child's preferences and reactions. Additionally, DSPs are advised to take their time when offering the stimulus. Since children with PIMD often process information in a different way, it is especially important that DSPs act in accordance with the speed of their clients. Furthermore, an explicit description of the stimulus presented is necessary on the scoring form. Based on observations before, during, and after offering a stimulus, changes due to that stimulus can be recognized. As a result, scoring frequency will increase. Whereas alertness levels are noted every five minutes in Step 3, scores have to be noted every twenty seconds in Step 4. Finally, all observations then need to be summarized in an individual alertness profile (Step 5). During all of the observations, alertness is assumed to occur on four different levels: alert, drowsy, asleep, and agitated. For scoring purposes, every alertness level is associated with a color: green, orange, and red, respectively. To include the frequently occurring self-injuring behavior of children with PIMD, blue has been added as a fourth color. In the alertness profile, individual behaviors and reactions that are associated with the four alertness levels are described.

Before introducing the Alertness Observation List into clinical practice, its psychometric quality was investigated. The instrument was used in a children's special educational center, with a focus on establishing its reliability. In only five cases, were we able to determine sufficient reliability (kappa = .60) (Petitiaux, Elsinga, Cuppen-Fonteine, & Vlaskamp, 2006). We therefore decided to try to calculate the reliability for a larger sample (Munde, Vlaskamp, Ruijssenaars & Nakken, in press). A Dutch school for special education volunteered to use the list. Four classes were chosen at random and all 23 children in these four classes were included in the study. The observation list was completed for the children and observations of the fourth form were videotaped. Because a number of the videotapes were of low quality, they had to be excluded. A pool of 120 situations remained. Out of this pool, we chose 39 situations in order to calculate the inter-observer reliability. For another 39 situations, we determined the intra-observer reliability. Moreover, three (groups of) observers were involved in the study: the teachers, an external observer who received additional information about the children, and an external observer who was not familiar with the children at all. Reliability was calculated by employing the overall agreement formula: agreement/ disagreement+ agreement)*100. A criterion of 80% was applied (Mudford et al., 1997).

Based on the scores of the fourth form, the reliability of the observation list was then estimated. Calculations resulted in an inter- observer reliability of 81% (*Mdn* = 81,44; *M* = 81,46; *SD* = 13,88). The intra- observer reliability was 87% (*Mdn* = 86,79; *M* = 85,23; *SD* = 11.,75). Ddetailed results can be found in Tables 1 and 2.

Table 1. Results for inter-observer reliability

	T and E+	T and E-	E+ and E-	
	83,33	50,00	83,33	
	75,00	75,00	80,00	
	87,50	70,83	86,67	
	75,17	79,17	75,86	
	80,00	83,33	93,33	
	100,00	91,67	100,00	
	75,00	100,00	50,00	
	62,50	100,00	64,86	
	100,00	87,50	81,82	
	87,50	91,67	94,74	
	62,50	79,16	64,44	
	100,00	66,67	100,00	
	87,50	75,00	76,00	TOTAL
M	*82,77*	*80,77*	*80,85*	81,46
Mdn	*83,33*	*79,17*	*81,82*	81,44
SD	*12,80*	*13,98*	*14,86*	13,88

Note. The letters refer to the different (groups of) observers. Teachers are "T", the external observer who received additional information about the children is "E+" and the external observer who did not know the children at all is "E-."

Table 2. Results for intra-observer reliability

	T	E+	E-	
	70,83	95,83	91,07	
	70,83	66,67	96,77	
	91,67	76,67	63,64	
	100,00	93,10	72,88	
	79,17	93,55	95,16	
	83,33	100,00	82,98	
	70,83	88,89	100,00	
	70,83	61,11	90,48	
	100,00	87,10	91,53	
	70,83	78,95	86,05	
	100,00	86,36	97,73	
	91,67	100,00	86,84	
	83,33	85,00	72,22	TOTAL
M	*83,33*	*85,63*	*86,72*	85,23
Mdn	*83,33*	*87,10*	*90,48*	86,97
SD	*12,15*	*12,02*	*11,09*	11,75

Note. The letters refer to the different (groups of) observers. Teachers are "T", the external observer who received additional information about the children is "E+" and the external observer who did not know the children at all is "E-."

Because the results exceed the formulated criterion, we may conclude that the Alertness Observation List reveals reliable information for determining alertness in children with PIMD. But, besides this general result, the data show additional information. One striking fact is the differences in reliability scores for the different (groups of) observers. Calculations of the inter-observer reliability revealed higher percentages for those observers who had more information about the children, while intra-observer reliability was higher for the observer who did not know the children at all. These differences in results may be explained as follows. Firstl, as research shows, proxies tend to be influenced in their judgment by their knowledge and daily experiences (Hogg, Cavet, Lambe, & Smeddle, 2001; Swennenhuis, Vermeer, Rispens, Teunissen, & Wensing, 2004). When they are in doubt about the correct interpretation of the child's behavior, they may decide differently based on a recent experience with their client. In contrast, external observers, lacking this type of additional information, only judge based on visible behavior. This consequently leads to more consistent scores. Secondl, observations of children who remain in the same alertness state for a prolonged period of time were scored with a higher reliability. Total agreement was reached when the children observed were clearly focused on their environment for the entire session. Most children, however, showed frequent changes in alertness levels. As a result, changes between alert and drowsy states especially aggravated alertness observations, because expressions of these alertness levels are difficult to differentiate for some children with PIMD. We may therefore conclude that a large number of quick changes in alertness level will complicate the task of DSPs in making reliable observations as suggested previously by Guess and colleagues (2002) and Mudford, Hogg and Roberts (1997). Third, low reliability scores can be linked to the heterogeneity of the target group. Consequently, the ability of an individual to show a clear focus of the eyes and control over his or her own movement are the main influencing factors. It is far more difficult to give a reliable score about the level of alertness of individuals with visual impairments, since these individuals will not always show their focus on the environment by means of fixing on it with the eyes. Additionally, severe spasticity and difficulties in directing the movements towards the stimuli presented may be interpreted as low alertness or incapacity to control the body movements.

The results of our study underscore the complexity of alertness observations in individuals with PIMD. To clarify the issues discussed above, the alertness observations of a girl called Emily will be described in the following section. First, we will introduce Emily as well as the questions DSPs have concerning Emily's alertness. Then, the results of the Alertness Observation List for Emily will be presented. Finally, results of observations will be linked back to the DSPs' questions concerning the alertness of Emily.

An example: Emily

Emily is a ten-year-old girl with profound intellectual and multiple disabilities. She has attended a special education center from the age of three. Emily has a friendly and outgoing nature, but for quite some time now, Emily has had periods in which she is rather withdrawn. In addition, during these withdrawn periods, Emily has crying fits, apparently without any clear cause. These periods have increased in number and duration in the past six months. DSPs feel ambiguous about what the most appropriate reaction towards this behavior should be. On the one hand, they think that it is better to "let her be" when she apparently feels uncomfortable; on the other hand, they would like to keep offering a balanced educational program that supports and stimulates Emily's development. A central issue in this balanced educational program is the optimal moment for stimulation.

Active, focused on the environment (green)	Concrete examples of behavior:
Emily is mainly active and focused on her environment in the morning. Because of low vision, she shows activity by listening and touching. Her strongest reactions are to tactile stimuli. *Emily is mainly focused on the DSPs. When you stay close to her and do not interrupt tactile contact with her, she can keep her focus for about 1 to 5 minutes per activity.*	*Emily turns her face to the soun;, her eyes are open; she is smiling permanently. She produces sounds when you touch her. At the same time, she tries to touch you back. Emily clamps objects and touches them.*
Inactive, withdrawn (orange)	Concrete examples of behavior:
Emily is mainly inactive and withdrawn after mealtimes or after other activitie, such as physiotherapy. This condition can then last for long periods.	*Emily is focused on her hands; she fiddles and plucks. She picks at her clothing,(using her thumb and index finger), sucks her thumb, makes humming noises, and rubs her eyes.*
Sleeping, drowsy (red)	Concrete examples of behavior:
Emily does not fall asleep during the day. You can only see periods of drowsiness following therapy sessions or group activities.	*Emily sits very quietly; her eyes open and close slowly and repeatedly.*
Agitated, discontented (blue)	Concrete examples of behavior:
Emily sometimes bursts out crying when things are overstraiings her. Crying fits mainly occur in the afternoon.	*Emily cries in long exhalation of breath, but without tears. When you do not give her your immediate attention, she starts biting on the palm of her hand.*

Figure 1. Form D – the "traffic light" **Name:** *Emily*

To determine such an optimal moment, the Alertness Observation List was completed. Form A was filled in twice: a day before the observations and just before the observations. This form showed that Emily was not ill, nor was she unusually passive or active, it also showed that she wasn't in an unusual environment, that there had been no change in medication and that she had not had any unusual epileptic activities prior to the observations. With Form B, DSPs searched for alertness patterns that Emily normally shows. The DSPs observed Emily over a period of three whole days. From the observations it became clear that Emily's best time of day was the morning, and that she was most alert between nine and ten o'clock. Except for lunch, Emily was in the orange and red level for the remainder of the day. With Form C, a DSP offered Emily a preferred activity, and assessed Emily's level of alertness every five minutes for ten minutes. Before and after the activity, the DSP scored her for another fifteen minutes, giving a score every five minutes. The observations show that after about five minutes of the activity, Emily's alertness decreased from green to orange level. Observing Emily's reacties to an activity every twenty seconds during five minutes (with Form D) showed quick changes from being active and focused on the environment to being inactive and withdrawn during the five minutes When an activity was being offered. Additionally, observations with both forms showed that Emily became drowsy after the activity. The information that resulted from the observations of the Alertness Observation List was summarized in a "traffic light" for Emily (see Figure 1).

Based on the "traffic light", DSPs made a number of decisions about Emily's program. All activities were now planned for the morning and activities were presented for a short period (about five minutes). Moments of rest were planned between two activities (again of about five minutes). During the afternoon, DSPs created periods of sufficient rest for Emily. Therapy sessions were planned in the afternoon, and such sessions were followed by a period of rest. In a subsequent step, DSPs were able to evaluate Emily's reactions to her new schedule and were then able to make an attempt at trying to prolong the duration of Emily's alert periods.

7. Conclusion

The results of our study and the example given above show that the Alertness Observation List is a reliable instrument and one which may serve as a starting point in any further understanding of alertness. For example, does starting an activity when the child is in an alert state lead to more preferable reactions than using an activity to make the child alert? Which aspect of the activity evokes changes in alertness levels? Do children with PIMD react because of the stimulus itself, because of the interaction with the DSP, or because of something else, some unknown factor? In several studies, a number of factors that were expected to have an impact on alertness were included in the observations themselves (Arthur, 2004; Guess, Roberts, & Guy, 1999; Vlaskamp, de Geeter, Huijsmans, & Smit, 2003). These can be summarized as being aspects of the interaction, the activity, and the setting. Whereas interaction is described as a general precondition for increasing alertness, individually the frequency, type, and content of the activity can have a different impact (Guess et al., 1999). Settings with a limited number of stimuli have been found to lead to higher alertness levels in general terms (Belfiore et al., 1993; Green, Gardner, Canipe, & Reid, 1994). Even if all studies, including ours, were carried out for a relatively small number of participants with large individual differences involved in this target group, they still are important in terms of a better understanding of the meaning of contextual influence on individual alertness levels.

The use of the Alertness Observation List in clinical practice represents a challenge for DSPs. They act as proxies, while the literature yields conflicting results concerning the value of using a proxy approach. Several researchers have attempted to evaluate the consumer-proxy agreement by comparing the proxy responses concerning people who are able to respond for themselves with self-reports from the same people. In some of these studies that concern aspects of quality of life, the answers given strongly disagreed with one another (Cummins, 2002; Stancliffe, 2000); others found greater concordance (McVilly, Burton-Smith, & Davidson, 2000; Stancliffe, 1999). Though the use of proxies may negatively influence validity, the fact remains that children with PIMD are unable to speak for themselves directly. Indirectly, the use of the Alertness Observation List enables children with PIMD to speak out: when the results of the Alertness Observation List are valid, and children are offered appropriate stimuli at an appropriate time, the child with PIMD will show its validity to us by being alert.

REFERENCES

Arthur, M. (2004). Patterns amongst behavior states, sociocommunicative, and activity variables in educational programs for students with profound and multiple disabilities. *Journal of Developmental and Physical Disabilities, 16,* 125-149.

Arthur-Kelly, M., Bochner, S., Center, Y., & Mok, M. (2007). Socio-communicative perspectives on research and evidence-based practice in the education of students with profound and multiple disabilities. *Journal of Developmental and Physical Disabilities, 19,* 161-176.

Arvio, M. & Sillanpää, M. (2003). Prevalence, etiology and comorbidity of severe and profound intellectual disability in Finland. *Journal of Intellectual Disability Research, 47,* 108-112.

Belfiore, P. J., Browder, D. M., & Mace, F. C. (1993). Effects of community and center-based settings on the alertness of persons with profound mental retardation. *Journal of Applied Behavior Analysis, 26,* 401-402.

Bromley, S. M. (2000). Smell and taste disorders: A primary care approach. *American Familiy Physician, 61,* 427-436.

Chaney, R. H., Givens, C. A., Aoki, M. F., & Gombiner, M. L. (1989). Pupillary Responses in Recognizing Awareness in Persons with Profound Mental-Retardation. *Perceptual and Motor Skills, 69,* 523-528.

Cummins, R. A. (2002). Proxy responding for subjective well-being: A review. In L.M.Glidden & L. M. Glidden (Eds.), *International review of research in mental retardation, Vol. 25* (183-207). San Diego, CA US: Academic Press.

Dunn, W. (1991). The sensorimotor systems: A framework for assessment and intervention. In *Educating children with multiple disabilities: A transdisciplinary approach (2nd ed.)* (33-78). Baltimore, MD US: Paul H Brookes Publishing.

Evenhuis, H. M., Theunissen, M., Denkers, I., Verschuure, H., & Kemme, H. (2001). Prevalence of visual and hearing impairment in a Dutch institutionalized population with intellectual disability. *Journal of Intellectual Disability Research, 45,* 457-464.

Green, C. W., Gardner, S. M., Canipe, V. S., & Reid, D. H. (1994). Analyzing alertness among people with profound multiple disabilites: Implications for provision of training. *Journal of Applied Behavior Analysis, 27,* 519-531.

Grove, N., Bunning, K., Porter, J., & Olsson, C. (1999). See what I mean: Interpreting the meaning of communication by people with severe and profound intellectual disabilities. *Journal of Applied Research in Intellectual Disabilities, 12,* 190-203.

Guess, D., Roberts, S., & Guy, B. (1999). Implications of behavior state for the assessment and education of students with profound disabilities. In A.C.Repp & R. H. Horner (Eds.), *Functional analysis of problem behavior – from effective assessment to effective support* (338-394). Belmont: Wadsworth.

Guess, D., Roberts, S., Siegel-Causey, E., Ault, M., Guy, B., & Thompson, B. (1993). Analysis of Behavior State Conditions and Associated Environmental Variables among Students with Profound Handicaps. *American Journal on Mental Retardation, 97,* 634-653.

Guess, D., Roberts, S., & Rues, J. (2002). Longitudinal analysis of state patterns and related variables among infants and children with significant disabilities. *Research and Practice for Persons with Severe Disabilities, 27,* 112-124.

Hogg, J. (1992). The administration of psychotropic and anticonvulsant drugs to children with profound intellectual disability and multiple impairments. *Journal of Intellectual Disability Research, 36,* 473-488.

Hogg, J., Cavet, J., Lambe, L., & Smeddle, M. (2001). The use of 'Snoezelen' as multisensory stimulation with people with intellectual disabilities: A review of the research. *Research in Developmental Disabilities, 22,* 353-372.

Hogg, J., Reeves, D., Roberts, J., & Mudford, O. C. (2001). Consistency, context and confidence in judgements of affective communication in adults with profound intellectual and multiple disabilities. *Journal of Intellectual Disability Research, 45,* 18-29.

Janicki, M. P. & Dalton, A. J. (1998). Sensory impairments among older adults with intellectual disability. *Journal of Intellectual & Developmental Disability, 23,* 3-11.

Lancioni, G. E., O'Reilly, M. F., & Mantini, M. (1999). Activity arrangements with or without mobility and performance of persons with profound multiple disabilities over long sessions. *Irish Journal of Psychology, 20,* 124-135.

Lohrmann-O'Rourke, S. & Browder, D. M. (1998). Empirically based methods to assess the preferences of individuals with severe disabilities. *American Journal on Mental Retardation, 103,* 146-161.

McVilly, K. R., Burton-Smith, R. M., & Davidson, J. A. (2000). Concurrence between subject and proxy ratings of quality of life for people with and without intellectual disabilities. *Journal of Intellectual & Developmental Disability, 25,* 19-39.

Mellstrom, B. P., Saunders, M. D., Saunders, R. R., & Olswang, L. B. (2005). Interaction of Behavioral State and Microswitch Use in Individuals with Profound Multiple Impairments. *Journal of Developmental and Physical Disabilities, 17,* 35-53.

Mudford, O. C., Hogg, J., & Roberts, J. (1997). Interobserver agreement and disagreement in continuous recording exemplified by measurement of behavior state. *American Journal on Mental Retardation, 102,* 54-66.

Munde, V. S., Vlaskamp, C., Ruijssenaars, A. J. J. M., & Nakken, H. (2009). Alertness in individuals with profound intellectual and multiple disabilities: a literature review. *Research in Developmental Disabilities, 30,* 462-480.

Munde, V. S., Vlaskamp, C., Ruijssenaars, A. J. J. M., & Nakken, H. (in press). Determining alertness in individuals with profound intellectual and multiple disabilities: the reliability of an observation list. *Education and Training in Developmental Disabilities.*

Nelson, C., van Dijk, J., McDonnell, A. P., & Thompson, K. (2002). A framework for understanding young children with severe multiple disabilities: The van Dijk approach to assessment. *Research and Practice for Persons with Severe Disabilities, 27,* 97-111.

Oberlander, T. F., Gilbert, C. A., Chambers, C. T., O'Donnell, M. E., & Craig, K. D. (1999). Biobehavioral responses to acute pain in adolescents with a significant neurologic impairment. *Clinical Journal of Pain, 15,* 201-209.

Parsons, M. B., Rollyson, J. H., & Reid, D. H. (2004). Improving day-treatment services for adults with severe disabilities: A norm-referenced application of outcome management. *Journal of Applied Behavior Analysis, 37,* 365-377.

Petitiaux, W. S. D., Elsinga, G. M., Cuppen-Fonteine, H., & Vlaskamp, C. (2006). Alertheid van kinderen met ernstige verstandelijke en meervoudige beperkingen: een casestudy. [Alertness in children with profound intellectual and multiple disabilities: a case study]. *NTZ, 32,* 241-254.

Petry, K. & Maes, B. (2006). Identifying expressions of pleasure and displeasure by persons with profound and multiple disabilities. *Journal of Intellectual & Developmental Disability, 31,* 28-38.

Richards, S. B. & Richards, R. Y. (1997). Implications for assessing biobehavioral states in individuals with profound disabilities. *Focus on Autism and Other Developmental Disabilities, 12,* 79-86.

Robertson, I. H. & Murre, J. M. J. (1999). Rehabilitation of brain damage: Brain plasticity and principles of guided recovery. *Psychological Bulletin, 125,* 544-575.

Siegel-Causey, E. & Bashinski, S. M. (1997). Enhancing initial communication and responsiveness of learners with multiple disabilities: A tri-focus framework for partners. *Focus on Autism and Other Developmental Disabilities, 12,* 105-120.

Stancliffe, R. J. (1999). Proxy respondents and the reliability of the Quality of Life Questionnaire Empowerment factor. *Journal of Intellectual Disability Research, 43,* 185-193.

Stancliffe, R. J. (2000). Proxy respondents and quality of life. *Evaluation and Program Planning, 23,* 89-93.

Swennenhuis, P., Vermeer, A., Rispens, J., Teunissen, J., & Wensing, M. (2004). Quality of the care process for children with intellectual disabilities: A Delphi study. *European Journal of Special Needs Education, 19,* 241-253.

van Splunder, J., Stilma, J. S., Bernsen, R. M. D., & Evenhuis, H. M. (2006). Prevalence of visual impairment in adults with intellectual disabilities in the Netherlands: cross-sectional study. *Eye, 20,* 1004-1010.

Vlaskamp, C. (2005). Assessing people with profound intellectual and multiple disabilities. In J.Hogg & A. Langa (Eds.), *Assessing adults with intellectual disability: A service provider's guide* (Oxford: Blackwell Publishers.

Vlaskamp, C. & Cuppen-Fonteine, H. (2007). Reliability of assessing the sensory perception of children with profound intellectual and multiple disabilities: A case study. *Child: Care, Health and Development, 33,* 547-551.

Vlaskamp, C., Fonteine, H., & Tadema, A. (2005). *Manual of the list 'Alertness in children with profound intellectual and multiple disabilities'. [Handleiding bij de lijst 'Alertheid van kinderen met zeer ernstige verstandelijke en meervoudige beperkingen].* Groningen: Stichting Kinderstudies.

Vlaskamp, C., de Geeter, K. I., Huijsmans, L. M., & Smit, I. H. (2003). Passive Activities: the Effectiveness of Multisensory Environments on the Level of Activity of Individuals with Profound Multiple Disabilities. *Journal of Applied Research in Intellectual Disabilities, 16,* 135-143.

Warburg, M. (2001). Assessment of visual acuity. *Journal of Intellectual Disability Research, 45,* 424-438.

Woodhouse, J. M., Griffiths, C., & Gedling, A. (2000). The prevalence of ocular defects and the provision of eye care in adults with learning disabilities living in the community. *Ophtalmic Physiology and Optics, 20,* 79-89.

Woodyatt, G., Marinac, J., Darnell, R., Sigafoos, J., & Halle, J. (2004). Behaviour State Analysis in Rett Syndrome: Continuous data reliability measurement. *International Journal of Disability, Development and Education, 51,* 383-400.

Zijlstra, H. P. & Vlaskamp, C. (2005). The Impact of Medical Conditions on the Support of Children with Profound Intellectual and Multiple Disabilities. *Journal of Applied Research in Intellectual Disabilities, 18,* 151-161.

In: Learning and Memory Developments...
Editors: L. C. Eklund, A. S. Nyman, pp. 271-282
ISBN: 978-1-60876-397-9

Chapter 13

ASSESSMENT OF TIME PROCESSING ABILITY AND DAILY TIME MANAGEMENT IN CHILDREN WITH AND WITHOUT DEVELOPMENTAL DISABILITIES

***Gunnel Janeslätt* [1, 3*]*, Mats Granlund*[1,4] *and Anders Kottorp*[2]**
[1]School of Health, Care and Social Welfare, Mälardalen University, Västerås, Sweden.
[2]Department NVS, Division of Occupational Therapy, Karolinska Institutet, Huddinge, Sweden.
[3*]Centre for Clinical Research Dalarna, Nissers väg 3, SE-791 82 Falun, Sweden.
[4]School of Health sciences, Jönköping University, Jönköping, Sweden.

ABSTRACT

In the time-dependent society of today, those with limited ability to manage time will show a heightened dependence on others and more need for support, exacerbating their vulnerability. Children with developmental disorders e.g. intellectual disabilities or Autism Spectrum Disorders are reported to have problems in time perception, time orientation or time management, in this chapter all related to the suggested overarching concept: *time processing ability* (TPA). The aim of this short communication is to present a currently developed innovative assessment of TPA and its relation to daily time management (TM) in children with and without developmental disabilities, including intellectual disabilities. The new assessment of TPA; **K**it for **a**ssessing **Ti**me processing ability (KaTid) for children was based on current knowledge of information processing in children with cognitive disabilities e.g. using iconic symbols and concrete concepts. Using modern test statistics (Rasch analysis), the evaluation of the KaTid and a related Parent scale for estimating the daily TM presented acceptable psychometric properties. The results indicate that the items in KaTid, initially defined as time perception, time orientation and time management, all empirically support a potential uni-dimensional construct, TPA. In this TPA construct, time perception, time orientation and time management can be seen as different levels of complexity rather than as separate constructs. The Parent scale of daily TM also demonstrated acceptable psychometric properties. There is a relation between the parents' ratings of a child's daily TM and TPA in children with developmental disabilities. Thus TPA seems to be a factor related to children's daily TM that needs to be taken into consideration when planning and evaluating interventions designed to facilitate everyday functioning for children with ID. This is a step towards providing evidence-based instruments that, together with other information, can help the professional in structuring the intervention *planning* process for children with difficulties in daily TM.

INTRODUCTION

In the time-dependent society of today, those with limited ability to manage time will show a heightened dependence on others and more need for support, exacerbating their inferior role and vulnerability. Children with developmental disabilities, e.g. autism or intellectual disability (ID), are often reported to have problems in understanding and managing time. People with ID have demonstrated problems in time orientation [Arvidsson & Jonsson, 2006; Owen & Wilson, 2006] and in time management (Davies, Stock, & Wehmeyer, 2002; Granlund, Bond, Lindstöm, & Wennberg, 1995], yet the knowledge base in the area is scarce [Owen & Wilson, 2006; Sharp, Murray, McKenzie, Quigley, & Patrick, 2001]. Children with Autism Spectrum Disorders (ASD) and children with Attention Deficit Hyperactivity Disorder (ADHD) have been reported to exhibit problems in time perception/time sense as compared to typically developing (TD) children [Barkley, Murphy, & Bush, 2001; Peeters & Gillberg, 1999; Smith, Taylor, Rogers, Newman, & Rubia, 2002; Szelag, Kowalska, Galkowski, & Poppel, 2004]. Children and adolescents with ASD were found to have abnormal temporal processing of auditive and visual stimuli [Bebko, Weiss, Demark, & Gomez, 2006; Groen, et al., 2009] and difficulties in sequencing events [Boucher, Pons, Lind, & Williams, 2007]. Time sense deficit is suggested to contribute to difficulties in fulfilling a task within a given time period. Children with ADHD act as if they have more time available than they actually do, perceiving waiting time as long compared to TD children. They are therefore less likely than their peers to be on time for an appointment [Barkley, 1997]. Among persons with physical disabilities e.g. Myelomeningocele (MMC) cognitive impairments have frequently been reported, including impairments in *planning* and executive functions [Hunt & Oakeshott, 2003; Hunt, Oakeshott, & Kerry, 1999] as well as in perceptual and non-verbal abilities [Lindquist, Carlsson, Persson, & Uvebrant, 2005]. Impaired executive planning functions were also found in young people with autism [Hughes, Russel, & Robbins, 1994]. As individuals within all diagnoses presented were reported to demonstrate difficulties in time perception, time orientation and/or time management, a new assessment should include items measuring all three aspects. In recent research they are all part of the suggested overarching *time processing ability* (TPA) and related to problems in daily time management (TM) [Janeslätt, Granlund, Alderman, & Kottorp, 2008]. There is need for improvement in the clinical methods for planning and evaluating interventions designed to facilitate time management in daily life for children with developmental disabilities. A systematic assessment of TPA in children could increase knowledge in this area, generating evidence in methods for assessment and intervention. The aim of this chapter is to present a short communication on a currently developed innovative assessment of TPA and its relation to daily TM in children with and without developmental disabilities.

The first step in creating a new assessment is to formulate the purpose of the tool [Coster, 1997; Miller, 1989]. Our initial purpose was to develop an assessment to collect information needed for planning and evaluating the effects of interventions (including time aids) in children. One initial problem was to find a valid base for the new assessment, due to the lack of consensus surrounding concepts and definitions [Christiansen, 2005]. The International Classification of Functioning, Disability and Health - Children and Youth (ICF-CY)[WHO, 2007] was recommended for use as an integrated system to clarify constructs, and to improve communication and coordination of health services for children and young people [Lollar & Simeonsson, 2005]. In response to this need, an assessment was developed by the author and a colleague: **K**it for **a**ssessing **Ti**me processing ability in children (KaTid) [Sw. **K**artläggning **av Tid**suppfattning hos barn] using a method described by Benson and Clark [1982]. It was based on time related concepts defined in ICF-CY[WHO, 2007]. In the next section, the operational definition of each construct or function to be measured will be presented. The key concepts are: time perception, time orientation and time management, TPA, and functioning in everyday life, daily TM.

The Construct Measured, Definitions

Time Perception

Time perception is defined in ICF-CY as the experience of time, comprising the specific mental functions of subjective experiences related to the length and passage of time. These are part of the specific mental functions related to the awareness of one's identity, body, position in reality, environment and of time [WHO, 2001, 2007]. Time perception was chosen as the term for this construct. It is commonly used for research on time sense e.g. interval timing, and on experience of time. Time perception also includes the perceived duration of activities.

Time Orientation

Time orientation is defined in ICF-CY as Orientation to time, comprising the mental functions that produce awareness of today, tomorrow, yesterday, date, month and year [WHO, 2001, 2007]. It includes concepts of time units (day, month etc), frequency ("How often?") and sequence e.g. knowing the temporal order of activities in a morning routine. Other aspects of time orientation are our awareness of and ability to understand physical time and our location in time [W. J. Friedman, 1990; Levin, Wilkening, & Dembo, 1984; Piaget, 2006]. In this chapter time orientation includes units, frequency, sequence and location in time, quantification, awareness of physical time and telling the time from a clock.

Time Management

Time management is a super-ordinate concept, part of higher-level cognitive functions, also named executive functions. Time management is used to describe the mental function of ordering events in chronological sequence and allocating amounts of time to events and activities [WHO, 2001, 2007]. Time management is also referred to as the ability to know what tasks to do, when to do them and for how long e.g. to judge which activity to do in a set period of time [Davies, et al., 2002].

Everyday performance in a person's life is based on the ability to perceive and evaluate time information and the ability to use/process it e.g. 1) to collect information from my diary to know when the next event takes place, 2) what time is it now? 3) how long time do I have at my disposal until that next event and 4) what will I have time to do in that period? For this last step of information processing I need to know how long each activity normally takes, the duration of daily activities.

Time Processing Ability (TPA)

Time Processing Ability, TPA, is the concept chosen to define the product of the three concepts or subcategories of time, in this chapter named subcategories; Time Perception, Time Orientation and Time Management [Janeslätt, et al., 2008].

Daily Time Management (TM)

Children's actual performance in everyday life situations related to time is termed as daily TM in this chapter. This is considered equivalent to *Managing one's time*, defined as managing the time required to complete usual or specific activities, such as preparing to depart from the home [WHO 2007]. Daily TM is an important aspect of autonomy. Individuals need to manage time to be able to plan and execute actions in relation to personal goals and environmental demands. In other words, they must manage time in order to exhibit autonomous behaviour [Arvidsson & Jonsson, 2006; Davies, et al., 2002].

INSTRUMENTS

How to Measure TPA

Because there was a need for a tool for assessing TPA and daily TM in children, existing assessments for measuring cognitive functions in children were reviewed. No assessments solely focused on daily TM, were found, nor any validated assessment measuring the three subcategories of time perception, time orientation or time management in children. In some of the existing assessments single items were identified as assessing isolated functions within one or two categories of TPA [Janeslätt, et al., 2008].

The development of testing procedures in the new assessment of TPA for children, KaTid, was based on current knowledge of information processing in children with cognitive disabilities e.g. using iconic symbols and concrete concepts. KaTid was validated using data from children with (*n*=118) [Janeslätt, Granlund, & Kottorp, 2009] and without disabilities (*n*=144) [Janeslätt, et al., 2008] by using modern test statistics e.g. Rasch models. Models developed in modern test theory are suggested as preferable for reducing complex data of qualitative observations to unidimensional measures (Smith Jr, Conrad, Chang, & Piazza, 2002; Tesio, 2003; Wright, 1996]. One of the advantages of using Rasch models is the mathematical estimation of the difficulty of the items and of the ability of the persons separately, ordered on the same, unidimensional, latent trait continuum [Streiner & Norman, 2003].

The KaTid has a detailed manual describing how to implement assessment, how to pose each question/each item and how to score. It currently contains 51 items ranging from easy to hard in a flip-page format. The unique features in this new assessment are: a) the items in time perception, aimed at measuring the child's perception of the duration of daily activities and b) the items in time management for children and c) that items from all three different aspects of time; time perception, time orientation and time management are included and d) that it is adapted for persons with cognitive impairments using iconic symbols and concrete concepts.

Time Perception

The subcategory *Time perception*, contains thirteen items, most of them focusing on comparing the duration of everyday activities. The child is presented with pictures of two activities and asked to point at the picture of one activity that takes long time to do, e.g. "Point at the picture of the activity that takes long time to do, eating a banana or going to the swimming pool". The items are presented one at the time in increasing order of difficulty.

Time Orientation

The subcategory of *Time orientation* contains twenty-nine items. In three items the child is asked to place a picture sequence of a daily activity in temporal order. Also in this category the time concepts of (a) location, (b) frequency and (c) units are included, i.e. concepts of "educated time" [Nelson, 2002]. Examples of items in (a) - location in time: "Which season is it now" or "What day was it yesterday?" (Figure 1). An example of (b) - frequency concepts: "Which do you do more seldom, brush your teeth or go to the dentist?" Examples of items in (c) - units: "Which days are you free from school?" and "Say the names of all the days of the week in the correct order".

Eight items are about telling time from a clock with increasing levels of difficulty. This type of item is the traditional way of measuring time ability included in instruments like Griffiths Mental Developmental scale [Alin-Åkerman & Nordberg, 1980]. One item includes objective time and perceived duration using a timer, and a similar item is seen in LOTCA [Katz, Itzkovich, Averbuch, & Elazar, 1989]. When starting the assessment, a timer is set for

15 minutes, without telling the child. When the timer rings, ask the child "– For how long do you think we have been doing this? A minute, a quarter of an hour, or an hour?". This kind of item aims to measure retrospectively the subjective time in passing [W. J. Friedman, 1990]. Seven items are about time quantity with questions like "How many minutes are there in a quarter of an hour?".

Time Management

In the subcategory Time management, the nine items focus on allocating proper amounts of time to events and activities. There are questions about (a) what one would have time to do in a set period, (b) when to do it and (c) for how long to do it [Davies, et al., 2002]. In items about (a) -what one would have time to do in a set period- the skill of reading the clock is combined with the duration of activities. For example, "If the hands on the clock are like this, and a TV program you want to see starts at six o'clock, what would you have time to do? Make a sandwich or eat dinner?" Items about when and for how long to do it include calculation. For example, "If it takes ten minutes to go to the dentist and you should be there by twenty past eleven, when will you have to leave?"

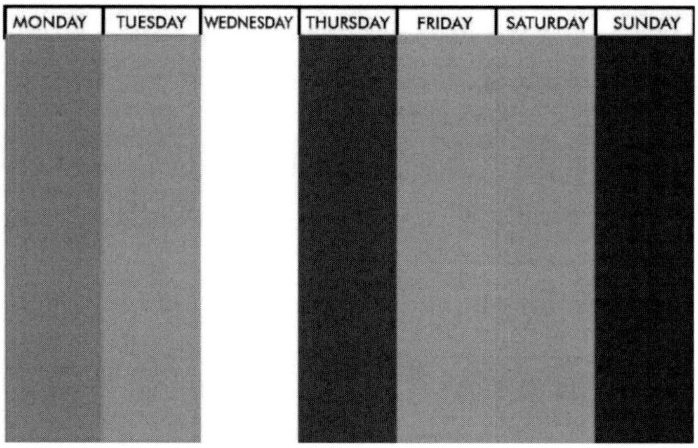

Manual. The KaTid-rater introduces the items.

Point at each weekday naming them in the correct order. Point at the day of today.

Item O8, say - This is today, what day was it yesterday?

Item O9, say - What day is it tomorrow?

Item O10, say - Which days are you free from school?

The child can point at the day or answer verbally. Note in protocol, a correct answer scores 1 point.

Figure 1. Items locating days of the week.

How to Measure Daily TM

No existing assessments usable for children for measuring only *daily TM* were found; possibly due to difficulties in defining what daily TM really is in children. Time problems might occur in any daily situation where you need to know when and for how long to perform an activity [Granlund, et al., 1995]. Also, because of the dependence on environmental factors, the daily TM of a person with cognitive disability will vary depending on the complexity and context of the activity.

The first author and her colleague created the *Parent scale*. It was designed to collect information about the parents' estimation of children's everyday functioning in situations that were possibly affected by difficulties in TPA. The Parent scale inevitably has its advantages and limitations. One possible limitation is parents basing their ratings on previous experiences of children's time management in daily life, for example with siblings. This means that other factors than children's observed daily TM may have an impact on what ratings they assign. Still, the information is of value since context is important for the child's opportunities to develop TPA and the parents themselves - and their motivation - are prerequisites for any support or intervention.

The Parent Scale was aimed at assessing everyday situations where skills in TPA are assumed to be needed. For example, it has been suggested that difficulties in time perception in children with ASD are related to limitations in daily rhythm/sleeping problems [Wimpory, Nicholas, & Nash, 2002], as implied by the statement "My child has a stable sleep-wake cycle...". Difficulties in time perception were assumed to be related to difficulties in adjusting activity level to the specific context (e.g. problems with waiting) [Barkley, 1997; Segal & Frank, 1998], thus generating two items in the scale. Many activities in daily living are done in a temporal sequence, e.g. making a snack, and since managing such activities is part of learning time management [Bambara & Ager, 1992; Davies, et al., 2002], one statement was designed to capture that ability. Another statement was added for information on whether the child understands time concepts in everyday situations [W. J. Friedman, 1990]. Time perspective, hindsight and forethought are aspects of psychological time [Barkley, 1997; Melges, 1990], and generated one item. The parent scale includes fourteen items based on a Likert agreement scale.

VALIDATION OF THE ASSESSMENTS

The evaluation of the KaTid, initially using data from 5 - 10 year old children with and without developmental disabilities, presented acceptable psychometric properties. The results indicate that the items in KaTid, initially defined as time perception, time orientation and time management, empirically support a potential uni-dimensional construct, TPA. In this TPA construct the subcategories can be seen as different levels of complexity rather than as separate constructs [Janeslätt, et al., 2008; Janeslätt, et al., 2009].

The psychometric properties of the Parent Scale were generally acceptable [Janeslätt, et al., 2008]. In a study aimed at the empirical investigation of the hypothesized relation between children's TPA, daily TM and self-rated autonomy, TPA was measured with the instrument KaTid, daily TM with a parent scale, and a validated scale for Self-rating of autonomy was used. Participants were children aged 6 – 11 years with disabilities: ADHD, ASD, mild or moderate ID, or with neurological disease such as CP or MMC (n=118). All data were transformed to interval measures using applications of Rasch models and then further analysed with correlation and regression analysis. The results demonstrate a moderate significant relation between parent ratings of daily TM and the TPA of the children (r= .513, p<.001), and between the self-rating of autonomy and TPA (r= .306, p<.001). There was also a significant relation between self-ratings of autonomy and parent ratings of the children's daily TM (r= .366, p<.001). The more skilled a child is in TPA, the more able s/he is in daily TM, regardless of whether s/he has a disability. When further investigating the relationship between parent ratings of the child's daily TM and the child's TPA, as measured with KaTid, a univariate regression analysis was used. The results indicated that the parent rating of children's daily TM was the strongest predictor for TPA, explaining 26% of the variation in TPA. In a backwards regression analysis parent ratings had almost as strong a predictive power as age [Janeslätt, et al., 2009]. The results indicate that the instrument for assessing TPA is also viable in children with disabilities, and that the ability measured by KaTid is relevant for daily TM and for self-rated autonomy.

Using the Assessments

Most of the least able 5- and 6-year-old TD children managed the items in *time perception* and also one of the items placing pictures in temporal order, confirming that young children usually have a general knowledge of the duration and temporal order of daily activities [Bylholt, 1997; E. R. Friedman, 1977; W. J. Friedman, 1990]. This result highlights the level of TPA acquired among TD children before they actually learn to read the clock. The methods used today for promoting TPA focus mainly on how to learn time concepts and to tell the time from a clock [Nelson, 2002]. Perhaps these findings and this assessment reveal opportunities to develop methods of promoting time perception – in a playful way – by comparing the duration of different activities. Children learn to process time information in interaction with the family and significant others [Adler & Holmgren, 2000; Guralnick, 1997; Owen & Wilson, 2006; Piaget, 2006; Wachs, 2000]. Therefore this result suggests a possibility for developing methods that can help parents and significant others to promote TPA in children with ID already at pre-school age.

Adults with ID commonly demonstrate problems in everyday life related to *time orientation* (e.g. using information about the hour/date/week/month) and time management (e.g. knowing when and for how long to perform an activity) [Davies, et al., 2002]. Our studies confirm that this is also applicable to *children* with ID, as suggested by Owen & Wilson [Owen & Wilson, 2006].

The results of using KaTid in the sample with children with typical development show that time management is processed already by children aged 5 – 10 [Janeslätt, et al., 2008]. The KaTid offers an option of assessing time management as part of TPA in children. This opens up possibilities for gathering new knowledge of what can be expected at this ages, for promoting and (where necessary) for supporting children at risk of delayed development of time management, as related to problems in daily TM.

The regression analysis indicated that, in the sample of children with disabilities, the child's age and level of TPA are both of importance for daily TM [Janeslätt, et al., 2009]. The results support the idea that difficulties in TPA affect the children's daily life, possibly in a way that is not generally appreciated by people around them [Owen & Wilson, 2006; Peeters & Gillberg, 1999]. Also, the context for children varies particularly with age, possibly reinforcing problems for children of school age with delayed development in TPA.

Unified use of the Concepts TPA and Daily TM

One initial problem was to find a valid base for the assessment of TPA, due to the lack of consensus surrounding concepts and definitions [Christiansen, 2005]. Our studies therefore strive to operationalize the concepts of time in ICF-CY empirically, both on a body function level and an activity/participation level. The Parent scale for daily TM, together with the KaTid (a common tool for assessing time perception, time orientation and time management), actually provide professionals with a unified language to use when communicating with parents about TPA and daily TM, as suggested by Simeonsson et al [2006]. Many of the trained raters report that after using this assessment, new and better-informed discussions take place. This can also contribute to improving communication used within the family, and between parents, professionals and significant others. If everybody involved in interventions for children with developmental disabilities uses similar definitions for concepts of time, we can envisage setting concrete goals and planning how to reach them. The relation between TPA and daily TM emphasizes the importance of the context. This result is in line with recent studies stating that the context is crucial for a child's skills development (here in TPA) and for learning how to manage time in his/her everyday life. This, in turn, requires parents and significant others to acquire knowledge about how to promote/support the child to make development possible. Using concepts of TPA and daily TM in a unified way may also offer new opportunities to develop knowledge about daily TM and contribute to improved coordination of health services for children with restrictions in daily TM.

CONCLUSION

An assessment instrument: KaTid, with acceptable psychometric properties, is now available for measuring TPA [Janeslätt, et al., 2008]. The results of our studies indicate that the items in KaTid, initially defined as time perception, time orientation and time management, all demonstrate acceptable internal scale validity, and statistically support a potential uni-dimensional construct, TPA. Based on the results of two studies [Janeslätt, et al., 2008; Janeslätt, et al., 2009] and a preliminary Principal Component Analysis [Janeslätt, 2009], we suggest that TPA is indeed uni-dimensional. It is indicated that the development of this ability is an ongoing process during childhood with expressions that vary over time.

KaTid can be used for assessment of the individual level of TPA, for children with or without developmental disability. Professionals - OT's, psychologists and teachers - can benefit from a validated assessment that generates linearized estimates of TPA from children. The findings also suggest that the Parent scale has potential as a valid assessment of a child's daily TM, useful in clinical and research work for children with or without cognitive disability.

The relation between TPA and daily TM indicates that the construct measured by KaTid is relevant for the daily TM of the child as rated by the parents, and that it can be used for defining possible causes of problems with managing time in daily life. The findings also suggest that TPA, as a factor related to children's daily TM, needs to be taken into account when planning and evaluating interventions designed to facilitate everyday functioning for children with cognitive impairments. Needs unmet may threaten childrens' rights to be active participants in family, school and community life.

In conclusion, this is a step towards evidence-based assessments that, together with other information, can help the professional in structuring the intervention *planning* process for children with difficulties in daily TM. The model for assessment can contribute to a common language for communicating with parents about TPA and daily TM. KaTid may reveal possibilities for new methods in promoting and supporting TPA and daily TM.

REFERENCES

Adler, B. & Holmgren, H. (2000). *Neuropedagogik-om komplicerat lärande [Neuropedagogics - about complicated learning]*. Lund, Sweden: Studentlitteratur.

Alin-Åkerman, B. & Nordberg, L. (1980). *Griffiths' utvecklingsskalor I och II: manual för administrering och utvärdering [Griffiths Developmental Scale I and II]*. Eskilstuna, Sweden: Psykologiförlaget ab

Arvidsson, G. & Jonsson, H. (2006). The impact of time aids on independence and autonomy in adults with developmental disabilities. *Occupational Therapy International, 13*(3), 160-175.

Bambara, L. M. & Ager, C. (1992). Using self-scheduling to promote self-directed leisure activity in home and community settings. *Journal of the Association for Persons with Severe Handicaps, 17*(2), 67-76.

Barkley, R. A. (1997). Attention-deficit/hyperactivity disorder, self-regulation, and time: toward a more comprehensive theory. *Journal of Developmental and Behavioral Pediatrics, 18*(4), 271-279.

Barkley, R. A., Murphy, K. R. & Bush, T. (2001). Time perception and reproduction in young adults with attention deficit hyperactivity disorder. *Neuropsychology, 15*(3), 351-360.

Bebko, J. M., Weiss, J. A., Demark, J. L. & Gomez, P. (2006). Discrimination of temporal synchrony in intermodal events by children with autism and children with developmental disabilities without autism. *J Child Psychol Psychiatry, 47*(1), 88-98.

Benson, J. & Clark, F. (1982). A guide for Instrument Developement and Validation. *The American Journal of Occupational Therapy, 36*(12), 789-800.

Boucher, J., Pons, F., Lind, S. & Williams, D. (2007). Temporal cognition in children with autistic spectrum disorders: tests of diachronic thinking. *J Autism Dev Disord, 37*(8), 1413-1429.

Bylholt, C. (1997). A review of the literature on the acquisition and development of time concepts in children. *CAEDHH Journal/La Revue ACESM, 23*(2-3), 119-124.

Christiansen, C. (2005). Time use patterns of occupation. In C. H. Christiansen, C. M. Baum & J. Bass-Haugen (Eds.), *Occupational Therapy: Performance, Participation, and Well-Being* (3 ed.). Thorofare, NJ: SLACK inc.

Coster, W. (1997). Occupation- Centered Assessment of Children. *American Journal of Occupational Therapy, 52*(5), 337-344.

Davies, D. K., Stock, S. E. & Wehmeyer, M. L. (2002). Enhancing Independent Time-Management Skills of Individuals With Mental Retardation Using a Palmtop Personal Computer. *Mental Retardation, 40*(5), 358-365.

Friedman, E. R. (1977). Judgements of time interval by young children. *Perceptual and Motor Skills, 45*, 715-720.

Friedman, W. J. (1990). Children's Representations of the Pattern of Daily Activities. *Child Development, 61* (5), 1399-1412.

Granlund, M., Bond, A., Lindstöm, E. & Wennberg, B. (1995). Assistive technology for cognitive disability. *Technology and disability, 4*(ala research foundation), 205 - 214.

Groen, W. B., van Orsouw, L., Huurne, N. T., Swinkels, S., van der Gaag, R. J., Buitelaar, J. K., et al. (2009). Intact Spectral but Abnormal Temporal Processing of Auditory Stimuli in Autism. *J Autism Dev Disord.*

Guralnick, M. J. (1997). Second Generation Research in the field of Early Intervention. In M. J. Guralnick (Ed.), *The effectiveness of Early Intervention*. Baltimore: P.H. Brookes.

Hughes, C., Russel, J. & Robbins, T. W. (1994). Evidence for Executive Dysfunctioning in Autism. *Neuropsychologia, 32*(4), 477-492.

Hunt, G. M. & Oakeshott, P. (2003). Outcome in people with open spina bifida at age 35: prospective community based cohort study. *BMJ, 326*(7403), 1365-1366

Hunt, G. M., Oakeshott, P. & Kerry, S. (1999). Link between the CSF shunt and achievement in adults with spina bifida

J Neurol Neurosurg Psychiatry 1999;67:591-595

Janeslätt, G. (2009). *TIME FOR TIME; Assessment of time processing ability and daily time management in children with and without disabilities.* Unpublished Doctoral, Karolinska Institutet, Stockholm.

Janeslätt, G., Granlund, M., Alderman, I. & Kottorp, A. (2008). Development of a new assessment of time processing ability for children, using Rasch analysis. *Child: care health and development, 34*(6), 771-780.

Janeslätt, G., Granlund, M. & Kottorp, A. (2009). Measurement of time processing ability and daily time management in children with disabilities. *Disability and Health Journal, 2*(1), 15-19.

Katz, N., Itzkovich, M., Averbuch, S. & Elazar, B. (1989). Loewenstein Occupational Therapy Cognitive Assessment (LOTCA) battery for brain-injured patients: reliability and validity. *American Journal of Occupational Therapy, 43*(3), 184-192.

Levin, I., Wilkening, F. & Dembo, Y. (1984). Development of Time Quantification: Integration and Nonintegration of Beginnings and Endings in Comparing Durations. *Child Development, 55*(6), 2160-2172.

Lindquist, B., Carlsson, G., Persson, E. K. & Uvebrant, P. (2005). Learning disabilities in a population-based group of children with hydrocephalus. *Acta Paediatrica, 94*(7), 878-883.

Lollar, D. J. & Simeonsson, R. J. (2005). Diagnosis to function: classification for children and youths. *Journal of Developmental and Behavioral Pediatrics, 26*(4), 323-330.

Melges, F. T. (1990). Identity and Temporal Perspective. In R. A. Block (Ed.), *Cognitive models of psychological time*. Hillsdale, NJ: Lawrence Erlbaum.

Miller, L. J. (1989). Developing Norm-Referenced Standardized Tests. *Physical & Occupational Therapy in Pediatrics, 9, Number 1.*

Nelson, K. (2002). *Language in Cognitive Development: The Emergence of the Mediated Mind.* Cambridge: Cambridge University Press.

Owen, A. L. & Wilson, R. R. (2006). Unlocking the Riddle of Time in Learning Disability. *Journal of Intellectual Disabilities, 10*(1), 9-17.

Peeters, T. & Gillberg, C. (1999). *Autism, medical and educational aspects* (2 ed.). London: WHURR publishers Ltd.

Piaget, J. (2006). *The child's conception of time* (A. J. Pomerans, Trans. 2 ed.). London: Routledge and Kegan Paul Ltd.

Segal, R. & Frank, G. (1998). The Extraordinary Construction of Ordinary Experience: Scheduling Daily Life in Families with Children with Attention Deficit Hyperactivity Disorder. *Scandinavian Journal of Occupational Therapy, 5*(3), 141-147.

Sharp, K., Murray, G. C., McKenzie, K., Quigley, A. & Patrick, S. (2001). A matter of time. *Learning Disability Practice 3*(6), 10-13.

Simeonsson, R. J., Scarborough, A. S. & Hebbeler, K. (2006). ICF and ICD codes provide a standard language of disability in young children. *Journal of Clinical Epidemiology, 59*, 364-372.

Smith, A., Taylor, E., Rogers, J. W., Newman, S. & Rubia, K. (2002). Evidence for a pure time perception deficit in children with ADHD. *Journal of Child Psychology and Psychiatry, 43*(4), 529-542.

Smith Jr, E. V., Conrad, K. M., Chang, K. & Piazza, J. (2002). An introduction to Rasch Measurement for Scale Development and Person Assessment. *Journal of Nursing Measurement, 10*(3), 189-206.

Streiner, L., D. , & Norman, G., R. (2003). *Health Measurement Scales. A practical guide to their development and use* (3 ed.). Oxford Oxford University Press.

Szelag, E., Kowalska, J., Galkowski, T. & Poppel, E. (2004). Temporal processing deficits in high-functioning children with autism. *British Journal of Psychology August, 95*(3), 269-282.

Tesio, L. (2003). Measuring behaviours and perceptions: Rasch analysis as a tool for rehabilitation research. *Journal of Rehabilitation Medicine, 35*(3), 105-115.

Wachs, T. D. (2000). *Necessary but not sufficient. The respective roles of single and multiple influences on individual development.* Washington DC: American Psychological Association.

WHO (2001). *International Classification of Functioning, Disability and Health, ICF.* Geneva, Switzerland: World Health Organization.

WHO (2007). *International Classification of Functioning, Disability and Health, ICF for children and youths (ICF-CY).* Geneva, Switzerland: World Health Organization.

Wimpory, D., Nicholas, B. & Nash, S. (2002). Social timing, clock genes and autism: a new hypothesis. *Journal of Intellectual Disability Research, 46*(part 4), 352-358.

Wright, B. D. (1996). Comparing Rasch measurement and factor analysis. *Structural Equation Modeling, 3*(1), 3-24.

In: Learning and Memory Developments...
Editors: L. C. Eklund, A. S. Nyman, pp. 283-292
ISBN: 978-1-60876-397-9

Chapter 14

A GEOGRAPHY OF INTELLECTUAL DISABILITIES

Andrew Power
Centre for Disability Law and Policy, National University of Ireland, Galway.

ABSTRACT

People with intellectual disabilities have had a long history of exclusion and enforced dependency. As this commentary examines, the uncertainty regarding their definition and an acknowledgement that a person with an intellectual disability can be particularly vulnerable to dependency, has led to a very hidden geography for this group. From the middle of the last century, geographers examined the locational separation of people committed to the 'idiot' asylums of Victorian Britain and Canada. It was clear that the asylum had a symbolic influence in the community well beyond its rather narrow role as the place of residence. More recently geographers have traced the movement of people with intellectual disabilities to group homes, co-operative housing, residence with parents and independent housing. It was hoped that the relocation from isolated stand-alone institutions would help to get rid of, or diminish stigmatisation. However, Hall[1] urges us to move away from assuming that marginalisation equates solely with exclusion from mainstream social activities and spaces, and constructing inclusion as a process of incorporation into these activities and spaces. This commentary therefore forces us to take a critical approach on today's geography of care, where we move beyond narrow binaries of institutionalisation/ deinstitutionalisation, isolation/integration and success/failure. We must be critical of the spaces of incorporation and not assume a place of incorporation is the best choice for a person with an intellectual disability. This is particularly the case if people with intellectual disabilities face a mix of patronisation, fear, an unwillingness to understand 'non-standard' forms of communication, and a strong sense of difference in public life.

---

[1] Hall, E. (1995) The entangled geographies of social exclusion/inclusion for people with learning disabilities. *Health & Place* **11**(1): 107-115.

INTRODUCTION

People with intellectual disabilities (ID) have had a long history of exclusion and enforced dependency. The study of intellectual disabilities, particularly in the medico-psychological literature, is a well-developed field. As early as the late nineteenth century, researchers and practitioners have examined the care and treatment of people with ID, particularly in institutional care settings[2]. Since the 1970s, the focus of study has reflected the move from congregated care to care in the community. Much of this has focused on the care of people with ID in the family home and has sought to identify best practice for maintaining people in the community.[3]

Throughout much of this research, evidence of the enduring paternalism still exists in the community. Arguably, much of the paternalism throughout the history of care was created by assumptions regarding the definition of ID and an acknowledgement that a person with an intellectual disability can be particularly vulnerable to dependency. Generally ID is characterised by intellectual functioning being significantly below average; having difficulties with everyday life skills; and the condition is present from early childhood. However, the meaning and interpretation of ID are negotiable and vary across time and place. For instance, assumptions and expectations regarding the independent living capabilities of people with Down's syndrome and Autism can vary between places.[4]

This paternalism shapes much of the lifeworld of the person with ID. The extent of it and the nature of care relationships involved have often significant geographical implications on the person with ID, such as where they live and the extent of their spatial network. Similarly, the place of care can shape the types of care and level of expectation on the person. For example, parents often pose much resistance to the closure of congregated care settings, as institutions represent a secure and safe option for the individual and their family. This suggests the need for more nuanced understandings of the care relationships involved and *where* they take place.

As this commentary shall examine, a closer look at the geography of ID reveals how care arrangements are shaped by real places. Despite the role of geography in shaping the organizational climate of disability support, within the broader ID literature there have been limited attempts to conceptualise geographical variation or the implications of space on the processes of care, dependency and exclusion. Indeed, much of the psychology and disability studies' fields have examined disability at the abstract non-contextualised level.

This commentary aims to trace the main concerns examined by geographers, and pinpoint their contribution to the scientific literature particularly in relation to the area of paternalism and the care of people with ID. The following section provides a quick introduction to the changing landscape of care, focusing on these main themes. In particular, the subject of advocacy from the turn of the last century is examined in order to better understand their experience of representation and the implications this has had on the geographies of their

---

[2] See Philo, C. (1987) "Fit localities for an asylum": the historical geography of the "mad business" in England viewed through the pages of the Asylum Journal. *Journal of Historical Geography.* **13**: 398-415.

[3] Robertson, J., Emerson, E., Hatton, C., Elliott, J., McIntosh, B., Swift, et al., (2007) Person Centred Planning: Factors associated with successful outcomes for people with intellectual disabilities. *Journal of Intellectual Disability Research.* **51**(3), 232-243.

[4] Lemon, C. and Lemon, J. (2003) Community-based cooperative ventures for adults with intellectual disabilities. *The Canadian Geographer* **47**(4): 414-428.

'care'. The paper then examines in more detail the spatial issues inherent in the care of people with ID. Finally, it considers the recent self-determination movement and its effects on the geography of ID. It suggests the need for a more extensive mapping exercise to capture the extent and quality of the spatial networks of people with ID.

MISUNDERSTOOD & OFF THE MAP

The geography of ID has been a relatively recent field of study, unlike that of mental illness, physical disability and the elderly population. Laws and Radford criticise the geographical community for its neglect of intellectual disability "...especially in comparison to studies of other marginalised groups such as the mentally ill"[5]. In any case, in terms of early geographic work, the focus of research became predominatly the location of people with ID in institutions. This shared many of the same themes found in the broader medical and social science literature. For example, Philo[6] and Radford and Tipper[7] examined the locational separation of people committed to the 'idiot' asylums of Victorian Britain. Similarly, in Canada, Radford and Park[8] studied the external catchment area geography of an early 'idiot' asylum and its internal geography of enclosing and therapeutic spaces. It was clear that the asylum had a symbolic influence in the community well beyond its rather narrow role as the place of residence. Park et al.'s research revealed that the asylum "exerted a symbolic influence well beyond its rather limited role as the place of residence of a small proportion of people diagnosed as 'mentally deficient' or 'feeble-minded''.[9] In acting as a 'container' for people deemed 'mentally deficient' it clearly stated that they had no place in society.

For much of this history, the advocacy of people with intellectual disabilities has been the source of contested debate regarding the roles of families, professionals, voluntary organisations, and people with disabilities themselves. Part of the reason for this contested debate is due to the fact that ID is not a unitary or homogenous category of impairment in itself. Furthermore, definitions have varied over time and place due to a particular society's values, wealth and culture.[10] Similarly the assumptions regarding their place in society and best care practices have varied over time. While Self Advocacy became a part of the disability movement generally in the 1990s[11], their continued lack of collective identity has expressed a

[5] Laws, G. and Radford, J. (1998) Place, identity and disability: narratives of intellectually disabled people in Toronto. In Gesler, W. (Ed). *Putting Health into Place: Landscape, Identity and Well-Being*. Syracuse University Press, Syracuse: 77–101.

[6] Philo, C. (1987) "Fit localities for an asylum": the historical geography of the "mad business" in England viewed through the pages of the Asylum Journal. *Journal of Historical Geography*. 13: 398-415.

[7] Radford, J. and Tipper, A. (1988) *Starcross: Out of the Mainstream – Plotted Catchment Area of a Victorian Asylum in the Context of Changing Policy*. Rocher Institute, Toronto.

[8] Radford, J. and Park, D. (1993) The asylum as place: an historical geography of the Huronia Regional Centre. In Gibson, J. (Ed.) Canada: Geographical Interpretations – Essays in Honour of John Warkentin, *Geographical Monographs*, 22, Atkinson College, York University.

[9] P. 223 in Park, D., (1995) *An imprisoned text: reading the Canadian mental handicap asylum*. Unpublished Ph.D. Thesis, York University, Toronto.

[10] Dorn, M. (1999) The moral geography of intemperance. In: Butler, R., Parr, H. (Eds.), *Mind and Body Spaces: Geographies of Illness, Impairment and Disability*. Routledge, London.

[11] The British Council of Disabled People was established in the UK in 1991

relatively fragile social composition, which has compounded this uncertainty. Dowse[12] also acknowledges that some people with ID have cognitive limitations which curtail a broader awareness of the social model concept. The tenuous and uncertain position that people with ID hold within disability politics and within society more generally has implications on their lives.

The recent landscape of care, made up of a range of community care living arrangements such as group homes and centres of independent living, arose largely from the 1940s and 1950s, where families became more involved as members of early pressure groups and as advocates for improved services. These organisations pushed local authorities to establish a less segregated landscape of care such as respite care services and employment opportunities as well as setting up day/occupation centres themselves in the community.[13]

Alongside these developments, there was evidence of families still trying to grapple with understanding the nature of ID and independent living. Many parent advocate groups were involved in stalling changes in attitude, such as those formally linked to institutions or parents whose siblings were patrons of them. For these people, deinstitutionalisation represented insecurity, a change from the assurance derived from knowing that one's relative was in lifelong institutional care to the uncertainty of a new and open service regime[14]. This form of opposition also articulated a view of the service user as vulnerable. This was frequently the mirror image of the other paradigm; the normalised (or 'socially valorised') subjectivity, imagined by supporters of community care.[15] Since this time, these two co-existing paradigms have been in conflict with each other.

Overall then, the 'care' and much of the advocacy of PwID people with ID was up to this point highly paternalistic and generally assumed the dependent status of a person with ID. Owing to the resettlement strategy that was emerging, families were increasingly becoming involved in the direct care of their children with ID. More recently, with neo-liberal government's focus on welfare pluralism, this trend has continued. This has taken advantage of opportunities to reduce funding for public social services, and as a result, community care services have relied increasingly on the unpaid help of families.[16] By the start of 1990s, according to the UK 1991 Census, 89 percent of adults with ID living in the community were being supported by members of their families in their home. In the following sections, the implications of this changing geography of care will be examined.

GEOGRAPHIES OF ID IN THE COMMUNITY

One common theme throughout the history and typology of care arrangements outlined above is that all aspects of care have been affected by the geography involved. Put simply, the local environment, and the dynamics operating in different spaces (types of places) and places

---

[12] Dowse, L. (2001) Contesting Practices, Challenging Codes: self advocacy, disability politics and the social model. *Disability and Society*, 16(1), 123-141

[13] Rolph, S. (2006) The Role and Perspectives of Families, in Welshman, J. and Walmsley, J. (eds.), *Community Care in Perspective: Care Control and Citizenship*, pp. 173-187.

[14] Ibid

[15] Gleeson, B. and Kearns, R. (2001) Remoralising landscapes of care. *Environment and Planning D: Society and Space* 19: 61-80.

[16] Clarke, J. and Langan, M. (1993) The British Welfare State: Foundation and Modernization. In Cochrane, A. and Clarke, J. (Eds). Comparing Welfare States: Britain in international context. Open University Press.

(specific sites) have had important and significant effects on the life of the individual. However, it is important in an analysis of this geography to move away from a static idea of geography as a one-dimensional backdrop towards a recognition of the multiple interactions between people and place.[17]

As the following sections show, geographers have recently begun to engage with the subject of ID in an attempt to unpack the geographies that have shaped (and been shaped by) the contested definitions and assumptions made of ID. With the changing geographies of care, people with ID continue to prove over and over that they are capable of far more independence than many had expected, and policy makers, researchers and 'advocates' gain a vision of greater changes that are possible. This section examines some of the key themes examined within the geography of ID literature and then identify some of the ways this literature can help unpack the dominant themes in the mainstream ID literature.

Since the move to less congregated settings, the focus of research has become predominantly the community based care locations and structures, which in many instances has meant multiple person accommodation with full-time staff presence. Wolpert's pioneering work[18] for example, traces the movement of PwID people with ID to group homes, co-operative housing, residence with parents and some independent housing. It was hoped at the time that the relocation from isolated stand-alone institutions would help to get rid of, or diminish stigmatisation. However, some researchers such as Parr[19], and Milligan[20] have refuted this, showing that there was little difference in a person's expectations of stigmatisation as a result of relocating them to the community. Similarly, Radford and Phillips[21] and Metzel[22] all conclude that invariably the large, spatially isolated asylum had been replaced by the apparent freedom of a life in the community which very often is life in an 'asylum without walls'.[23] With group homes, there was much antagonism and ignorance in communities at neighbourhood level. Many people still exhibited nervousness, fear, and basic ignorance to people with disabilities[24]. Similar problems have been outlined by geographic work done by Parr[25], who refers to accounts of people with mental illness who tried to reintegrate within mainstream society, pointing out that they have found new forms of marginalisation outside the institution.

In terms of case studies of the experiences of people with ID, Dear and Wolch[26] exposed the social exclusion and service dependency experienced by many people with ID,

---

[17] See Hubbard P, Bartley B, Fuller D, Kitchin R M. (2002) *Thinking Geographically: Space, Theory and Contemporary Human Geography.* Continuum, London.

[18] Wolpert, J., (1976) Opening closed spaces. Annals of the Association of American Geographers 66, 1–13.

[19] Parr, H. 1997 Mental health, public space, and the city: questions of individual and collective access. *Environment and Planning D: Society and Space* 15: 435-454.

[20] Milligan, C. (2000) Breaking out of the asylum: development in the geography of mental ill-health - the influence of the informal sector. *Health and Place* 6: 189-20

[21] Radford, J. and Phillips, D. (1985) Closure of major institutions for the mentally handicapped: geographical evidence from a case study in Southwest England. *South West Papers in Geography*, Occasional Series, 10.

[22] Metzel, D. S. (2004) Historical Social Geography. In Noll, S. and Trent Jr., J., W (Eds). *Mental Retardation in America.* New York University Press, New York: 420-444.

[23] Dear, M.J. and Wolch, J.R. (1987) Landscapes of Despair: From Deinstitutionalisation to Homelessness. Polity Press, Oxford.

[24] Wilton, R., Dear, M., Gaber, S. J. and Takahashi, L. (1997) Seeing people differently: the sociospatial construction of disability. *Environment and Planning D: Society and Space* 15: 455-480.

[25] Parr, H. (1997) Mental health, public space, and the city: questions of individual and collective access. *Environment and Planning D: Society and Space* 15: 435-454.

[26] Dear M. J., Wolch J. R. (1987) *Landscapes of Despair: From Deinstitutionalisation to Homelessness.* Polity Press, Oxford.

particularly in Toronto. The city's sole focus on deinstitutionalization, as opposed to setting up viable community based alternatives meant many people became isolated and homeless. Similarly, Radford[27] identified the extent of community opposition directed at the smaller-scale group home facilities and related services in Toronto as a result of anxieties about strange neighbours exhibiting unpredictable behaviours. This 'not in my backyard' (NIMBY) reaction hardly gives people previously in institutions a feeling of being welcomed back into the community.

As with the mainstream ID literature discussed above, over this time period, the uncertainty regarding their definition and an acknowledgement that PwID people with ID can be particularly vulnerable to dependency creation[28], also led to much debate within the geography of ID. For example, the exchange between Golledge, Imrie and Gleeson in the pages of Transactions[29] redefined the role of geography and geographers in ID research. Their exchange, largely based around a disagreement in advocating for changes in existing (disablist) structures versus broader societal changes, led to a recognition amongst geographers of the wider debates within disability studies regarding the social model of disability and its subsequent critiques.

This renewed research agenda was also profoundly influenced by the publication of a paper in Health & Place by Hall and Kearns entitled 'Making space for the ''intellectual'' in geographies of disability'.[30] It kickstarted a special issue in the same journal on the geographies of intellectual disability[31]. Its timing was fortunate, as despite community care being accepted as the strategic vision of most government's ID policy, evidence of isolation, lack of jobs, and impoverishment had increased within the ID population[32]. Geographers have since attempted to provide more nuanced readings of the complex geography of ID whilst being aware of the contested definition and assumptions regarding the 'most suitable' place of care. This literature was influenced by the rapid growth of disability studies and by the developments in social theory concerning the body.[33] An inherent guiding principle has been to produce a geography more representative of disabled people's experiences in order to better understand how they relate to their environment, and what their spatial and environmental needs are.[34]

Metzel illustrates this lack of understanding of people's spatial needs through a case study of a voluntary service organization in Baltimore, Maryland. In her analysis, she shows how the agency re/created service dependency and social poverty of people with intellectual disabilities through their residential location decision process. She found that service

---

[27] Radford, J.P. (1985a) Group homes for developmentally handicapped people in Toronto: policies and locational strategies. *Urban Studies*, Working Paper No.8, York University, Toronto.

[28] Swain, J., French, S. and Cameron, C. (2003) *Controversial Issues in a Disabling Society*. Open University Press, Buckingham.

[29] See (1996) *Transactions of the Institute of British Geographers*. 21 (2), 387–396

[30] Hall, E. and Kearns, R., 2001. Making space for the 'intellectual' in geographies of disability. *Health & Place* 7(3): 237–246.

[31] Special Section: Geographies of Intellectual Disability (2005) *Health & Place*. 11(2) 77-195.

[32] Emerson, E., (2007) Poverty and people with intellectual disabilities. *Mental Retardation and Developmental Disabilities Research Reviews*. 13(2), 107-113.

[33] Dorn, M. and Laws, J. (1994) Social theory, body politics and medical geography: extending Kearns's invitation. *Professional Geographer* 46, 106-110

[34] Posed research questions in Radford, J.P. (1985b) Some issues in the geography of mental handicap. Seminar, Department of Geography, University of Cambridge, January 1985 cited in Philo C, (2005) "Editorial: Introduction to theme section on geographies of intellectual disability: 'outside the participatory mainstream'? " *Health & Place* 11 77-85.

dependency and social poverty for people with intellectual disabilities rested directly with the large involvement of personnel in the process, including direct care staff, the service coordinator, the assistant director, the director of residential services, and the realtor. The small number of residents who were assisted by partners or friends outside of the service system underscored how most of the residents had few others whom they could involve in major decisions.

This more recent geographical work has provided a more nuanced account of the geographical lives of people with ID, their families, and the people involved in their care. The traditional binaries between spaces of institutionalisation/ deinstitutionalisation, isolation/integration and success/failure have also been challenged. Hall's work in particular[35] has scrutinised the entangled geographies of social exclusion/inclusion for people with ID. Drawing on group interviews in Scotland, he develops a nuanced account of the lives of people with ID, exploring their experiences of exclusion and seeming 'inclusion', and also the alternative spaces and networks of inclusion developed by many people with ID. His paper argues that we must be critical of the spaces of incorporation and not assume a place of incorporation is the best choice for a person with an intellectual disability. His analysis illustrates the extent of there being a socio-spatial *production* of disability, where the situations and experiences of exclusion/inclusion are shaped by the socio-spatial contexts within which people with ID live.

This is particularly evident in the public sphere, where people with intellectual disabilities often face a mix of patronisation, fear, an unwillingness to understand 'non-standard' forms of communication, and a strong sense of difference. In public space, Ryan[36] examined the effects on family caregivers of caring for an adult with ID. Her illustration of the reactions to disability in public life, such as stares, pity and negative comments, and parent's consequential coping strategies, serves to demonstrate the importance of geography in discussions regarding caregiving for people with ID such as deciding on places to go and how to act in these places.

Similarly, Power's study[37] examined personal interactions between family carers and their young adult children with ID in Ireland within the home, public space, and the in-between spaces they used, such as day care centers, parent groups or other family homes with a child with a disability. The study found that all these sites were affected by the impairment effects of ID; and in turn led to complex geographical lifeworlds where parents grappled with promoting independence on the one hand, and the risk of overprotection on the other.

Mapping the Social Ecology of ID

The more nuanced understandings of the geographies of ID discussed above are increasingly proving more necessary, as the self-determination movement has begun gaining momentum in western countries. This movement has seen a move towards more

[35] Hall, E. (2005) The entangled geographies of social exclusion/inclusion for people with learning disabilities. *Health & Place* 11(1): 107-115.

[36] Ryan, S. (2008) "I used to worry about what other people thought but now I just think... well I don't care": shifting accounts of learning difficulties in public places, *Health & Place*. 23(3), 199-210

[37] Power, A. (2008) 'Caring for Independent Lives: Geographies of Caring for Young Adults with Intellectual Disabilities'. *Social Science and Medicine*. 67 (5), 834-843

individualised services, based on the idea of self-determination and person-centred planning. Welfare programs are becoming organised around the concept of 'money follows the person' and the idea that the individual receives a personalised budget. This decentralised form of 'care' has led to a new geography of ID and geographers have begun attempting to map the effects of this.

Services for people with ID are being reconfigured to provide the individual more choice in their own care. In the UK, direct payments are given with wrap around support provided by a Resource Allocation System (to provide support in using and accounting for the budget) and support brokers (to provide care management and life coaching advice). Similarly, in many states in the US, personalised Medicaid budgets are given with the assistance of fiscal intermediaries and independent consultants. In this model, social support may be derived from different sources, both informal (family, friends, neighbours) and formal (paid carers).

Geographers have thus had to examine the additional complexity in the spatial lives of individuals with ID. They also have had a role in assessing the benefits or pitfalls involved in this decentralised form of support, as well as identify the main barriers and success factors involved in making care systems such as these work. To meet this challenge, geographers have recently begun turning to social ecology models to assess the extent and quality of personal networks across scale. These have attempted to map the networks of support from different service providers, care staff, friends, family, and mainstream support in the community, across the many different places in the everyday life of the person with ID. For example, the Social Network Guide (SNG)[38] maps the components of individuals' networks. These are structural, (size, membership and density), interactional (reciprocity, frequency, duration and closeness) and functional (e.g. companionship, decision making). Participants define the members of their social network using a 'wheel of life'; people are included if they are considered important in the respondent's life and they can either name them (by first or second name) or reference them situationally (e.g. the grocer). For each identified member, information is collected on the type of relationship (e.g. family, staff, neighbour, volunteer, friend), and the area of life from which they were derived (e.g. household, residential home, retail, such as cafe's and pubs). Thus, a 'friend' might be a local publican or a member of staff.

In terms of different locations of care, people in small group homes and supported accommodation and, to a lesser extent, hostels were significantly more likely to report companiable relationships than those in residential and nursing homes. Relationships in these three settings were more likely to be described as 'close' compared with relationships in residential and nursing homes. The type of accommodation in which people were living therefore had a strongly significant effect on the types of social support which they received. Unfortunately, low scores for personal support were associated with living in hostels, small group homes and especially supported accommodation. However, considering material support, the situation is reversed: here living in hostels, small group homes and supported accommodation is associated with higher scores for material support; people living in

[38] Forrester-Jones R. (1998) Social Networks and Social Support: Development of Instrument. Departmental Working Paper, Tizard Centre, University of Kent at Canterbury.lectual disability. *Disability and Society* 13, 389–413.

residential and nursing homes reported lower levels of such support[39]. In a study by Emerson et al.[40], the size of the network was found to differ according to where people lived, with an average network size of 6.7 for people living in village communities, compared with 4.4 for those in residential campuses and 6.8 for community-based residences.

For those living in the community, a small literature is developing that explores relationships between disabled people and their family caregivers, formal service providers, and others who contribute to creating their social space. From bus drivers to family members, these social networks are integral to creating or eliminating barriers for those with various impairments.[41] Walker[42] and Erevelles[43] suggest that we take seriously the relational aspects of disability service provision and the ways that institutional and professional practice can foster progressive alliances. For example, Smith et al. examined the social ecology of a residential special school for young people with challenging behaviours[44]. The methodology includes an analysis of staffing ratios, levels of staff assistance and attention and resident activity in two different settings. Although little difference was found in comparable adult community services, the methodology has the potential to reveal the social ecology of different care sites. Masucci has argued that geographers can lead the way in mapping new networks of power, exposing structured gaps and barriers within existing technologies. They can also suggest innovative ways to meet people's needs and demonstrate that enabling environments can be created in multiple ways including innovative transport arrangements; an important issue for transportation-dependent people. Kasnitz[45] for example, examined the effective use of a 'rural employment transportation voucher' model by people with mobility impairments who wish to pursue paid or volunteer employment. Specifically, the programme offered disabled rural residents the financial resources to recruit family and friends as paid taxi providers, helping to overcome enduring barriers to social participation.

Studies such as these illustrated above are paving new ground in understanding the everyday networks of people with ID across space and scale. As people with ID approach adulthood, many move from the family home to living independently in rented or owner-occupied housing. This is held up as the key marker of social inclusion policy for people with ID, yet can be a complex experience and geographers must again look at the relational aspect of this changing geography of ID. With government policy currently advocating more de-centralised forms of care, for example with the recent Valuing People Now report promoting

---

[39] Forrester-Jones, R., Carpenter, J., Coolen-Schrijnerà, P., Cambridge. P., et al., (2006) "The Social Networks of People with Intellectual Disability Living in the Community 12 Years after Resettlement from Long-Stay Hospitals " *Journal of Applied Research in Intellectual Disabilities* **19** 285–295

[40] Emerson E., Robertson J., Gregory N., Hatton C., Kessissoglou S., et al. (2000) The quality and costs of village communities, residential campuses and community-based residential supports in the UK. *American Journal on Mental Retardation* 105, 81–102.

[41] Crooks, V. A., Dorn, M. and Wilton, R., (2008) Emerging scholarship in the geographies of disability. *Health & Place*, 14(4), 883-888.

[42] Walker, P. (1999) From community presence to sense of place: community experiences of adults with developmental disabilities. Journal of the Association for Persons with Severe Handicaps 24 (1), 23–32.

[43] Erevelles, N. (2001) Disability and the political economy of place: case study of a voluntary organization in South India. *Disability Studies Quarterly*. 21 (4).

[44] Smith, K., Powlitch, S., Little, D. and F. Furniss. (2007) Social Ecology of a Residential Special School for Young People with Challenging Behaviours: A Preliminary Report. *Journal of Applied Research in Intellectual Disabilities*, 20, 99–104

[45] cited in Crooks, V. A., Dorn, M. and Wilton, R. (2008) Emerging scholarship in the geographies of disability. *Health & Place*, 14(4), 883-888.

the closure of traditional day care services and the reappropriation of mainstream spaces[46], the mapping of people with ID's networks will become a crucial form of analysis in understanding the extent of isolation or integration caused by the particular social care policy and extent of supports in different sites in the community.

Conclusion

This commentary has identified the main developments in the geography of ID. As ideas of care and welfare have changed over time, geographers have attempted to examine the spatial implications of these changes on people's lives. They have sought to identify the effects of the gradual move from congregated care to individualised supports in different places.

As well as giving a background to the sub-field of geography, this commentary has sought to explicate its contribution to the broader debates within the ID literature on best practice in the care of people with ID. While the broader literature has identified the current social issues facing people with ID, appreciating the geographical effects of isolation, paternalism and different forms of care can enrich the study of ID by contextualizing debates in real communities and caregiving sites, as well as revealing variations across different places in how people with ID live. As the last section has illustrated, the challenges facing people with ID and the potential for isolation are greater than ever, as people are increasingly being called upon to navigate less centralised services and self-determine their own support.

[46] Department of Health. (2009) *Valuing People Now: a new three-year strategy for people with learning disabilities 'Making it happen for everyone'*. UK Stationary Office, London.

INDEX

A

B

C

D

E

F

I

J

K

L

M

N

O

P

Q

R

S

T

U

V

W

X

Y